The Healing Landscapes of Central and Southeastern Siberia

David G. Anderson, Editor

Patterns of Northern Traditional Healing Series
Volume 1

Series Editor: Earle Waugh

CCI Press
2011

Library and Archives Canada Cataloguing in Publication

The healing landscapes of central and southeastern Siberia / David G. Anderson, editor.

(Patterns of Northern traditional healing series ; v. 1) (Occasional publications series, 0068-0303 ; 71) Papers originally presented during the Idioms of Indigenous
   Health and Healing Conference at the University of Tromsø,
   Norway, June 2010.
Co-published by: Centre for the Cross-Cultural Study of Health and Healing, Dept. of Family Medicine, Faculty of Medicine and Dentistry,
   University of Alberta.
Includes bibliographical references and index.
ISBN 978-1-896445-58-8

   1. Traditional medicine--Russia (Federation)--Siberia. 2. Alternative medicine--Russia (Federation)--Siberia. 3. Integrative medicine--Russia (Federation)--Siberia. I. Anderson, David G. (David George), 1965- II. University of Alberta. Centre for the Cross-Cultural Study of Health and Healing III. Title. IV. Series: Occasional publication series (Canadian Circumpolar Institute) ; 71 V. Series: Patterns of Northern traditional healing series ; v. 1

GN477.H42 2012   306.4'610957   C2012-901304-8

All rights reserved.

© 2011 CCI Press in cooperation with the
Centre for the Cross-Cultural Study of Health and Healing,
Department of Family Medicine, Faculty of Medicine and Dentistry,
University of Alberta

ISBN 978-1-896445-58-8

ISSN 1927-9671
Patterns of Northern Traditional Healing, Volume One
Series Editor: Earle Waugh, University of Alberta earle.waugh@ualberta.ca

ISSN 0068-0303
Occasional Publication No. 71

Printed in Edmonton, Alberta, Canada by art design printing, inc.
Cover design by CCI Press and art design printing, inc,

Cover photo: Nikolai Aruneev and Nastya. Photo credit Donatas Brandišauskas. Used with permission of the photographer and the subjects of the photograph.

Table of Contents

Preface to the Series v
Earle Waugh

Acknowledgements vi

Introduction: *Local Healing Landscapes* 1
David G. Anderson

Chapter One: *Symptoms as Signs in Buriat Shamanic Callings* 13
Justine Buck Quijada

Chapter Two: *Medical Pluralism and Expert Knowledge in Buriatiia* 29
Katherine Metzo

Chapter Three: *The Development of Tibetan Medicine in Buriatiia* 45
Vindarya N. Gololobova (translated by Ol'ga Pak)

Chapter Four: *Healing Springs in the Lake Baikal Region* 63
Janice Brummond

Chapter Five: *The Paradox of Alcohol in Western Buriat Communities: Vodka and Ritualized Commensality in Ekhirit-Bulagat Raion* 87
Joseph J. Long

Chapter Six: *Idioms of Health and Healing in Central Siberia* 95
David G. Anderson

Chapter Seven: *Spirits, Taiga Medicine, and the Practical Engagement of the Landscape among Orochen-Evenkis* 111
Donatas Brandišauskas

Chapter Eight: *Public Health and Folk Medicine Among North Baikal Evenkis* 129
Vladimir N. Davydov

Chapter Nine: *The Categories of Ket Spiritual Healing* 147
Edward Vajda

References 159

Glossary 171

Notes on Contributors 177

Index 179

Preface

Earle Waugh, Series Editor

This volume has had considerable gestation. Indeed, the series itself, of which this is the first, began as an initiative of my University of Saskatchewan colleague Andrei Vinogradov and I during the late-1980s to examine contemporary folk healing and shamanism in Siberia. We were partially responding to the claim made by Eliade and others that Siberian shamanism was the locus of all ancient forms of healing and the central motif of the genre. Our reasoning was that, were this claim correct, we should still see impressive artefacts today.

Andrei sought out many folk healers, all of them Russian-speaking, and requested short descriptions of their activities. Unfortunately folk healers are not usually writers, so it became obvious that much more local academic study would be needed to authenticate any shamanic activity. The project languished as we moved on to other interests. It has been revived under the husbandry of the Centre for the Cross-Cultural Study of Health and Healing (CCCSHH) in the Department of Family Medicine at the University of Alberta. After discussion with David Anderson from the University of Tromsø, Norway, we decided to re-configure it and give it its current design.

This, then, is volume one of a planned five-book series. The series is designed to survey important local and regional healing traditions within roughly conceived geographic areas: Siberia, Central-Northern Asia, Scandinavia and the Sami People, North Western Canada and Alaska and North Eastern Canada and Iceland. A central focus of the series is on the 'therapeutic landscape' and its ramifications for understanding medical alternatives. We have joined forces with our colleagues in the Canadian Circumpolar Institute at the University of Alberta to develop and bring to fruition this project over the next decade.

This first collection of essays arose out of a conference held at the University of Tromsø June 3-5, 2010 entitled 'Idioms of Indigenous Health and Healing.' It was jointly sponsored by the Department of Archaeology and Social Anthropology of the University of Tromsø and CCCSHH of the University of Alberta. Papers delivered there formed the backbone of this collection along with other solicited contributions.

Our hope is to address a long-standing need for a closer look at the way health care is mediated in northern regions, most of them rural and relatively difficult places of access. This volume focuses on how the peoples of Siberia construct and foster health processes when they lack the resources and the skills located in major cities. When one examines the actual practices in these environments, one comes to the conclusions that both the notion of health and the means of maintaining and fostering it are very diverse; that there are several different pathways that people utilize to address health issues. Some of these pathways are very old, and some reflect hybridization and modification. Our concern is to encourage a new generation of scholarship to address the actual and concrete structures by which healthcare is known and conceived in the north. This is the maiden volume of the series.

Many people have contributed to the successful publication of this first volume. First, our scholars and their commitment to research in areas little canvassed until now. Second, our respective universities and institutions that have not only supported the research that made the articles possible, but have undertaken to assist us in countless ways in promoting this project and providing funding to launch this book. Third, our colleagues at CCI, Marianne Douglas and Elaine Maloney have been excellent co-workers for this project. Fourth, both the University of Tromsø and the University of Alberta have willingly assisted in making this a success.

Acknowledgements

This collection came about as the result of a number of meetings over the past ten years. Without the encouragement of Earle Waugh at the Centre for Cross-Cultural Health and Healing, much of the material here would have remained in our notebooks and would not have been collected here. We would all like to thank the University of Tromsø for providing an International Symposium grant allowing many of us to meet together to assemble the manuscripts. We are especially grateful to Marit Myrvoll for organizing a panel on Sami traditional healing which led to a fruitful discussion as to what was unique in Siberian healing paradigms, and to Roald Kristiansen for hosting us on a tour of Sami healing landscape in the Tromsø region. Several of the chapters (Anderson, Brandišaukas, Davydov, Long) here benefited from fieldwork funding in part provided from the School of Social Sciences, University of Aberdeen and from the Social Sciences Research Council of Canada through its grant MCRI 412-2005-1005. A number of people helped bring this manuscript to completion. Olga Pak provided an excellent translation of Vindarya Gololobova's article from Russian. Mary Moffet, at the University of Aberdeen, copy edited the text, helping to standardize terms and improve the flow of the text. Finally we are thankful to Elaine Maloney and the Canadian Circumpolar Institute Press for turning this manuscript into a book.

Introduction

Local Healing Landscapes

David G. Anderson

Edited volumes each have different histories, but most begin with significant conversations. When I began my fieldwork in Siberia in 1989, I never thought I might end up writing about health or on the interface between differing medical traditions. However, at that time when Soviet civic structures were beginning to change, or crumble, this was clearly the issue that most people living in rural areas wanted most to talk about. My own fieldwork came to be interspersed with requests for medicines that had suddenly become prohibitively expensive, questions about prescription pills that could 'cure' alcoholism, and an engaged interest in the everyday lives of Canadian native people who my Siberian hosts suspected lived a much more secure and healthier life.

In trying to answer these questions for my friends, I began to read different literatures. Not surprisingly, there was no magical solution on how to improve health in the Northern communities of a North American late capitalist society. The Canadian Arctic was characterised by a better subsidized yet similarly over-centralized approach to health care. Indeed, when looking at Siberia from the point of view of a Cree or a Dene community, people in Siberia seemed to be one step ahead due to their confidence in their own healing traditions. Each context seemed to offer a small part of the answer for which the other community was searching. If before I had assumed that there existed a 'Western' medical tradition lying in crisp contrast to an 'indigenous' tradition, these conversations led to the conclusion that there were different ways of combining healing intuitions to solve particular problems. Two important themes also came out of this conversation. The first was that although local healers were flexible in what treatments they would accept, they had to temper their creativity with a canny knowledge of which medical solutions might be tolerated by the state agents who controlled access to resources. The second, related theme was that what I had lazily labelled as an 'indigenous' approach to health and healing was better described as a conviction that communities should be able to heal themselves. Whether this second goal was achieved by recruiting a doctor from 'outside' to live in the community, or by assembling a treatment out of locally recognized cures and prescription pills, the emphasis was nevertheless upon an autonomous model of healing. This volume is an attempt to address this call for a 'local healing landscape' that seeks to make Northern communities healthy and autonomous by combining insights from various healing traditions.

The volume follows on a seminar held at the University of Tromsø in June of 2010 entitled *Idioms of Indigenous Health and Healing*. The goal of the seminar was to compare Eastern Siberian and Sami ways of approaching community health. My colleague, Dr. Marit Myrvoll, suggested that the seminar be held in Tromsø with the deliberate aim of raising the profile of community-controlled ways of organizing health and healing. Northern 'health problems' occupy a very prominent place on government agendas in Scandinavia. However, much of the research on these issues tends to be epidemiological and focussed on the 'peculiarities' of small, rural, and often ethnically distinct communities when compared to urban settings. Our goal, instead, was to speak about the strengths of these communities. Through our meetings and correspondence with Prof. Earle Waugh at the Centre for Cross-Cultural Health and Healing at the University of Alberta, we realized that this worry over the lack of a place to discuss local idioms of health was a common one internationally. This led to the production of this book, and indeed, this book series.

Central and Southeastern Siberia

This particular volume documents healing traditions in Eastern Siberia in a geographical area roughly surrounding Lake Baikal and then extending northward to the Arctic Ocean (Fig. 1). The collection of papers came about through the happy coincidence of there being a large number of young scholars completing their first fieldwork in the region in the period immediately following the worst dislocations of a shift to a neo-liberal market economy (roughly 2002-2008). On the one hand, our definition of this region was fortuitous—governed by the specialists we were fortunate to attract at the time this project was developed. On the other hand, the region shows an interesting unity in healing traditions extending across a wide range of landscape types—from the open tundra of Taimyr, to the larch forests of Evenkiia and Irkutsk oblast', and the northerly steppe zones around Irkutsk, Ulan-Ude and the Tunka Valley. The mountainous shoreline of the world's largest lake, in turn, reminds one of the coastal landscapes of the northwest coast of North America or Northern Norway. Due to this diversity, this region provides a strong point of comparison to ecologies in other parts of the circumpolar North and an appropriate volume with which to launch this series.

One can understand these diverse regions to be one through the action of political and geographic factors. The Enisei River, linked to Lake Baikal through the Angara, is a natural corridor through which ideas of health and healing are shared. Russian colonization of this region proceeded from North to South, upstream along the Enisei River, eventually reaching Lake Baikal. The city of Irkutsk for several centuries served as the administrative capital for both Eastern Siberia and Russian America. This river-mediated North-South colonial structure created opportunities for local people to travel and trade, sharing both their furs and ideas about the land and of health.

In writing the history of this region today it is all too easy to over-emphasize the role of the Russian state and Russian state-building in creating trade links and infrastructure. It is important not to forget that the peoples of this region also had a long experience in conducting trade and regulating relationships with the Mongol and Manchurian Chinese Empires. The impact of the Russian state seems to have had an important impact upon the contemporary topography of biomedicine, and in particular on the present understanding of what is a regional medical 'center' and what is an 'outlying' medical district. However, local healing protocols have not only been highly influenced by these older Tibetan and shamanic traditions, but it seems that these ideas also flowed back to influence the unique mix of healing traditions used by urban Russians today. As Katherine Metzo and Vindarya Gololobova document in their chapters, Russian biomedicine was heavily influenced by ideas from Tibetan medicine, which, in turn, was influenced by Indian *ayurveda* healing.

Neither should one underestimate the power of the landscape to recommend certain cures. There are strong continuities in local folk healing 'shamanic' practices that extend North-South throughout the region. An orthodox ethnologist might explain this away as the effect of cultural diffusion along this corridor. However, local healers might prefer to emphasize that the spirits in this Eurasian landscape are as closely linked to each other as the local mountain ranges and rivers that link the top of the continent to the polar sea.

In the local idioms of healing, power flows from the landscape and is rooted within it. As both Brandišauskas and Davydov powerfully illustrate through their fieldwork with Orochens and Evenkis in a region that had been heavily repressed in the 1930s, contemporary hunters can relearn relationships with the land spirits by observing how animals move and use the landscape, and by watching what animals eat.

This volume contains chapters reporting from the most significant landscapes in this region. In the first part of the book, the five chapters by Justine Buck Quijada, Katherine Metzo, Vindarya Gololobova, Janice Brummond and Joseph Long present recent ethnography from the taiga-steppe borderlands to the south of Lake Baikal. They represent a culture area most heavily influenced by Tibetan and Russian medicine and are a laboratory for a particularly strong type of medical pluralism that finds its expression not only in healing practice but in published books and manuals. The four chapters in the latter part of the book by David Anderson, Donatas Brandišauskas, Vladimir Davydov and Edward Vajda represent different types of taiga healing practices along the northern arm of this corridor. Here, the idioms of Tibetan medicine are not as strong but one finds a stronger voice from the shamanic landscape traditions of the region, and many types of healing that may be unfamiliar to readers from other parts of the world. The chapter by Edward Vajda, on Kets living on the left bank of the Enisei, makes links to healing traditions further westward in Siberia. Joseph Long's chapter, on the use of alcohol rituals, addresses a sensitive topic that is common throughout the North. His fieldwork amongst Pribaikal Buriats is from a region where local cultural traditions represent a sort of bridge between northern taiga medicine and Tibetan steppe healing traditions. His call for a critical yet nuanced understanding of alcohol offering rituals is an important illustration of how ethnographic insight can inform a critical understanding of health. Vodka cures are also analyzed in Chapter 7 by Brandišauskas and Chapter 8 by Davydov.

Medical Pluralism in Post–Soviet Siberia

The 'mixing' of healing traditions is usually described as 'medical pluralism.' The origins of this term dates back to the very foundation of medical anthropology in the early 1970s (Hsu 2008) and is associated most closely with the work of Charles Leslie (1976, 1980) in South Asia. Leslie's pioneering work was devoted to showing that alternate 'local medical systems' were not only possible but often could work alongside officially recognized systems. At heart, the term 'medical pluralism' is a challenge against the asserted dominance of what has come to be known as 'clinical' or 'cosmopolitan' medicine, or 'biomedicine' (Lock and Gordon 1988; Baer 2001).

Biomedicine is defined as a set of empirically proven and closely guarded sets of healing protocols financed and policed by powerful centralized institutions—most often government agencies, but also large international pharmaceutical companies. Sociologists of science have tracked the rise of a cosmopolitan biomedical system with the rise of a global capitalist system, and the term is tailored best to fit a Marxist account of how social institutions are distorted to assist a dominant class to reproduce itself and the capital resources upon which it depends (Han 2002; Hsu 2008:319). There is a wide debate in the literature as to how 'monolithic' this system can be (Hsu 2008:319-320; Gordon 1988). Many medical anthropologists have documented national varieties of biomedicine in different parts of the world which have seemingly accepted different styles of healing (Lock and Gordon 1988; Baer 2001). Historians of science have similarly pointed out that so-called Western societies once supported much more diversity in healing practice in the 18th and 19th centuries, and that the post-war emphasis on hospital-based authorized care is a recent disruption to European healing traditions (Baer 2001:Ch1; Arnold 1988). These contextualizing studies have led scholars to question what 'pluralism' really means. Leslie's original work spoke of the co-existence of differing 'systems' which can be understood as relatively deeply rooted, and somewhat autochtonous, healing traditions. Following his lead, many anthropologists have come to focus empirically on how individuals choose between different and competing cures in a marketplace of healing strategies. This empirical strategy has enriched the literature but has had the disadvantage of making healing look more like a consumer strategy. In an era when the public health literature has increasingly come to recommend that governments dismantle public healthcare bureaucracies to allow 'choice,' medical pluralism has lost its shine as a critique and instead come to look like an apology for neo-liberalism. In the words of Elisabeth Hsu (2008:317):

> [Since] its inception the notion [of] medical pluralism has been criticized for being grounded in an overly simplistic concept of culture; for conceptualizing health care from the professional's, rather than patient's, perspective; for engendering an overly behaviorist account of health seeking; for generating a false consciousness of choice; for underplaying the importance of financial, structural, and other political economic considerations; for insufficiently attending to issues of power, authority, and policy, or working with naive notions of them; and for implicitly reproducing a monolithic concept of (bio-)medicine. In summary, the concept is unsatisfactory as it is not grounded in social theory.

The term is best used heuristically to capture the diversity of formal and informal strategies of healing, and perhaps still as a critique of dominant systems, as we have used it in this volume. However, it seems that once one evokes the term 'medical pluralism' or its evil twin 'biomedicine,' one is locked into a critical sociological debate that quickly obscures the voices of existing communities and the choices they have made. The purpose of this volume is to draw attention to those voices.

In reviewing the literature on medical pluralism, it is striking how strongly it is based on examples taken from 'Great' medical traditions such as *ayurveda*, Chinese, or Tibetan medicine, and the near lack of any published work on pluralism within Russia, state socialist countries in general, or indeed across the circumpolar North. Given the powerful influence of Marxism embedded in the history of the concept, what could be the fate of this concept within a region that for several generations was so avowedly anti-capitalist? Should one not expect a large and powerful state socialist country like the former Soviet Union to have been more tolerant of healing traditions that united peasants and workers together in local communities?

One of the conclusions of this volume, as ironic as it may seem, is that both terms—biomedicine and medical pluralism—seem to hold their heuristic analytical power when viewed from the perspective of small, rural villages located a long way from central medical institutions. Without even entering into the debate on whether or not the former Soviet Union was actually a 'state capitalist' social formation, the highly centralized manner in which infrastructure was imposed on rural areas to improve them created many of the same hierarchical divides that one can find in other capitalist contexts. Medical care in the former Soviet Union may not have been intended to help the shareholders of international pharmaceutical companies prosper, or to disaggregate human beings into fractal sets of medical conditions, but it was clearly organized to benefit urban-based professional elites. The way in which this professional corps behaved was very similar in other parts of the world in the way that teams of specialists would be assembled to address health problems (and not communities) and that resources were redistributed from regional centres. Given that rural communities were located, by definition, farther from the centres of expert power, they often had to cultivate local resources and healing traditions to solve their own problems. These centrifugal pressures only increased after the collapse of the Soviet welfare state through what became a complete rupture between the urban centres and the rural peripheries. The structural brittleness of the centralized state created a 'pluralist' healing environment by default. Here, individuals may not have had the luxury to 'shop around,' but communities were nevertheless able to draw upon formal and informal sources of medical care. Centrally-based specialists similarly recognized the regional limits of their authority, often tolerated these cures or even prescribed these home remedies.

It is important, however, not to overstretch the homology between Soviet biomedicine and European or North American biomedicine. It must be remembered that during the Soviet period, biomedical treatment in the Siberian North was provided free of charge whether or not that care involved helicopter evacuation flights or expensive courses of medications supervised within a regional hospital. Unlike in many other state-financed medical systems, Soviet physicians were not asked to weigh the cost of a particular course of treatment for a patient whether they lived near the hospital or thousands of kilometres away. Although this point is not made all that clearly in the chapters in this collection, medical systems in the Soviet period behaved like total social institutions which provided, along with treatment, a way for people to move back and forth between the city and village or even a way for people to find some respite from work in the village in a heated, urban hospital environment.

Hospitals, in turn, did not have solid boundaries, but served as locations for healing as the patient's kinsmen would bring food and even medicines into the hospital. Thus, like in Europe or North America, this Soviet biomedical system was also not monolithic. It was, however, fractured in a different way. It was hampered from achieving total medical control of the population by a lack of resources and perhaps by a lack of vision over incorporating the rural periphery. However, it was also open to change from within through its curiosity with Eastern medicine, herbal medicines, and tolerance of home remedies.

The chapters in this collection document what can be described as a blossoming of autonomous healing traditions in post-Soviet Siberia due to the effects of the unique crisis suffered by rural residents in the aftermath of the collapse of this centralized system. This is a type of 'medical pluralism' only in a very general sense, since it refers to the growth of the popularity of alternate, non-clinical treatments due to the abdication of the biomedical system. However, the sudden upsurge in autonomous cures also speaks to the silent survival of these knowledge traditions in a context where only official medical practice dominated the public sphere for seventy years.

Describing Soviet biomedicine as dominant makes this process seem more peaceful than it was in fact. Soviet biomedicine fought for dominance. At the start of the Soviet period, many traditional healers appeared to early Soviet organizers as threats to their authority. Many self-professed shamans were labelled 'enemies of the people,' initially having their civic rights restricted and often being arrested and executed in the repressions of the 1930s. This tragic history forced all self-taught healing experts to work silently behind the scenes, but also confined folk remedies to the security of the home, guarded by kinship networks. Despite this brutal history, many contributors to this volume remind us that the Soviet biomedical system had a place for traditional healers as long as they were not shamans. As Katherine Metzo, Vladimir Davydov and Donatas Brandišauskas document in their chapters, traditional healers could represent themselves as traditional Russian *znakary* ['one who knows'] or *tselitely* ['one who makes whole']—designations which seemingly put them above politics. Further, Soviet organisers often could not understand that individuals did not choose to shamanise but that spirits chose them. Arresting and repressing these individuals created an impossible atmosphere for the healing community, but it did not stem the flow of healers. This meant that even professional shamans survived well into the deep Soviet period, as Edward Vajda documents. Justine Buck Quijada's ethnographic account of the shamanic organisation Tengeri in Ulan-Ude brings this story a full circle as Tengeri sees its goal to make shamanic healing a 'public health initiative' within existing public health institutions.

One of the strongest examples of the resilience of a local healing system is Vindarya Gololobova's detailed and nuanced account of the development of Tibetan medicine with Buriatiia (Chapter 3). Here, she places her accent upon the long pedigree of this healing system which, despite a hiatus in the 1930s, nevertheless steadily adapted itself to Buriat folk healing and has developed a clinical 'scientific' branch as well. Adaptations came through the replacement of traditional Tibetan plants, animal products, and rocks with raw materials offered by the local landscape in the Baikal region. However, to compensate for the repression of the *datsan* [Buddhist monastic] centres of learning, the Russian Academy of Sciences has sponsored a programme of reinscribing pulse diagnostics and pharmacology within the language recognised by the biomedical profession.

The chapters which illustrate local ingenuity in the face of economic adversity are those documenting primarily Evenki and Orochen healing in villages that were cut off from access to urban institutions. The contributions by Katherine Metzo (Chapter 2), David Anderson (Chapter 6) Donatas Brandišauskas (Chapter 7) and Vladimir Davydov (Chapter 8) document the local landscape medicines used by rural pastoralists and hunters who traditionally lived autonomously from urban centres and that became extremely important again in the post-Soviet transition period. All of these chapters document an unofficial kind of alliance between biomedical institutions and local experts in harbouring this knowledge. While the nursing stations and hospitals of the Soviet period had no official category or prescription that relied upon traditional cures, the fact that they employed local people as nurses or nurse-practitioners [*fel'dshery*] gave local people with a healing gift a chance to occupy a healing 'slot' within a local community, and thereby unofficially collect and reproduce healing knowledge. During the collapse of biomedicine at the end of the Soviet period, rural patients did not find a ready-made shaman who needed to be dusted-off and employed, but they found fragments of ecological knowledge held by women, nurses, and hunters which could be reassembled. On the one hand, one could argue that had the Soviet system been more tolerant of traditional cures, these communities might have been more autonomous and resilient against changes to the global economic order. On the other hand, seventy years of direct investment in rural institutions had a clumsy yet measurable effect in supporting local knowledge systems. In comparison to other parts of the world, that effect seemed stronger than not investing in rural infrastructure at all.

Landscape Medicine

In his overview of alternative healing systems in the United States, Baer (2001) noted a tendency for corporate or state-sponsored biomedicine to recognise and accept some healing strategies and to reject others. Similarly, he noted a disturbing tendency for the practitioners of alternate healing systems to change their practice to make them appear to be more clinical and thus more attractive to the biomedical community. This local adaptation or translation of healing strategy across medical idioms is undoubtedly an important step in the dialogue that leads to a functional, pluralistic environment. But by definition it also silences some of the history behind local healing traditions. One of the goals of this volume was to document Siberian healing legacies in their own terms.

Across this North-South corridor one can find certain broad similarities in preparing and applying the use of unrefined natural materials for healing, as well as in a concern over the 'spiritual' foundations of health. The focus of healing tends to be a holistic and a personal one, and is governed by a relationship between a particular healer and a 'patient' (who is often a kinsman). More often than not, both patients and healers emphasize what makes them strong or well without much talk of particular named diseases or conditions. What unites healers and patients across the region is a concern with how forces, spirits or 'masters' rooted in particular places in the landscape affect health. While the combination of the use of herbal and spiritual remedies can be found in many rural communities around the world, this accent upon the land is an important dimension to healing in central and eastern Siberia. For this reason, many contributors to this volume focus on what can be called 'landscape medicine,' or as Brandišauskas calls it 'taiga medicine.'

One of the reasons for choosing this term is to emphasise the broad nature of the remedies used in the region. Perhaps stemming from the processes of accommodation and translation that Baer criticised, alternative therapies are often reduced to 'plant medicine.' The ratification and refining of plant medicines was one of the earliest forms of collaboration between European medics and indigenous peoples creating, over time, the pharmaceutical industry. In Russia, the history of the 'plant pharmacies' [*zelenaia apteka*] is also quite deep. The study of the aboriginal use of plant medicine specifically extends as far back as the Second Kamchatka expedition of 1740 (Lukina 1982). A quick search of the catalogue of the American Library of Congress turned up over 200 books published in Russian in the last century alone on the topic of plant medicines. As many of the contributors to this volume illustrate, plant medicines are also an important part of the pharmacopeia in Eastern Siberia. This pharmacopea is not limited to plants, however, and even plant medicine is contextualized within a culture of attention.

As Vindarya Golobova points out, the effectiveness of herbal cures lies not in the fact that they come from plants but that they come from plants growing in significant places, and which are collected and processed with care (and often with gifts given back to the land). Vladimir Davydov provides a good example in his illustration of the local economy of *ianda*—a type of Evenki plant medicine held to be useful in a wide variety of contexts. *Ianda* is associated with a particular plant species, but not all representatives of that species are *ianda*. The efficient aspect of the plant is identified through its bitter taste and partially through the careful way in which it is gathered and shared.

Katherine Metzo takes a more critical approach to this question through her fieldwork in the Tunka Valley. Here she observed the paradox that rural residents in the post-Soviet period made a radical switch to the use of plant medicines, but that they preferred to use packaged plant medicines since they distrusted both their own skills to gather plants and those of the traders in street markets selling medicinal plants. On the one hand, she identifies deference to expert knowledge in the way that rural residents approach plants which speaks to a lack of autonomous healing power in these regions. On the other hand, she points to the fine discrimination of these rural residents who choose to recognise those companies or 'brands' in the post-Soviet plant pharmaceutical industry which have successfully combined traditional forms of knowledge with commoditised forms approved by and monitored by the state.

Janice Brummond's account of healing springs in the Lake Baikal region provides a classic case of the co-evolution of a traditional form of 'landscape medicine' with official medicine. The springs that she documents are all very old traditional sites of healing as well as having long histories of being incorporated into public medicinal practice from before the Revolution to the present. As Kathleen Wilson (2003:85) observes, spas, baths, and healing springs seem to have a privileged path of access into Euro-American medical systems due to the fact that they are easily mapped, measured and quantified. However, Brummond documents the important rituals that Buriat healers must perform to keep certain springs 'alive' as well as the complex links between altitude and environment which alter the properties of particular types of springs. In her account, healing springs, just as with plant medicine, are not a pre-packaged healing force. They must also be activated by conscious and deliberate action and be treated with care.

In David Anderson's account of a cross-cultural healing dialogue between Canadian Crees and Denes and Siberian Evenkis, the issue of plant medicine comes up as one of the 'misunderstandings' that structured these meetings. Northern Siberian Evenki were happy to talk about healing plants, but they were much more articulate about powerful healing rocks, touched by lightening, or forms of animal medicine. As with the other examples in this volume, the point of the healing exercise was not the easily-commodified thing in itself, but its relationship to the healing power which flows from the landscape. The fact that Enisei River Kets do not have many words for plants, as documented by Edward Vajda, might be considered a negative proof of this northern type of healing.

The chapters by Gololobov, Brandišauskas and Davidov document the use of a particular substance translated here as 'stone-oil' [*kamennoe maslo*; *mumeo*] which presents itself as an interesting example of a creolisation of landscape healing traditions. The term 'stone-oil' refers to a type of dark, liquid-like mineralization that one finds on cliffs and rock-outcroppings. It is known as mineral pitch in the Tibetan tradition. It is a type of medicine that Evenkis and Orochens understand that one has to 'hunt' and which reveals itself only to those who treat it properly. An entire discussion was devoted to the proper way the name of this substance, which is neither mineral nor liquid, neither plant nor animal, translated into English during our seminar in Tromsø. It appears to be a substance of the landscape itself.

In this volume we use the terms 'landscape medicine' and 'healing landscapes' as ethnographic concepts that capture the diversity of healing protocols which are nevertheless grounded in particular evocative places. However, the landscape metaphor has recently been put forward prominently as a way to resolve some of the dizzying polarities created by the contrast between the terms biomedicine and medical pluralism. Elisabeth Hsu (2008:320) sees the concept of a medical landscape as a way of decentering the role of the 'culturally adept healer' and encourage us to focus all of the social processes surrounding both the healer and the patient in the way that the subject of a painting is constructed by that painting's background. Kathleen Wilson (2003) in her review of the literature on health geography argues that the term 'therapeutic landscape' holds a special relevance for Canadian First Nations people by emphasizing the way that dearly held ordinary landscapes help keep communities healthy. This close nexus between people and land that she identifies overlaps very closely with the material in this volume.

Conclusion

All of the chapters presented here were written by ethnographers with a long-term connection to particular communities. It is a particular privilege of ethnographic writing to let real life examples stand as metaphors for larger debates in the sociological and philosophical literature. Here, these examples of 'local healing landscapes' show the creative way that individuals in central and southeastern Siberia have managed to heal their families and communities within the context of one of the more abrupt economic crises suffered by any society. The examples are indeed special to this particular place and time. However, the intuition of how to balance locally accessible knowledge with centrally financed expert knowledge is a common problem throughout the North, if not throughout the world. In a context where the academic literature is dominated by examples of local healing traditions from India or Latin America, we hope this volume will encourage more interest in the local healing solutions devised by people in living in the circumpolar North.

The Healing Landscapes of Central and Southeastern Siberia

Chapter One

Symptoms as Signs in Buriat Shamanic Callings

Justine Buck Quijada

For Buriat shamans at the Local Religious Organization of Shamans, Tengeri in Ulan-Ude, Buriatiia, a shamanic calling is experienced through the physical symptoms of illness.[1] This formula should be familiar to students and scholars of shamanism, or readers of Mircea Eliade (1964): the prospective shaman becomes ill, and through the process of healing him or herself, he or she 'masters' the illness and learns to heal others. The way that the shamans at Tengeri understand and describe a shamanic calling can be summarized by this process. However, when removed from the specific context of practice, this formula tells us little, if anything, about becoming a shaman, nor does it tell us anything about how illness in this context is to be defined or understood.

There is a long tradition in the academic literature, Eliade included, of analyzing the illnesses that herald a shamanic calling as varieties of mental illness, thereby rendering plausible to non-believers the possibility that healing can be effected through shamanic intervention. However, these interpretations are external, and do not reference the understandings of those afflicted. Drawing on field research with Tengeri in Ulan-Ude, Republic of Buriatiia, this chapter examines how the shamans at Tengeri understand the illnesses that come to be defined as shamanic callings. I argue that they see their afflictions as, but not limited to, bio-medical conditions. Their definition of illness includes bio-medical physical symptoms, but expands the boundaries of illness beyond the causes and symptoms recognized by bio-medical illness. I describe the process of diagnosing a shamanic calling as a semiotic process of learning to correctly read physical symptoms as signs of hidden social relationships. I argue that the process of accepting a shamanic calling is a process of re-interpreting physical symptoms of illness as signs of the will of *ongonuud* ancestor spirits (sing: *ongon*). Both the physical symptoms and their original misdiagnosis come to be seen as signs that the prospective shaman is not sufficiently integrated into Buriat kinship networks and Buriat traditional knowledge. Healing is effected not only by removing the symptoms, but also by changing their significance from signs of illness, to signs that embed the shaman in new social, kinship and historical relationships. In doing so, however, they do not cease to remain signs of illness. Healing is possible because the physical symptoms are now both signs of illness and of kinship obligation. Approaching illness in this way allows us to think about illnesses not as *a priori* physical conditions which are understood differently in different cultural contexts, but rather to ask, what kinds of bodily states are defined as illnesses, under what conditions? It also enables us to broaden our understanding of healing and illness from a body-centered approach to one that considers how bodies are incorporated into social networks.[2]

---

[1] The legal title of the organization is *Mestnoe religioznoe organizatsiia shamanov Tengeri*. Hereafter it will be referred to simply as Tengeri.

[2] Viewing possession as a system of communication is not a new idea. Lambek (1980) for example, presents possession in Mayotte as a tripartite process of communication between spirit, host and intermediary. "Communication," Lambek argues, "is a major theme of the curing process; that is, of the development of a stable and

The Republic of Buriatiia is a semi-autonomous republic within the Russian Federation in south-central Siberia, on the Mongolian border. The Republic's western border is Lake Baikal, which is the largest freshwater lake in the world, and a UNESCO world heritage site due to its stunning biodiversity and unique beauty. The ethnic group for whom the Republic is named, Buriats, are closely related to Mongolians, and comprise approximately 28% of the Republic's population. Ulan-Ude, the capital city, was founded in 1666 as a Russian trading post. Previously named Verkhneudinsk, the city was re-named Ulan-Ude in 1934 as part of Soviet nationalization initiatives [*korenizatsiia*], and over the next five decades the Soviet government invested heavily in transforming the former Russian trading post into the capital of an indigenous republic. Today, the city has approximately 400,000 residents, and although Buriats are a statistical minority, they constitute a majority of those employed in government, education, cultural and medical professions. Urban Buriats are, for the most part, a highly educated population employed in professions which, in the post-Soviet period, are severely underpaid but still prestigious. At first glance, this urban population may seem like an odd place to look for traditional healing methods, but urban Buriats share many of the same health problems as rural indigenous populations world-wide, including high rates of alcoholism, and the shamans at Tengeri believe that shamanic healing can address these problems (Fig. 1.1).

The organization Tengeri is a group of practicing shamans committed to reviving what they call 'traditional Buriat shamanism' and establishing shamanism as a religion on par with Tibetan Buddhism, which is the dominant institutional religion in Buriatiia. Monastic Tibetan Buddhism spread widely throughout Buriatiia in the 17th century, but many Buriats continue pre-Buddhist shamanic practices in addition. Both Buddhism and shamanism were repressed and continued in attenuated form under socialism. Both religions, as well as Russian Orthodox Christianity, are experiencing a strong revival in the post-Soviet period, but for shamanism, this revival is increasingly taking an institutional form. Tengeri was registered as a religious organization by the Republic government in 2003, and is the third registered shamanic organization in the Republic.[3] Their offices are located in Ulan-Ude. In 2005, the organization had a core group of thirteen practicing shamans, led by Bair Zhambalovich Tsirendorzhiev, the Director of the organization and the teacher/mentor of the other shamans. It has since expanded considerably, and opened an entire ritual complex on the outskirts of the city.[4]

---

mutually satisfactory relationship between host and spirit" (1980:322). Like members of spirit possession cults documented elsewhere in the ethnographic literature (Boddy 1989; Bourguignon 2004; Crapanzano 1973; Lewis 2003; Masquelier 2001), shamans at Tengeri progress from inchoate symptoms of illness to maintained relationships with possessing spirits. This process can be understood as an ever-increasing degree of communication between spirit and host. However, this analytic approach usually stresses the way in which spirit possession enables types of communication (protest, critique, satire) that would not be acceptable if voiced by the spirit's host (*see* for example, Boddy 1989; Lambek 1980). Communication, in this context, centers on verbal communication, on the content of speech. Spirits are only able to speak after the relationship between host and spirit is established. Verbal communication can occur only after the spirit and host have successfully communicated well enough to establish a relationship. My interest here lies in the preceding non-verbal communication, in indexical physical signs that establish the shamanic relationship in the first place. As I shall argue, these physical symptoms bear much greater meaning than merely indexing the presence of a possessing spirit..

[3] The organization is described further in Jokic (2008) and Quijada (2008, 2009).

[4] Personal communication, Bair Tsirendorzhiev 4/6/2010.

Chapter One: *Symptoms as Signs in Buriat Shamanic Callings*

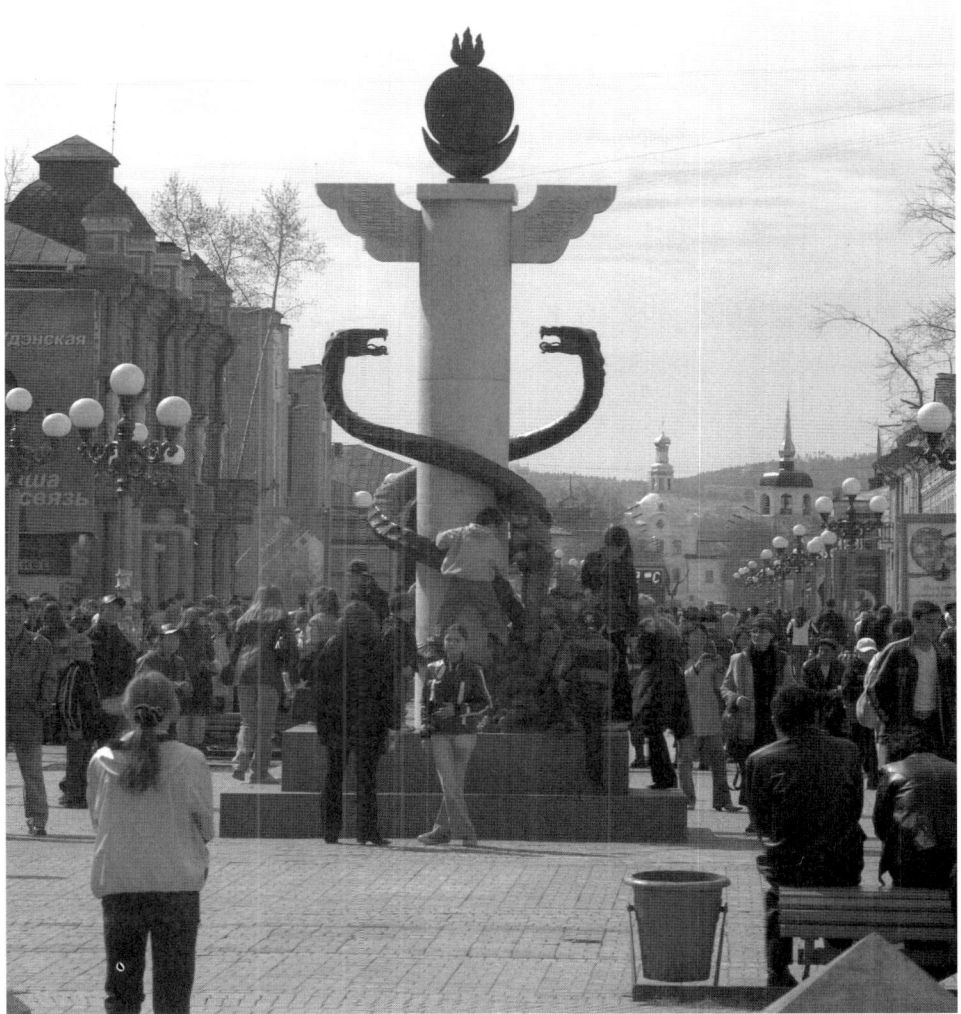

Figure 1.1 *Downtown Ulan-Ude, 2005.* Photo by Roberto Quijada.

In addition to the core group of shamans, the organization's membership comprises a much larger and fluid group of initiates, patients and their supportive family members, who come and go at the offices. The information in this chapter is based on my experiences and conversations with the members of Tengeri over 12 months of fieldwork in 2005. Although I sometimes quote specific conversations, many of my explanations are compiled from multiple conversations. As with any group that tells the same narrative on many occasions, the members of Tengeri echoed and quoted each other, and above all, their director, Bair Zhambalovich Tsirendorzhiev, so certain phrases and explanations were repeated often.

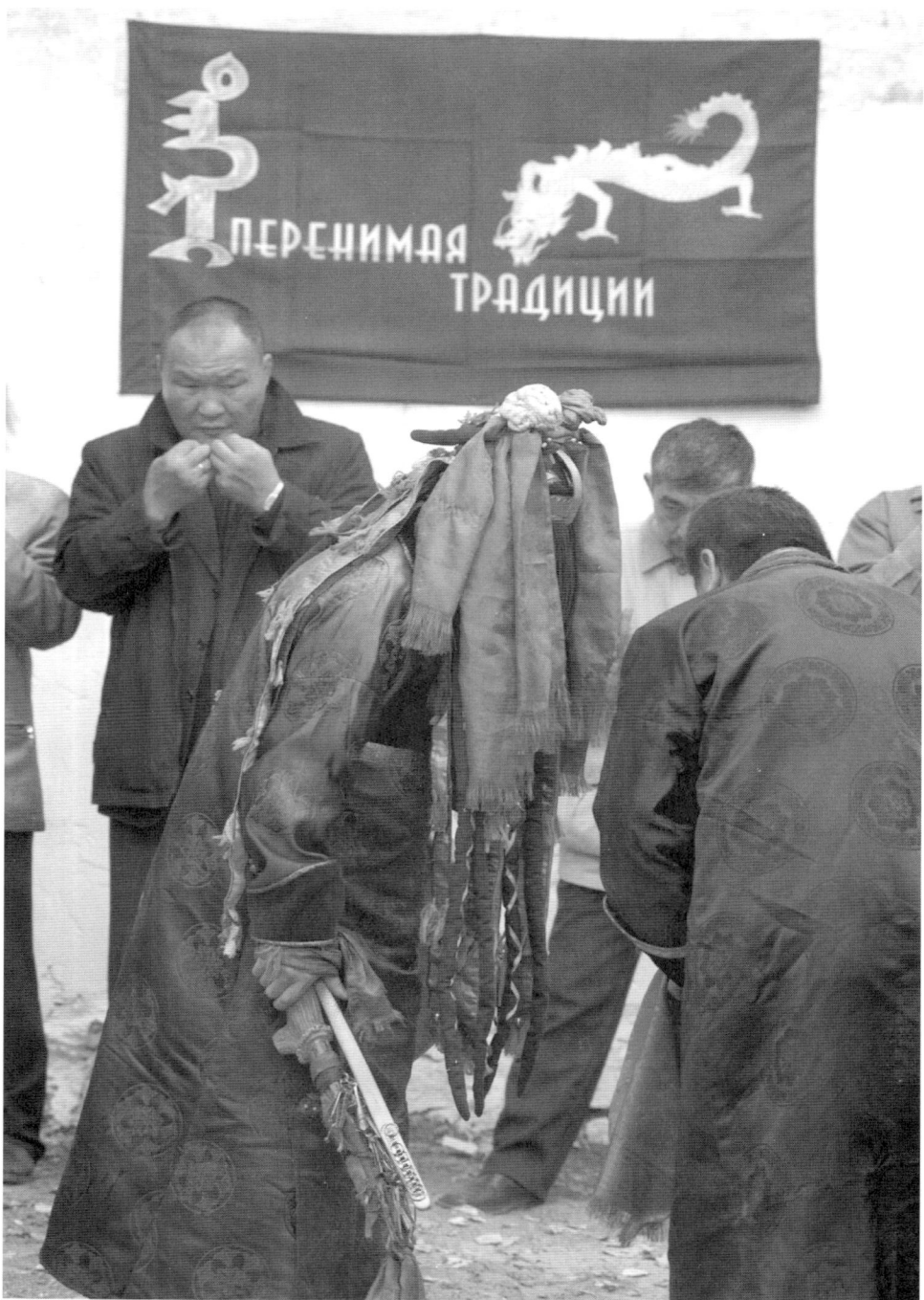

Figure 1.2 *The opening ceremony of the Tengeri offices in 2005. The banner on the wall reads 'adopting traditions' and bears the organization's name, Tengeri, in a stylized version of the old Mongolian script. Members of the organization wear the Buriat national costume, the* degel, *during ceremonies.* Photo by Roberto Quijada.

The shamans at Tengeri are not 'traditional' shamans, in the sense that 'traditionally' Buriat shamans were not part of organizations; nor do they match Western images of wise, indigenous shamans in remote villages. Bair Zhambalovich, is, by training, a veterinarian. Many of the other shamans once worked, or are still employed as scientists or teachers, and came to their callings late in life. They are sometimes criticized by others, including other shamans, for incorporating ritual practices learned in Mongolia, or from ethnographic accounts, but they are increasingly popular, and are seen as authentic, reliable and 'true' shamans by the many people who have come to them for healing. They are offended by the term 'neo-shaman,' because they argue that what they do is part of a long-standing indigenous tradition, even if much of that tradition was lost during the years of Soviet repression.[5] There is a great deal of debate in Buriatiia, and especially among shamans and local intellectuals about whether or not Buriat shamanism should be considered a 'living' tradition, or one that is 'recovered' (Fig. 1.2).

Jakobsen draws a useful distinction between shamanism and neo-shamanism (Jakobsen 1999). Traditional shamanism, despite wide variations in practice, is considered a burden by the chosen individual, entails a responsibility to heal others, and deals with a range of spirits who can be both benevolent and malevolent. She defines neo-shamanism, in contrast, as the use of shamanic techniques in a way that is predominantly focused on personal spiritual growth, open to all, and notes that the spirits called upon in these techniques are generally perceived as benevolent. If one accepts this distinction, then the shamans at Tengeri are definitely not neo-shamans.

As I will show, for the shamans at Tengeri, the shamanic calling is a burden and a responsibility that cannot be denied. But they are modern shamans, who acknowledge and constantly negotiate the practical exigencies of working in a multi-ethnic, urban environment, with a multi-ethnic clientele possessing a wide range of cultural knowledge.[6] They improvise and experiment as they seek to re-build a body of knowledge about shamanic practice that has been fractured by a century of Soviet repression. They argue that Soviet repression, combined with modernization campaigns, produced a loss of cultural knowledge, and the resulting spiritual imbalance has produced a profound public health crisis in Buriatiia. This sense of crisis motivates them to collaborate with scientists and disseminate information about their practices in ways that might be controversial in other indigenous communities.

Most of the shamans at Tengeri came to their shamanic callings through illnesses that they originally misrecognized as bio-medical illnesses, but that failed to respond to standard bio-medical treatment, until the underlying spiritual causes were remedied. Making shamanic information public knowledge, they argue, can save lives, just as their own were saved. Shamanic healing, as they see it, complements and completes other forms of medical intervention.

I will begin with my friend Viktor's account of his shamanic calling. Viktor Dorzhievich is a founding member of Tengeri, and has been a practicing shaman for over a decade, but like many of his colleagues at Tengeri, he was trained as a Soviet scientist. He

---

[5] I use the term 'tradition' here, not as a description of a static state of being that has been lost, but rather in the sense Talal Asad argues for, of a body of knowledge and a tradition of interpretation and debate about that knowledge, which references its own past, which is both continuing and therefore continuous, without being static (Asad 2003:222).

[6] *See* Humphrey (2002) on urban shamanism, landscape and innovation in Ulan-Ude. See Zhukovskaia (2004), Quijada (2008), Jokic (2008) and Metzo (2008) for discussions about 'tradition' and innovation in Buriat shamanism.

has an advanced engineering degree. As Viktor explains it, when a person is chosen by his ancestors to be a shaman, he or she is marked before birth by a thread that connects him to the gods, and the gods look for that person after they are born. When he was twenty, he was told he was meant to become a shaman, but he thought it was all foolishness [*irunda*]. He knew he had blacksmith ancestors, but he didn't think it was important. His family didn't think it was important. It was the 1980s and there were no shamans. When he was twenty-eight, around the time of *perestroika*, he was attacked on the street by drunk hooligans, who beat him severely with a metal bar, probably a tire iron. He lost consciousness and was taken to the hospital. He lost his sight as a result of his injuries. Doctors told him that there was blood on his brain. He was taken to Moscow and St. Petersburg to be treated and the doctors said there was nothing they could do, that the trauma had been too great to be healed. Although he wasn't completely blind, he was legally blind, and could not see enough to function in daily life or work in his previous profession.[7] He visited every doctor he could, and all the doctors said the same thing, that they couldn't help him. So he started visiting *lamas*, and they too couldn't help him. Then a friend took him to a shaman in Mongolia, who helped him, released some of the blood on his brain, and told him he needed to become a shaman. He visited one shaman after another until he met Bair Zhambalovich, the Director of Tengeri. At that time, Bair was living in Aga, and studying with a shaman in Mongolia. Bair was able to help him.

After his first protective initiation, Viktor's vision began to improve. Bair channelled Viktor's family spirits who told him he had been selected to be a shaman. His ancestral spirits are blacksmith shamans [*kuznetsi*] and they sent the drunks to attack him and change the course of his life. He and Bair read the metal bar with which he was attacked as a sign that the attack was motivated by his blacksmith ancestors. Under Bair's tutelage Viktor began to learn about and accept his calling, and his vision steadily improved with each initiation. Viktor and his friends brought Bair Zhambalovich to Ulan-Ude and they set up Tengeri together. When I met him, Viktor wore very thick glasses and held things very close to read, but his vision did not seem otherwise impaired. I am not qualified to evaluate the optical signals that Viktor's brain receives. However, it was clear from our discussions that he considers his eyesight to have improved, and he understands this improvement to be a direct result of his activities as a shaman.

It would be easy to argue that Viktor no longer considers his blindness an illness, that instead of indexing physical illness, his vision problems index his relationship to the spirits, and that healing has occurred through this re-signification. To a certain degree that is true, but it is also overly facile. As Viktor explains it, in order to achieve a cure, the cause of an illness must be treated. If the cause is physical in nature, then bio-medical treatment is sufficient. If the cause is spiritual in nature, then bio-medical treatment will not relieve physical symptoms. For Viktor, the physical relief of symptoms, the fact that his eyesight has actually improved, is an indication that the diagnosis of a shamanic calling was correct, and validation that he has learned to read his symptoms, that he has learned to communicate properly. This communication has established a healthy relationship between Viktor and his ancestors. The health of his relationship with his ancestors is evidenced by the health of his eyesight.

Further, however, he reads his cure as a sign that he has become the kind of person capable of reading the signs correctly. The attack occurred in the first place because he

---

[7] As in the United States, in the Russian Federation 'legally blind' is a state-recognized disability category. Many of the shamans at Tengeri are, as a result of the illnesses that provided their callings, registered under one of the many state-recognized disability categories.

dismissed his shamanic calling as 'foolishness.' As a young engineer from an atheist family, he lacked the knowledge to recognize the signs his ancestors were sending him. They were required to send a sign he could not ignore—the attack which left him legally blind. His ancestors literally 'hit him over the head' with his calling. In response, Viktor was led to re-configure his relationship to what he sees as 'traditional' Buriat knowledge and values, and to accept the kinship obligations imposed by his dead ancestor shamans [ongonuud]. These interpretations, and the life-choices he has made based on these interpretations, are validated by the improvement of his physical symptoms. Instead of just being a sign of physical illness, his blindness has been re-signified as communication with his ancestors. But it also remains a sign of illness. It is precisely because it is both that the experience has become so meaningful and powerful to Viktor.

For the shamans at Tengeri, the path to becoming a shaman invariably begins with physical illness. Many describe their calling as a matter of life or death. Budashab Purboevich, another founding member of the organization told me, "I finally realized, I could die or I could become a shaman. What could I do? I have kids. So I became a shaman." All of the shamans experienced serious illnesses. Some also experienced family tragedies, including the deaths of relatives that they attribute to the wrath of ignored ancestors. Many were at some point so sick that they receive permanent disability pensions, and rather than explain their illness, they would tell me their state-registered disability pension category. While at first I found this frustrating, I eventually realized that it was precisely because their illnesses defy standard medical categories that they come to be diagnosed as a shamanic calling.

For most Buriats, as well as members of other ethnic groups in Buriatiia, the primary recourse in the event of physical illness is Russian bio-medicine or, depending on the illness and the interests of the patient, Tibetan herbal medicine. Most people only begin to consult a shaman when their illness does not respond to either of these treatment methods. Nor would the shamans want them to. No one at Tengeri disputes the efficacy of either Russian state-run medicine or the Tibetan herbal medicine offered at Buddhist temples, in treating physical illnesses. It is precisely when an illness does not respond to standard medical treatment that alternative causes begin to be suspected. In their view, Russian bio-medicine, and Tibetan herbal medicine treat the body. If the causes of illness are purely physical, then this is enough. However, as they see it, many forms of physical illness are merely symptoms of an underlying spiritual cause. If the cause of the illness is spiritual, then bio-medical and herbal treatments may treat the symptoms, but they will not heal the illness, because they cannot treat the cause.

Many individuals first come to Tengeri to be treated for physical symptoms of illness.[8] As I have explained, usually these are symptoms that have not responded well to bio-medical treatment. Treatment begins by determining a diagnosis. Diagnosing a shamanic calling is a long and complicated process that sometimes takes years from the onset of symptoms to the first protective initiation [zashchita]. Not all forms of spirit-caused illness are shamanic callings. Symptoms can be caused by possession, by curses [porcha], soul loss or inflicted by angry ancestors. Treatment depends on the cause. Tengeri shamans, and many other Buriats I have spoken with, recognize several types of possession. Individuals can be possessed by a wide range of spirits, usually malevolent, with whom no accommo-

---

[8] Clients also visit Tengeri for divination, to make routine offerings to their ancestors, or to treat spirit-caused ailments that have been diagnosed by other shamans, but which the diagnosing shaman did not feel qualified to treat. Usually these clients are people who are already embedded in shamanic forms of practice. Other clients may be experiencing 'bad luck' or seeking advice for a variety of problems.

dation can or should be reached. Alcoholism and other forms of addiction are sometimes explained through possession by a malevolent spirit whose desires override the will of the possessed individual. These spirits must simply be exorcised. A shamanic calling is not considered to be possession in quite the same way.

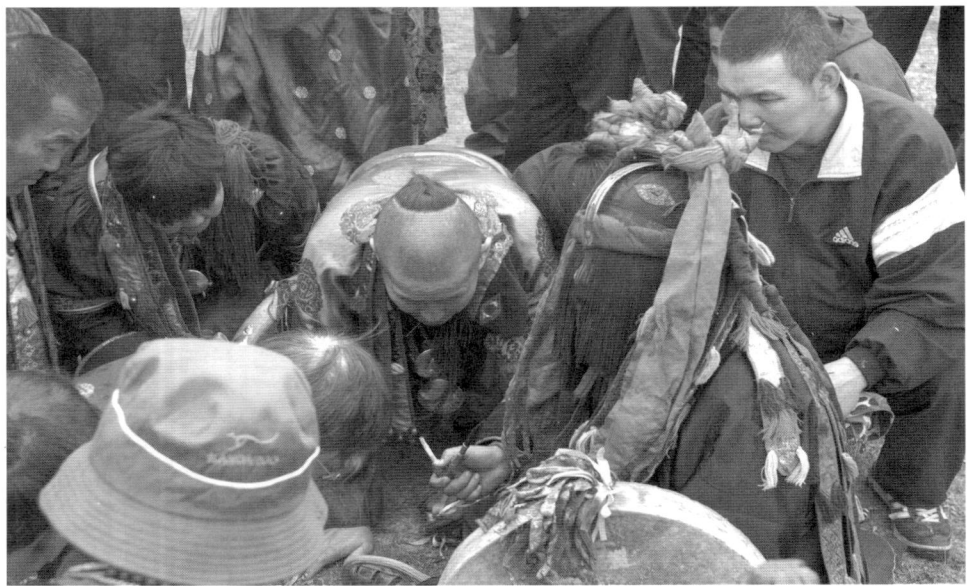

Figure 1.3. *Asking questions of the* ongonuud*: The shaman in the center, wearing the headdress, is in trance. The* ongon *has 'settled down' and accepted a cigarette from the attending shamans, signaling that he or she is ready to communicate. The people surrounding him are other shamans, who are asking the* ongon *questions. Everyone is careful not to look the* ongon *directly in the eyes.*
Photo by Roberto Quijada.

In many cases, a shaman may determine that symptoms are caused by ancestors who are angry because their living descendents have not maintained the proper ritual relationship with them. As documented in Russian ethnographic sources (Banzarov 1997; Dugarov 2002; Galdanova 1987; Gerasimova *et al.* 2000; Mikhailov 1990, 2004a, 2004b) and as described by the shamans at Tengeri, 'traditional' Buriat shamanism is clan-based, meaning that the shaman's primary responsibility is to maintain the proper relationship between the living and dead members of a kinship group. During the Soviet period, however, clan designations became less important, shamanism became politically dangerous, and as a result, many families did not maintain ritual obligations to their clan ancestors. Now that some families have resumed these ceremonies, those whose descendants were not making offerings might become jealous, and afflict their living descendants with familial problems, illnesses, alcoholism, and bouts of bad luck. Sometimes having a shaman perform regular offerings is enough to relieve physical symptoms and other related conditions. In this case, the patient is not called to become a shaman.

A shamanic calling is perceived to be a considerable burden and the diagnosis is not made or accepted lightly. As it was explained to me by the shamans at Tengeri, individuals are chosen to be shamans by their ancestor shamans [*ongonuud*]. An *ongon* is an ancestor shaman.[9] Ancestors can influence the lives of the living, helping them if they choose to,

---

[9] *See* Humphrey and Onon (1996:183-193) for an excellent description of *onggor* among Daur Mongols. Humphrey describes *onggor* as "the soul-spoor of previous

harming them if they are neglected and angry. Although all ancestors affect the living, only ancestors who were shamans become *ongonuud*. These ancestral shamans select the member of the family who will receive the clan's shamanic gift at birth. The individual is marked before birth, and connected to their ancestors by a thread. Over the course of a lifetime, signs are sent to indicate that the individual has been called to be a shaman, and is to be 'harnessed' [*zalozheno*] to their ancestors.[10] Sometimes individuals are told, by other shamans or healers, that they are meant to be a shaman, sometimes not. Sometimes the information is imparted in dreams, sometimes there are no semantic indications at all. If the candidate does not recognize, acknowledge or accept the gift, the ancestor shaman or shamans will track them down [*dogoniat'*] and inflict suffering. In most cases, at this point, the prospective shaman will become very ill, and the symptoms will not respond to biomedical treatment. However, as we shall see, symptoms can include physical and mental illnesses, as well as the misfortune, injury or death of family members. The symptoms, whatever they are, will continue until the prospective shaman either accepts their calling or dies. Only in rare cases will the *ongon* allow the gift to be transferred from one family member to another.

Diagnosing a shamanic calling is usually a long and complicated process. In several cases I have been told that the treating shaman could tell immediately that the patient had a calling, but even in these cases confirming a diagnosis is complicated. If a calling is suspected, the patient is instructed to start asking family members about relatives who were shamans, and to trace the family's genealogy to determine which ancestors may be afflicting the patient. During a diagnostic ceremony, the treating shaman goes into a trance, embodying his or her own *ongon*. The shaman's assistants and the patient ask the shaman's *ongon* to communicate with the patient's ancestors to find out whether the patient has a calling, and which ancestor is inflicting the symptoms. Pre-existing genealogical information helps the questioning process, because *ongonuud* speak in old dialects of Buriat, and in verse, and their answers may be difficult to interpret (Fig. 1.3).

Once the diagnosis has been established, and the possessing ancestor identified, the patient undergoes their first initiation, a *zashchita* [protection] during which the patient must make an offering, and promise to accept the calling and begin training. In return, the *ongon* agrees to stop tormenting the afflicted. Performing the *zashchita* should relieve the symptoms of illness. If it does, the initiate has a period of physical recovery during which he or she can begin to learn how to be a shaman. When Bair Zhambalovich determines that the candidate is ready, and they have saved enough resources for the ceremony, the initiate must complete a second initiation in order to learn to go into trance and embody his or her *ongon*(*-uud*). However, if they wait too long to take the next step, the *ongonuud* will express their displeasure by causing the initial symptoms to return. Sometimes the *zashchita* does not relieve all the symptoms. In these cases, further diagnostic ceremonies often reveal that the initiate has inherited a shamanic gift from more than one side of the family, and must undergo a second *zashchita* for the other lineage.

By this point in the process, the initiate has already learned to read their physical

---

and now dead shamans" (1996:185). Although the Tengeri shamans spoke about their *ongonuud* as individual persons, the way in which they discussed their calling implied that the (singular) shamanic force of a clan had been embodied in each of these individual ancestral shamans, and the living shaman was the current holder of this power, which is referred to as *onggor* by the Daur Mongols described by Humphrey and Onon.

[10] [Editor's note] The modern meaning of *zalozhit'* means 'to be built into' or 'in debt to.' The root, *zalog*, is related to an old Slavic word for 'to lay' (Vasmer 1986 vol.2:509). This secondary meaning may come from a regional dialect of Russian.

symptoms not as signs of illness, but as signs of a social relationship with their ancestors. They are no longer a patient, but an initiate. During the diagnostic and protective ceremonies the initiate's *ongonuud* communicate verbally through the treating shaman's *ongonuud*. However, this form of communication is, as I have mentioned, limited, often difficult to interpret and necessarily conducted through several mediators—the treating shaman's *ongonuud* and the shaman's assistants. The only way that an initiate's *ongon* can speak directly to them is through physical symptoms and in dreams. The initiate is healed not because the symptoms have gone away (although sometimes this is the case) but because they have learned to read their symptoms as a means of communication. When and if the symptoms return, they are interpreted as signs that the relationship between the shaman and his or her *ongon* needs adjusting.

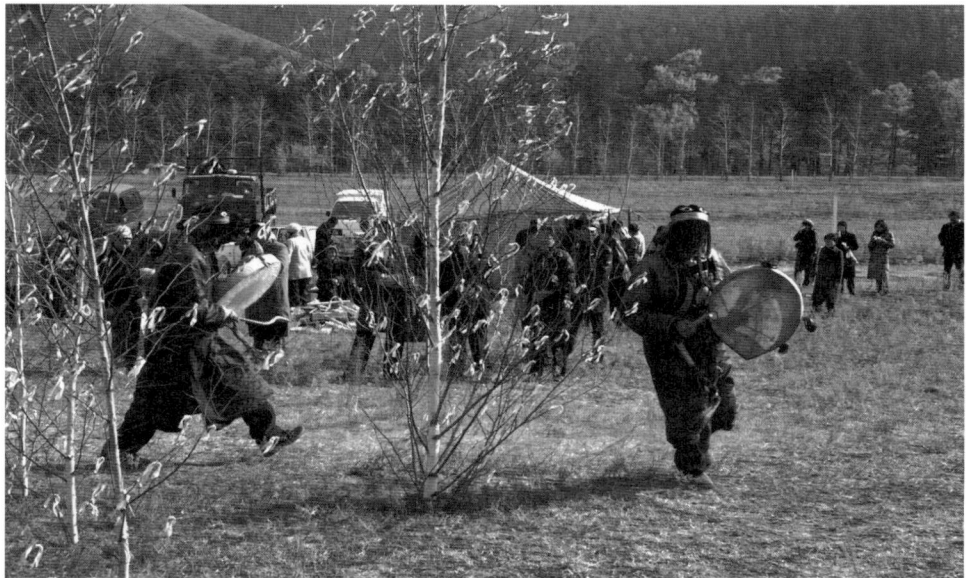

Figure 1.4 *Birch trees, decorated with fabric strips, are erected at the center of a ceremonial site. Yellow and red fabric symbolizes gold, blue and white symbolizes silver, and are intended as a gift to the* ongonuud. *Shamans run around the grove of birch trees while drumming, or shaking bells, to induce trance. The trees are burned at the end of the ceremony. Spring* tailgan *ceremony, Verkhne Beriozovkhe, 2005.* Photo by Roberto Quijada.

The Tengeri shamans describe the shamanic calling as a physical imperative, as a demand placed on them both by their bodies and their ancestors. Everyone I spoke to emphasized that they did not have a choice, that this was not a question of choosing a profession, but rather diagnosing a physical condition—the state of being a shaman. I met Tuiana on a trip to Olkhon Island.[11] Tuiana had suffered from various un-diagnosable illnesses, including pain in her joints and unexplained fevers, as well as family tragedies. Tuiana told me that she inherited her gift from her mother. Her mother had been sick her

---

[11] Tengri, in cooperation with another Tengeri organization from the Aga Buriat Okrug, has been conducting an annual 'International Shamanic Conference' on Olkhon Island since 2003. This includes a *tailgan* [offering] ceremony to the spirit master of Lake Baikal and is intended to re-sanctify the island, which they believe is an *axis mundi*. They envision the conference as an event where indigenous shamans from other areas of the world can come and exchange ideas and techniques. To date there have been visiting shamans from California, Germany, and Buriat shamans from Inner Mongolia.

entire life. Back in 1968, when Tuiana was a year old, her parents drove people to visit a Russian folk healer, and on a whim, decided to go hear what the woman had to say. Her mother took one step over the threshold and the Russian healer told her "You know why you've been sick your whole life? Because you were supposed to help people, and you didn't. But now it's too late, and your gift has passed to one of your daughters."

When she was younger, Tuiana had been told that she was the daughter who had inherited the gift and needed to become a shaman. By the time I met her, she had undergone the first initiation [*zashchita*] but had been postponing the second, in which she would finally embody her possessing *ongon*, because the prospect of becoming a full-fledged shaman and going into trance frightened her. However, another relative had recently died, and Tuiana was convinced his death was caused by her *ongonuud* because she had postponed the ceremony. She was determined to go through with the initiation before any further calamities befell her family. The shaman she was working with suggested that she go along to Olkhon Island and participate in order to get acquainted with other shamans and more comfortable with trance states. She told me that her first initiation went smoothly, but it was frightening because her hands and legs moved on their own, without her volition, in response to the drumming. When she told the initiated shamans this, they always laughed, and said, "Yes, those are the *ongonuud* coming," and assured her she would get used to the feeling. These sensations were a sign of her prospective ability to go into trance and become possessed, another sign of her relationship with her *ongonuud*.

Tuiana's shamanic calling cannot be understood in the standard bio-medical sense of a physical condition experienced by her body. It was indeed manifested through physical states of being, in high fevers that had no bio-medically discernible cause and which left her completely debilitated, with pains in her joints, but also in the way her hands and feet vibrated when she heard the shaman's drums. But her illness, as she came to understand it, was also her mother's illness, and the cause of a relative's death. All were equally symptoms of the same underlying disease—her (and her mother's) shamanic calling. Her body is only one part of an entire family of bodies that suffered from the same illness, and could be cured only by her initiation. Tuiana's story gives us a sense of the weight borne by those who are 'harnessed' [*zalozheno*] to their ancestors.

In the Tengeri understanding, shamanism is a kinship obligation. Every family needs someone who can intercede between the living and the dead, and the obligation to do so is an obligation to both living and dead family members. If the calling is refused, the entire family can and does suffer. Likewise, both living and dead members of the family must support the initiate. If the initiate is to become a shaman, the *ongonuud* must accept the initiate's offering, and they must agree to communicate, through physical symptoms, through dreams, by sending omens,[12] and eventually they agree to enter the initiate's body and communicate verbally, through the use of the shaman's body. The shaman's living relatives must also accept and support the initiate, through participation in initiations, and by providing the resources necessary to conduct the appropriate ceremonies. If either of these groups of relatives refuses their assistance, the initiate will not be able to become a shaman. His or her symptoms will continue. A shamanic calling, in this sense, is an illness that afflicts an entire family, but is manifested in the body of the prospective shaman. Iuri,

---

[12] The most common form of omen that I was told about was the appearance of particular species of birds, usually ones that are linked to the initiate's clan in mythology. For example, an eagle circled above an initiation ceremony which I attended, and was immediately noted as a good sign. Another shaman's wife told me that when her husband had reached an important decision about his training, a flock of ravens took up residence outside their house and would not leave.

who successfully passed his second initiation in 2005, told me that before an important ceremony, all the men in his family developed fevers, because the *ongonuud* were always worried that they would back out. "As soon as the trees go up" he said, referring to the birch trees that are erected at a ceremonial site, "we all feel better, because they [the *ongonuud*] know the ceremony will take place" (Fig. 1.4). For both Iuri and Tuiana, physical symptoms of illness are not confined to a single physical body, but rather index the relationships between bodies of common descent. Particular bodily states of being are given new interpretations. These interpretations are grounded in the obligations and dependencies of kinship relations. But learning to read these symptoms correctly involves a transformation in subjectivity, from the kind of person who sees physical symptoms as signs of a biomedical illness, to the kind of person who can see that the cause of that illness is rooted in kinship obligations denied.

Interpreting physical symptoms as communication from *ongonuud* is only the first layer of signification. Bair Zhambalovich and his students see the prevailing inability of contemporary urban Buriats to properly recognize shamanic signs as a sign of social degeneration. Viktor explained to me:

> If you ignore these signs, your ancestors make you sick, but if you don't know the signs, if you can't recognize them, how will you know that is what is wrong? That's why, during the Soviet period, many people ended up in mental hospitals; doctors thought they were schizophrenic, or they died, because they didn't know. The knowledge had been lost and so they suffered. When you think of all the people who died unnecessarily because they didn't know what was happening to them. There is a young man here who was in a mental hospital for two years, and now he's fine. You see all the social problems we suffer from now—alcoholism, broken families, depression. Alcoholics are possessed by evil spirits, *sabdaguud*. You can see them, they have no control over their actions, the *sabdak* controls them. Once you know you can see it. We can treat that, exorcize them, but people don't know this. Other people think if their grandfather was a shaman, they are one too, and just set up shop. They don't know that it doesn't work that way. If the information is out there, and people have a centre they can turn to for help and for information, then some of these problems can be solved. We have to educate people about their traditions.

Tengeri's mission, as an organization, is to provide a resource people can turn to for education and treatment in all matters shamanic. They see the inability of many people to recognize the symptoms of a shamanic calling, the fact that these symptoms are first interpreted as signs of bio-medical illness, as a sign of broader disconnection from traditional culture, traditional knowledge and traditional kinship obligations. In order to become fully initiated, embody *ongonuud* in trance, and begin to work as a shaman, the initiate has to learn a great deal, and in effect, fundamentally transform themselves. They must learn, and sometimes re-create through oral history, archival research and dream-guidance, their family and clan history. They must learn to communicate in Buriat, at least enough so that they are able to perform the chants that call down the *ongonuud* to the ceremony [*kamlanie*] and into their body and to communicate with the spirits of other shamans during the ceremonies. Many urban-born and educated Buriats speak only Russian. Although modern Buriat is written in the Cyrillic alphabet, Buriat is an Altaic language whose grammatical and phonological system is fundamentally different from Russian. Many of the new initiates struggled with the language. Those who grew up in families where Buriat was spoken at home had a significant advantage, but others, who had the discipline to practice were also those who succeeded in other areas.

Transformations were not only required by the initiate themselves, but also by their spouses and relatives. Spouses, especially the wives of male shamans, often offered the most dramatic accounts of how they became convinced of their spouse's calling. Spouses have an intimate view of the initial illness, failed medical treatments, relief of symptoms and, once the shaman is able to embody their *ongonuud*, of direct communication with the spirit. They are therefore often better able to narrate the transformation than the shaman. When the shamans discussed their callings, spouses and other relatives often presented themselves as impartial witnesses who could attest that, indeed, all other possible diagnoses and treatments had been tried. Only if the spouses, parents and other relatives of the initiate are willing and able to support the process, are willing to supply resources and take part in ceremonies, can the initiate become a shaman. Although relatives do not need to learn to read the signs sent by the ancestors, they must be willing to accept that what appear to be bio-medical symptoms are indeed something more.

When speaking about their callings, most of the shamans at Tengeri draw a sharp distinction between the person they were before their calling and the person they became afterward. The physical symptoms of illness that brought them to shamanism were often severe, but they all stress the ways in which they were not connected to what they see as Buriat traditions. "I thought it was foolishness. It was Soviet times, there were no shamans then." "I did not understand." "I wasn't able to see the signs."

Misdiagnosed shamanic callings, are, in this instance, a sign that the initiate, and in many cases, their family, are insufficiently integrated into 'traditional' forms of Buriat knowledge and ritual behaviour. When they speak about the organization's mission, they describe an almost utopian vision of the past, in which ritual obligations between ancestors and the living were always maintained, and as a result the lines of communication between ancestors, deities and living humans were open. In such a world, shamanic callings would be communicated between *ongonuud* and the living without invoking pain or suffering. That world, should it ever have existed (and I think most of the shamans at Tengeri would agree it is more an ideal than an actually existing historical period), has been corrupted by the presence of Buddhism, Russian colonization and the Soviet government, all of which have made communication between ancestors and the living more complicated, by providing alternative forms of signification, alternative frames of meaning, and alternative possible diagnoses for physical symptoms. Within this narrative, undiagnosed and misdiagnosed shamanic callings are an illness caused by the fact that pre-Buddhist and pre-Soviet forms of knowledge and communication have broken down. This is an illness which, while manifested in the body of the prospective shaman, is an illness from which whole families, and the whole Buriat nation, suffer.

However, although Tengeri is committed to reviving what they call 'traditional' Buriat shamanism, and they are explicitly committed to improving the health of the 'Buriat nation', they do not define Buriat in an exclusive way. As Bair Zhambalovich explained to me, they chose the name 'Local Religious Organization of Shamans Tengeri' because 'local' was more inclusive, and recognized the multi-ethnic nature of their constituency, as well as acknowledged that other ethnic groups residing in the area also have shamanic traditions. Buriats have been part of Russia for over 300 years, and Tengeri's vision of shamanism as a public health initiative acknowledges that after 300 years of intermarriage, a shamanic calling may pass to an individual who may not otherwise think of themselves as Buriat. In addition, like many of the shamans at Tengeri who were, before their calling, unable to recognize shamanic signs, those who identify as Buriats have widely varying degrees of embeddedness in pre-Soviet kinship and ritual structures. In Tengeri's view, spirits are tied to places and to bodies. Therefore, if you live in Buriat places, or have 'Buriatness' in your body, you may need to maintain relationships with Buriat spirits in order to be healthy.

The process of becoming a shaman requires that an individual recognize the claims that their family and their nationality make on their body. In understanding this claim, it is useful to turn to Povinelli's distinction between the genealogical society and the autological subject (Povinelli 2006). The autological subject is the western post-enlightenment ideal of the free individual, while the genealogical society stands for the social, familial and cultural ties that render certain types of individuals, usually indigenous individuals, less than fully 'free.' In Povinelli's analysis, she argues that the value of this distinction is not merely the idea of society contrasted with the idea of the free individual, but the way in which these ideas manifest in bodies and in bodily experience. In her analysis, different kinds of sociality produce different kinds of bodily risk. Bio-medical approaches to illness take the autological individual, a single person within a single body, as the base-line from which to approach illness. Genealogical society, the kinds of social bonds represented by indigenous kinship networks are, from a bio-medical point of view, more likely to be seen as causing illness, than in producing a cure. This attitude was certainly a mainstay of Soviet educational projects throughout the 1920s and 30s, within which traditional practices, typified by shamanism, were considered to keep people in ignorance, dirt, and disease.[13]

When they speak about the process of diagnosing their shamanic calling, the shamans at Tengeri speak very differently about the relationship between self and kin, between autological subject and genealogical society. They begin their stories as free individuals, autological subjects who are ill because they are not properly embedded in kinship relations and genealogical society. Kinship obligations exist. The free individual does not see them, does not value them, does not honor them, and is therefore ill. The individual initiate is healed by recognizing and accepting their genealogical relationships, by recreating themselves as subjects of their ancestor's will, 'harnessed' to their *ongonuud* and in service of the living. Healing is achieved through an ever increasing degree of communication between *ongonuud* and shaman that begins with, and is maintained through, reading physical symptoms of illness as a means of communication. This interpretation of illness is necessarily also a critique of the forms of social life, originating in Soviet modernization projects, that predominate in post-Soviet Ulan-Ude, advocating a return to what they see as more 'traditional' forms of Buriat sociality. They should not, however, be interpreted as a rejection of 'modernity' as a whole. Rather, the shamans at Tengeri seek to integrate shamanic healing into modern, urban life.

As I have argued in relation to Viktor's calling, it would be too facile to assume that just because they have learned to read physical symptoms as a form of communication from their ancestors, that these physical symptoms cease to be signs of bio-medical illness. This is not the case, and to interpret healing in this way runs the risk of inviting a romanticized vision of Siberian indigenous peoples as somehow subject to cultural interpretation in a way that those of us raised in bio-medical spheres of interpretation are not. The shamans at Tengeri are just as embedded in bio-medical forms of knowledge as any American anthropologist, and in the case of Bair Zhambalovich Tsirendorzhiev, who was a veterinarian before he became a shaman, probably more so. The physical symptoms of illness, the fevers, the aching joints, the headaches, the bouts of blindness, the seizures and

---

[13] A good example of this discourse is in early Soviet research on syphilis and the spread of syphilis through traditional religious practices (Solomon 1993). This rhetoric is also discussed in Slezkine (1992, 1994).

blood sugar levels that index communication from *ongonuud* are also and always will be signs of bio-medical illness to the shamans who suffer from them. Bair Zhambalovich does not tell his students to stop taking their medicine. He tells them that the medicine will not work unless they have addressed the underlying spiritual cause of the illness. The fact that ritual action ameliorates these undeniably bio-medical physical symptoms is what makes the diagnosis of a shamanic calling compelling and convincing to both shaman and patient.

The shamans at Tengeri are healed through a process of re-signifying bodily symptoms as signs of communication by ancestor spirits. Learning to read these signs is a process that embeds the initiate in kinship relations and in forms of traditional knowledge and sociality that give bio-medical symptoms additional meaning. The boundaries of illness in this context are not limited to the individual body. The body of the individual shaman is merely the locus of an illness that afflicts an entire family, and indeed, the entire Buriat nation. However, as I have argued, it is important to see this not as an alternative way of understanding illness that must be contrasted to a purely bio-medical approach to illness, but one that is embedded within, and yet exceeds a purely bio-medical interpretation. The shamans at Tengeri and their patients do not see shamanic knowledge and bio-medical knowledge as fundamentally distinct and potentially conflicting spheres of knowledge production. Rather, they consider shamanic treatment to provide the spiritual and social context that renders bio-medical healing meaningful for modern, urban Buriats.

Acknowledgements

The research for this chapter was supported by a Leiffer Grant from the Department of Anthropology, University of Chicago, a Fulbright-Hays Doctoral Dissertation Fellowship, IREX Individual Advanced Research Opportunity Grant and a Charlotte W. Newcombe Doctoral Dissertation Completion Fellowship, as well as the generous cooperation of the Local Shaman's Organization Tengeri. All conclusions are my own.

Chapter Two

Medical Pluralism and Expert Knowledge in Buriatiia

Katherine Metzo

My interest in medicinal plants and healing emerged after a series of coincidences. While carrying out my dissertation research on the domestic economy of post-socialist, rural Buriatiia in 2000, I researched the household use of non-timber forest resources. I sought to understand the full range of paid and unpaid labour, cultivated and wild food production, and other entrepreneurial activities that helped families make ends meet. What I found was a kind of 're-peasantization' of the countryside, where people became increasingly dependent on subsistence production and kin networks to improve the stability of household economies (Metzo 2003, 2006). My colleagues in Ulan-Ude, the Buriat capital, delighted in pointing out the 'obvious' answers to the questions I was asking. Their answers often did not match up with my data, raising new questions about how people think about plant-based resources and how they act on their knowledge and perceptions.

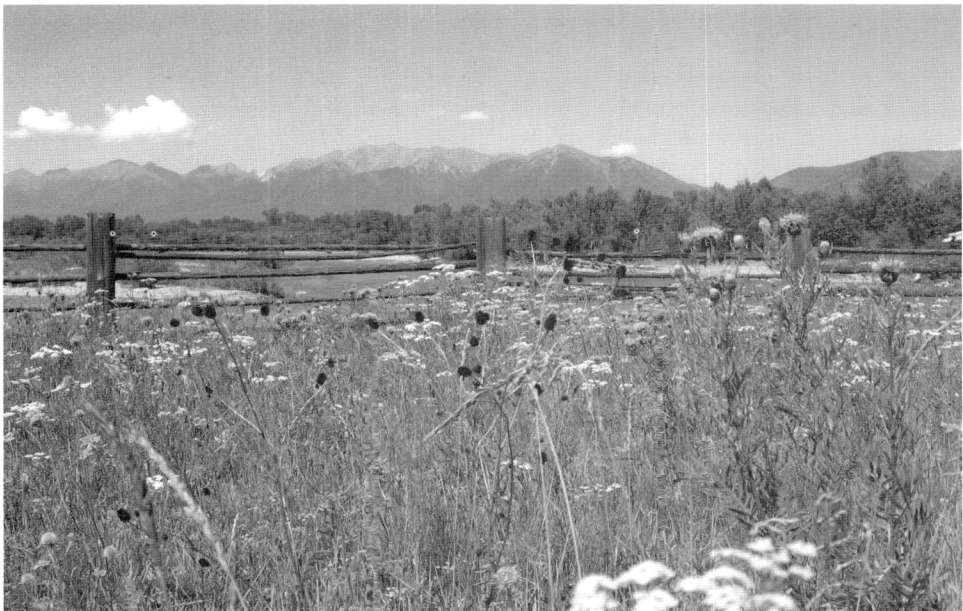

Figure 2.1. *Medicinal plants growing in private pasture, Tory, Tunka Valley, Buriatiia, 2005.*
All photos by author.

The first coincidence arose when I compared my survey data on plant collections to the 'common sense' impressions my interlocutors held about forest resources. My urban colleagues expected that since the countryside was full of natural herbal resources, that local villagers collected medicinal plants widely. For example, when I reported with gravity that the medical clinic in one of the villages was closing down, my urban colleagues and friends replied that "They don't need a clinic," or "They can get by without a clinic," because of the 'pharmacy' right under their feet (Fig 2.1). However, my initial survey results showed that very few locals actually collected medicinal plants. This paradox led me to pay closer attention to the actual treatments that people used when I returned to the Tunka Valley, southwest of Lake Baikal, in 2005.

When I returned, a second coincidence alerted me to the existence of a complex, pluralistic medical system. Although not many people gathered medicinal plants, I noticed that a nurse regularly drank herbal teas as a supplement to allopathic treatments. My own weak health in the field led my friends to recommend that I prepare teas to combat my survey-recording-induced laryngitis. When surveying kitchen cupboards, I discovered boxes of industrially prepared herbals sharing shelf space with pharmaceuticals. Prepared medicinal plant teas were at least as pervasive as pharmaceutical treatments. Ironically, many of these industrially produced teas boasted that their contents originated in the Tunka Valley, where my consultants lived.

It turned out that residents of the Tunka Valley do not gather medicinal plants despite their widespread availability, yet purchase medicinal teas made from these same plants. Stated another way, people are paying to buy back plants from their own backyards. A key to understanding this puzzle comes from the revival of Buddhism in the Lake Baikal region because many of the teas produced commercially make use of Buddhist *ayurveda* 'recipes.'

The disconnection between what I knew and what urbanites thought they knew about rural healthcare motivated me to figure out what was really going on. This chapter addresses a number of questions related to the collection and use of medicinal plants in Buriatiia, on the basis of research conducted primarily in the Tunka Valley. First, are medicinal plants displacing pharmaceuticals in the treatment of illness? If true, this folk hypothesis has some significant implications for the relationship between individuals or families and biomedicine.[1] There would also be a great economic potential for the employees of Tunka National Park,[2] or other local entrepreneurs to harvest and create value-added products from non-timber forest resources for regional and global markets. I argue that pharmaceuticals are not being displaced and that what exists is a pluralistic medical system in which the state has co-opted or absorbed elements of traditional and folk medicine, especially Tibetan Buddhist medicine. Second, why do people in Tunka Valley choose not to collect the medicinal plants growing 'under their feet?' Certainly, the entire range of plants needed for a comprehensive inventory of Buddhist medicines is not available in the restricted spaces where people spend their daily lives, but a number of important plants used to treat common illnesses are available nearby.

The use of medicinal plants in Tibetan Buddhist medicine is viewed as a specialized skill, despite the availability of published literature on plants and their uses. Tunka residents maintain a folk understanding of health that is limited to the Buddhist emphasis on a healthy diet and lifestyle. Therefore, one of the reasons people do not collect special plants is because their diet and climate provides them the necessary nutrients and energy to remain healthy. In cases where a specialized treatment is required, I argue that they see this as expert knowledge that can only be learned through formal training, and which they lack.

---

[1] I cannot explore these implications here, but they may include things like tracking epidemiological information on the region which has high rates of tuberculosis and hepatitis.

[2] Tunka National Park, at the time of my research, shared co-terminous borders with Tunkin district, the administrative unit I also refer to as the Tunka Valley. Several settled areas have been excluded from strict park management and there have been efforts to include a portion of neighbouring Oka district into the National Park.

Chapter Two: *Medical Pluralism and Expert Knowledge in Buriatiia*

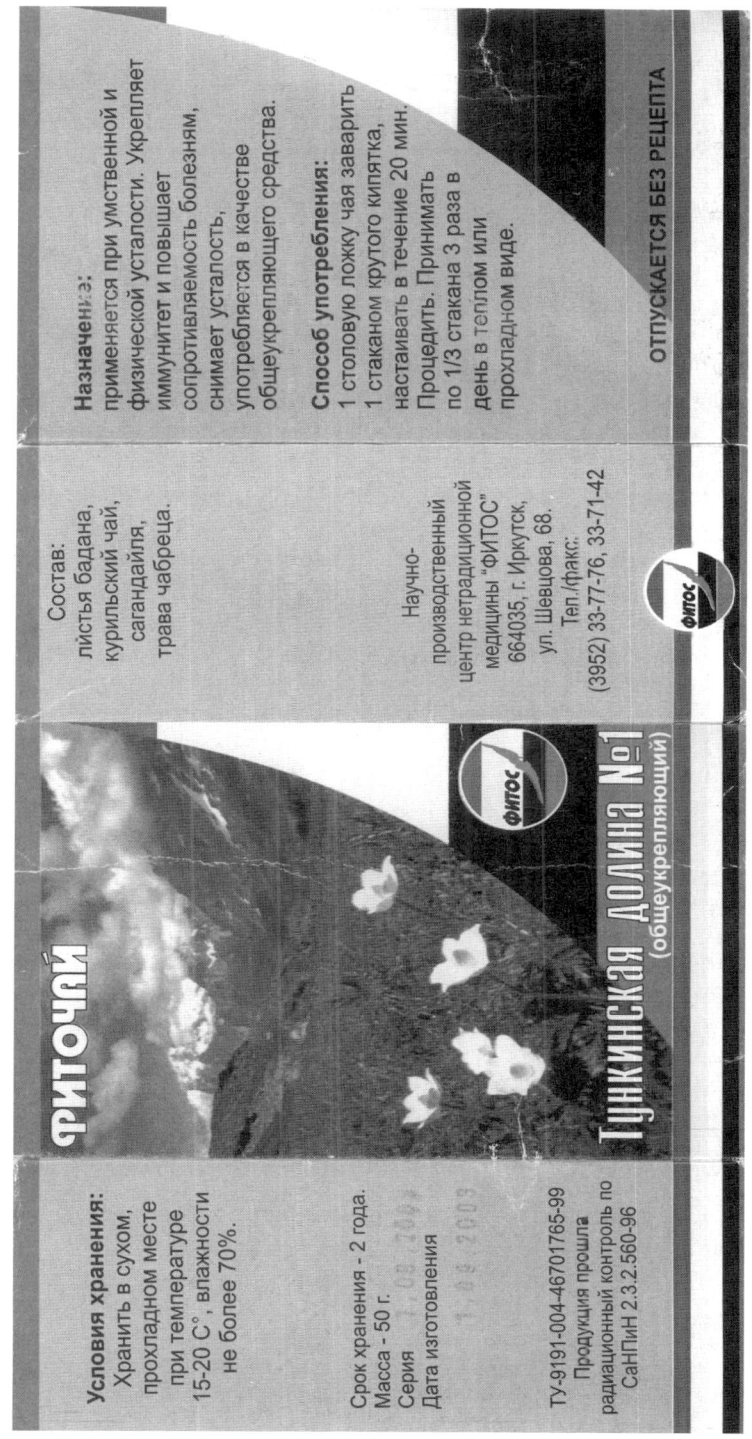

Figure 2.2. *Tunka Valley Tea No. 1 'General Health.' This is a scanned package of a medicinal tea from the Tunka valley giving the contents, storage instructions, dosage instructions, and the address of the factory in Irkutsk.*

Medicinal Plants and Medical Pluralism

Herbal remedies have been part of both Russian and Buriat cultures for several centuries. The renewed interest in medicinal plants is illustrated by the proliferation of publications (books, pamphlets, brochures) on home remedies, traditional healing, healing herbs and other topics, as well as by the availability in shops of herbal teas and herbal balsam made from local plants. In Russian culture, the preparation of herbal treatments is associated primarily with female folk healers [Rus. *tselitely*], while in Buriat culture, medicinal plants are associated with Buddhist monasteries and *emchi-lamas* [healers][3] who meet with patients, prepare and dispense treatments.

Russian use of medicinal plants has a place in the discussion of Buriat healing because of the long history of interaction between these cultures in the Baikal Region. I focus on this tradition briefly here in order to highlight the contrast between folk traditions and the Indian medical tradition *ayurveda* (discussed in more detail in Chapter 3 by Gololobova).

Russian folk medicine was primarily an oral tradition until the nineteenth century. Based on a cursory search of contemporary written sources available at my field sites and interviews, it is also a non-unified tradition. While there are clearly connections to Russian Orthodoxy in the practices of contemporary Russian folk healers (e.g., using incense, making the sign of the cross, reciting prayers, lighting candles before icons), the church's official position on herbalists and folk healers is that they are heretics. Among published sources, it is not unusual to see books by Russian authors that fuse 'traditional' Russian folk healing with Eastern medical practices, such as Slavo-Tibetan medicine by a self-named 'white *lama*' whose training in Tuva included apprenticing with 'top' Tuvan shamans (Vostokov 2003). The openness to alternative treatments across ethnic groups in the region helps explain the popularity and availability of medicinal plant products.

Buddhist *ayurveda* medicine in the Baikal Region dates to the 14-15th centuries as an oral tradition. Buriats practice the Mahayana form of Tibetan Buddhism and use medicinal plant teas within a naturalistic medical system that also includes pulse diagnosis, moxibustion,[4] cupping, and acupuncture. In the 19th Century, Buriat *lamas* went as far away as Lhasa Tibet for their medical training. Locally, *lamas* could receive training at several monasteries [*datsanuud*], most famously at Atsagat Datsan in the Aga district.[5] Tibetan medicine was familiar to European Russian audiences as well, through the work of the Buddhist temple in St. Petersburg. By 1924, there were 440 *lama* doctors across 44 temples (Danzanova *et al.* 2001). At the all-Buriat spiritual gathering in 1924, Agvan Dorzhiev made recommendations to the communist party to use Tibetan medicine doctors to supplement medical doctors and nurse-practitioners [*fel'dshery*] in rural areas where there were not a sufficient number of personnel to serve all citizens (Danzanova *et al.* 2001). However, an NKVD [State Secret Police] document from October 1, 1929, forbade all types of religious activity, including medical help (Danzanova *et al.* 2001).

The *ayurveda* medicine practiced in the Baikal region corresponds well with the already existing ideas about illness and disease within Buriat traditional culture. Buriats embrace the concept of balance [Bur. *tegsh*] as important for physiological and spiritual

---

[3] The term *emchi-lami* is derived from the Mongolian word *emchi* meaning doctor, healer.

[4] Moxibustion is a traditional Chinese medicine technique that involves burning cones [*moxa*] of the bitter herb mugwort (*Artemisia vulgaris*) on acupuncture points.

[5] In the Aga district of the former Aga Buriat Autonomous Okrug, since March 2008 now one of three separate districts within Zabaikal' Krai.

health, although it has been argued that the emphasis on balance in Tibetan *ayurveda* is more of a Western interpretation (Janes 2002). According to Tibetan medical theory, there are three humors—*lung* [air], *tri-pa* [bile], and *pe-ken* [phlegm]—at work in the body. Shamanic approaches to healing do not necessarily involve the ingestion of medicinal plants, though it is one of the tools used by shamans in some lineages. Plants, and specifically the smoke of juniper or the local variety of thyme—*chabrets* [Rus.] or *aia-ganga* (Bur.)—are used to clear a space or assist in the process of divination. Ritual offerings, diet, and behavioral modification are most commonly used as ways to return an individual to a state of balance (Fig 2.3).

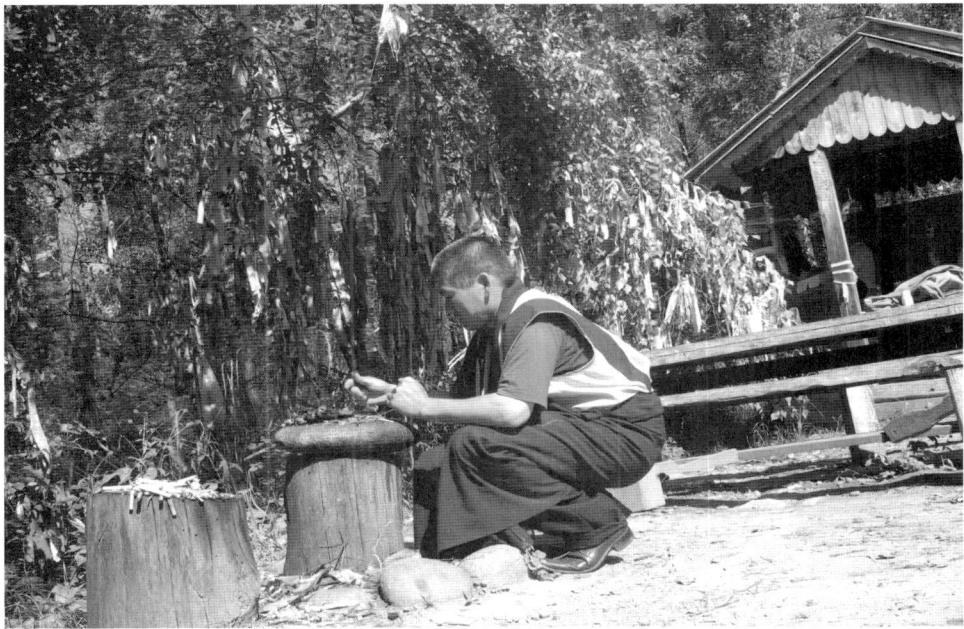

Figure 2.3. *A* lama *burning incense at the* Khongor-uula spring, *Tunka Valley, 2007.*

Buddhist *ayurveda* medicine operates at three levels, according to a senior physician at the Center for Eastern Medicine in Ulan-Ude. First, Tibetan medicine deals with lifestyle [Rus. *obraz zhizni*], which includes responses to seasonal changes in climate as well as behavior and worldview. "The Asian way of thinking [Rus. *myshlenie*] differs from the European." Ecological understanding is critical to this difference. "We don't kill animals for sport, we don't break branches off trees just because" or things like that, he stated. The second level of Tibetan medicine is diet, which I will discuss in greater detail below. The third level is what most people associate with Tibetan medicine—the work of doctors. Medical interventions start with herbal medicines, moving to massage and manual therapy, and ultimately to surgery. Thus, the use of herbal medicines is an important, but limited aspect of Buddhist *ayurveda* as understood, or used more broadly. The goal of Tibetan medicine is to prevent a patient from getting to this level of imbalance and Tibetan doctors encourage people to think about the preventative aspects of medicine and to come in before they are sick.

Well before the introduction of universal biomedical care, shamans, *lamas*, and herbalists co-existed in the Baikal region in a "many-layered, pluralistic medical system" (Garmaeva 2001:9). Baer (2001:3) describes medical pluralism as the coexistence of, "multiple, often antagonistic medical systems." Baer (2001:5) further notes that, in the

American case, "the relationship between biomedicine and alternative medical systems has been characterized by processes of annihilation, restriction, absorption, and even collaboration." While various medical systems coexist, they often borrow from one another, and as one system gains power they absorb elements of other medical systems. Drawing on White (2001), Janes (2002:269) noted that medical pluralism, "reflects as much about how people—patients and healers—position themselves in regard to powerful regional, state, and global discourses of modernity. At the same time, healing articulates with the brute realities of life and, as such, is a form of social action that rests in important ways on entirely, if not solely, pragmatic considerations." Treatment decisions, then, reflect more than simply the decision to return to a state of health. In the case of Buriatiia, the pragmatism of the late 19th and early 20th century included introducing Eastern medicine to the dominant Russian culture, via the St. Petersburg temple, as a legitimate health care practice. In the Soviet era, folk healing, rather than be eliminated by the state, went underground. "Alternatives to biomedicine, when they cannot be set aside as inefficacious or simply labelled as quackery, are often co-opted or 'tamed' by state-supported biomedicine" (Baer 2001).

The state's goal in seeking to achieve universal health care was more utilitarian and economic than it was altruistic. Low life expectancy (29 years) in rural areas in the late 19th century "was a definite liability in terms of return on investments, since the longer a person lived, the greater could be his contribution to society and to the welfare of the population" (Field 1957:6).

In the 1970s and 1980s, medical doctors began experimenting with alternative medical practices, setting up 'private practices' to work with patients through social networks (Lindquist 2002). Acupuncture, homeopathy, herbal treatments, and bio-energy had particular appeal. The end of socialism brought with it the opportunity for all types of alternative medicine to emerge from the shadows and offer their service under market conditions. In Russia, as in China, Eastern traditional medicine became attractive to state authorities because of its ability to treat chronic diseases and was quickly integrated as a therapy within biomedical practice (*see* Janes 2002). In both contexts, the state, as represented in biomedicine, began standardizing care, using Tibetan medicine to deal with those illnesses that biomedicine could not support (Janes 2002).

To make sense of the particulars of the contemporary situation in Buriatiia, I also draw on recent work by Galina Lindquist. A crucial question in a pluralistic medical environment is the question of how individuals, families, or households chose from among the available treatment options. Lindquist rightly argues that post-socialist citizens seeking out health care are, "vigorous agents who challenge and contest the 'experts,' actively seek and discard alternatives, select components that suit them and combine them into their own idiosyncratic versions of treatment regimes" (Lindquist 2002:338). This is equally true in the provinces as it is in Moscow. Lindquist looks at how efficacy is constructed by patient and healer. She suggests that "therapeutic efficacy, a sensory process of betterment, is (especially in non-biomedical treatment) connected with the acceptance of the healer as a person with 'power' or 'charisma': with the recognition of his or her 'charismatic legitimacy'" (Lindquist 2002:338). Lindquist's focus in her Moscow research is specifically on such independent folk healers—some who apprentice with established folk healers, others who draw from a variety of traditional, folk, and new age practices.

In Buriatiia, Buddhist *ayurveda* medicine and shamanism dominate the public consciousness. For healers in these traditions, legitimacy is derived in part from the ancient practice of this knowledge. Russian folk healing, while also ancient, is more idiosyncratic in comparison. Across all types of alternative healing, charisma has a central place in choosing from among individual health care providers as the patient seeks transformation, rather than a mere treatment (Csordas 1994). Biomedicine, which is the standard form of treatment, is often said to address symptoms rather than causes of illness. Nevertheless, biomedicine benefits from scientific legitimacy, the type of legitimacy promoted by the Soviet state which allowed the state to repress other forms of healing. A fascinating consequence of the emphasis on scientific legitimacy is that alternative forms of healing emerge from the shadows in the 1980s and 1990s, scientists begin to study their efficacy (Lindquist 2006). Buddhist *ayurveda*, with its meticulous documentation in the *Tibetan Book of Medicine*[6] and long history of scientific research outside Soviet borders is, then, accessible and much more readily studied, verified, and integrated with biomedicine than other 'alternative' medicines.

Methods and Data

The data for this chapter comes from a variety of sources. I draw on survey and economic diary data from my 2000-01 dissertation research as well as interviews I conducted in 2005 with householders, traditional healers and herbalists, physicians, and plant collectors. I also incorporate a pilot study I arranged in 2007 when I employed a research assistant to ask 18 respondents in the city of Ulan-Ude to assemble 'freelists' of medicinal plants. Those replies were organized in order of 'salience' by using a specialized software programme.[7] Some of the data of these freelists is presented here in Table 2.2. In 2001, I also asked about medical plants during interviews in the villages of Kyren and Tory, a handful of interviews in Arshan, as well as in the village of Zhemchug and the city of Ulan-Ude. Because I already had baseline data for Tory, I wanted to better understand what distinguished households that collect from those that do not. Therefore, I returned to several of the households from my original sample, while adding a handful of new families, as well as interviewing residents with medical training, shamans, and herbalists. I also took walks with several herbalists, who pointed out meadow and forest plants with medicinal properties growing in the village.

My attention was drawn to medical pluralism while living in Tory because the Soviet-era clinic closed in the late 1990s. Without a clinic, residents began relying on a number of strategies. They continued to consult with a visiting/retired nurse-practitioner [*fel'dsher*] from a neighboring community and made use of emergency medical services and hospital care in the regional center of Kyren. They made extensive use of commercially produced medicinal teas sold in local shops. In addition, they also consulted with local shamans, and, as I would learn in 2005, a number of female herbalists who were using and adapting family recipes. In this chapter, I use primarily the insights gained from interviews from the Tunka Valley, with the exception of the free listed data in Table 2.2 collected from 18 individuals by a research assistant in the city of Ulan-Ude.

---

[6] *See* Parfionovich (1994) for an overview of the historical material available in the Baikal Region and how they are analyzed by local scholars. Lama Tenzin-Khetsun (Feodor Samaev) oversaw the reprinting of a late 19th Century textbook on Tibetan Medicine used in the Atsagat Datsan (Pozdneev 1991).

[7] A 'freelist' is a list of words associated with a research topic, in this case, the names of plants. The analysis of 'salience' was calculated using Anthropac software (Anthropac 2010). Salience is a measure both of the frequency with which an item was mentioned by respondents as well as the average ranking given to that item on the freelists.

When I designed my original household survey in 2000, I assumed, like my urban interlocutors, that households would collect a variety of non-timber forest resources, including medicinal plants, and bring them to market. Before beginning the survey, however, I suspected that the collection of medicinal plants would be neither a universal nor a comprehensive practice. First, I was aware that people were already combining salaried activities with subsistence activity, which would logically restrict the amount of time they could spend away from home. These salaried workers, I thought, would be unlikely to collect plants that grew at some distance from their homes or that matured during peak periods at work. Second, I suspected that people would avoid collecting medicinal plants that were easily accessible within a few hours. Instead, I thought, they would concentrate their efforts on gathering important sources of food from the forest such as berries or mushrooms. Third, I was aware that collecting medicinal plants would be simply complicated by the fact that they may not grow in close proximity to other forest resources of interest, and might not be ready to harvest at the same time as such important subsistence resources as berries. Finally, since medicinal plants grew in very specific places because of the variation in terrain and microclimates, gatherers of medicine might have to devote time to extract exactly what was needed. For example, if one were seeking out a variety of plants to make a blended tea, this may require traveling to multiple locations at different times of the year.

I had expected that some households would specialize in plant collection, and then trade the plants for other forgone resources, much like today where people share or trade berries or mushrooms with neighbors, friends, and relatives. However, I was surprised by the results. Based on a survey of 91 households in 2000, only about 2% gathered medicinal plants. The number of households that dried medicinal plants gathered by family members was likely closer to 5%, and some households occasionally bought dried plants from vendors at the open air market in Arshan.[8] Almost all households have pre-packaged medicinal teas on their shelves. My challenge during the repeat survey in 2005 was to make sense of the resulting paradox that householders did not collect even those medicinal plants that were convenient for them, yet almost universally used medicinal plants to treat ill household members.

Medical Pluralism in Tunka

Each household navigates the pluralist terrain of health and healing in its own way. I outline some general characteristics, but with the caveat that there is broad variation even within small villages. Based on questionnaires[9] and interviews, decisions about health care are regularly made in consultation with other household members. The most knowledgeable individual about health care decisions, the person most regularly consulted by other household members, is most often a senior female. Simple illnesses are treated with folk remedies or over-the-counter medicines. For example, fermented dairy products are often

---

[8] The first figure is based on informal observations in households where I conducted follow-up interviews. In one case, I was suffering from laryngitis and was given 'camel tail' (*Caragana jubata* Pallas) that a family member had collected in the mountains the year before. The second figure is also based on informal observations and conversations with plant vendors in Arshan in 2001 and 2005.

[9] The questionnaire was a pilot, not a random sample. Because many are incomplete or filled out incorrectly, I have not analyzed them in a traditional manner, but use them here as semi-structured interviews. The failure of this pre-test raises interesting questions about how locals perceive illness and health which I cannot address fully in this chapter.

used to treat digestive problems. When an illness is deemed serious enough to seek external help, the treatment is often linked to the nature of the illness. The quickest route to relief is often biomedicine. In locations where there is no clinic, or a *fel'dsher*, the sick family member takes a bus ride to the district hospital in Kyren. There are no *emchi* or medical *lamas* in Tunka, and the only physicians with Tibetan or Chinese medical training in the region are located in Arshan. Sometimes people will also travel to Irkutsk or Ulan-Ude for either biomedical or Tibetan medical treatments.

For many, a shaman's help is sought only when nothing else has helped or when no diagnosis could be made. The shaman may be a 'last resort' for some individuals because they may have greater faith in the efficacy of other medical systems. For others, shamanic healing is the most powerful and consequently the most dangerous form of healing. A shaman may be sought out initially when the illness manifests more psychological than physical symptoms or to heal misfortune, often requiring the participation of entire kin networks. Sometimes, shamans are sought out as a complement to biomedicine, as in the case of the woman who phoned a shaman during an interview to seek advice on her husband's diagnosis of cancer (Metzo 2008b). Only one respondent on the questionnaires stated that his/her family seeks out a shaman for any and all illnesses. A medical doctor who also practices Tibetan medicine at the Center for Eastern Medicine in Ulan-Ude says that, "people go to conventional doctors for a quick remedy and if it is not working, they move onto a more holistic system." Thus, the illness does not have to be a long-term chronic illness, but may simply be one for which the biomedical treatment proved ineffective. The pattern I have described here is nearly as common among ethnic Russians as it is among ethnic Buriats in the region.

It is worth noting that traditional healing includes not only medicinal plants, but mineral springs and natural foods. Buriat folk medicine focuses on diet as a means of preventing illness. Buriats and Russians alike highlighted the nutritional value of the berries as sources of much needed vitamin C during the winter cold season. Nearly all households I surveyed in 2005 (86%) collected some type of berry, often based on personal taste of household members. *Brusnika*, (*Vaccinimu vitisidaea*) is especially valued for its additional medicinal properties of helping to reduce fevers. Based on a smaller group of households that filled out economic diaries, about half of the households who gather collect *brusnika* and about half of those households also sold their goods at local and regional markets (Irkutsk or Baikalsk) or shared with relatives in the valley and in Ulan-Ude. By and large, however, berries are actually used as a sweet snack or dessert. Another plant that constitutes an important ingredient in the winter diet is the wild leek or *cheremsha*. Finely chopped and salted for preservation, *cheremsha* is used as a condiment for soups and potato dishes. When asked follow up questions about medicinal plants, broadly defined as plants that contribute to overall health, people frequently mentioned *cheremsha*. Locally-collected wild foods are the most highly valued because they are 'cleaner,' followed by Russian made [Rus. *rossiiskii, otechestvennyi*] products (*see* Caldwell 2002).

Mineral springs are also central to folk healing, having been used by local Buriats before being discovered by *lamas* and later discovered by Russian geologists. During the 20th century, mineral springs have been analyzed for their mineral composition and, through the establishment of sanatoria and clinics, have been co-opted by biomedicine (Metzo 2008a). Several of the most regionally and nationally well-known and 'powerful' springs are located in the Saian Mountains, in Arshan and at Shumak (*see* Brummond Ch. 4, this volume). I have discussed the institutionalization of Arshan's springs elsewhere (Metzo 2008a) and there are several important ways in which the use of mineral springs differs from medicinal plants. In the local imagination, I suggest that mineral springs have a stronger association with shamanic traditions than they do with Buddhist traditions, even though the local monasteries in Tunka and Oka have long been caretakers of these sites. Water, like berries and mushrooms, has a quotidian, if not nutritional value. While the springs have the power to heal, drinking from springs that are not specific to your condition will not have negative side effects and some residents collect large canisters of water when they travel to springs, which is then shared with family, friends, and neighbors in the 24-hour period following their return home and used for tea and soups in subsequent days. Water from many wells throughout the valley shares some of the properties and mineral content of the springs. Residents of Arshan specifically mentioned that living in Arshan itself had a health-improving effect, both from the clean mountain air[10] and the energy that they derive from the mountains.

Diet as a preventative measure is important to a discussion of the collection and use of medicinal plants for several reasons. First, berries and wild leeks (and water), while thought of primarily as foodstuffs having nutritional properties, also have medicinal properties. Second, as one of my consultants said, dairy products have healing properties, too, not necessarily because they are derived from cattle, but because the cows eat in pastures of diverse flora. "It's like a multivitamin tablet" one woman said. Meat and dairy products from the Saian mountains are highly valued for their taste, especially Oka meat, which some residents joke is pre-seasoned with the wild leek and wild thyme [Rus. *chabrets*], that grow in vast quantities in the meadows in Oka. Traveling to regional markets in Baikalsk and Irkutsk, women vendors fetch higher prices than local farmers, making it worth the cost of travel. Finally, diet is important as a way of preventing disease because, as many interviewees and questionnaire respondents noted, "we don't get sick."

For weeks I heard and read the refrain of "we don't get sick" and it frustrated me beyond words. There were also a number of respondents who wrote "I don't know" on the questionnaire in response to questions about how household members treat common illnesses such as diarrhoea. Certainly, I thought, someone in one of these households has experienced diarrhoea in the past year. The piece that I was missing became clear as I intensely questioned a friend who had volunteered as a research assistant to distribute questionnaires in Arshan. She told me, "we're healthy and when we're not, we can't afford to go to the doctor." In fact, people rely on a handful of 'universal' medicines, such as an over-the-counter medicine called 'Dr. Mom,' rest, and traditional foods (especially sour dairy products) if they feel discomfort. They rarely take sick days and when they do, they still have to feed the pigs and milk the cows and thresh the hay for winter. Only when a condition becomes chronic do people seek outside help. Support for the general healthiness of Buriats is supported ethnography from the 17-19th centuries (Daribazarova 2001:38).

To Collect or Not Collect Medicinal Plants

The final piece to the puzzle of medicinal plant use is understanding the characteristics of people who gather medicinal plants and of those who do not. On the one hand, most residents of Tunka purchase teas—the kind of one-size-fits-all treatments available in pharmacies and kiosks that contain partly or exclusively plants gathered in the Saian Mountains. When I visited people's homes, I made note of what types of medicines they had stocked in their kitchens (usually the first room you enter in someone's home and often where people

---

[10] According to measurements from 1999 and 2000 taken by the state ecological inspector in Kyren, the air quality in the village of Arshan itself is of lower quality than in many of the neighbouring villages because of the use of coal to heat municipal buildings.

keep their medicines). All of the homes I visited generally had some kind of herbal/medicinal tea in addition to pharmaceuticals—tinctures, pills, or syrups. In several homes, people also kept dried medicinal plants which could have been gathered, gifted, or purchased.

The suggestion that medicinal teas are cheaper than pharmaceuticals and that is why these teas have become popular does not stand up to scrutiny. In 2001, and again in 2005, I spent time in several pharmacies examining medicines to treat specific ailments (using my own illness history to select medicines). While teas may be nominally cheaper, that is, a box of tea may cost less than a bottle of pills, the cost of treatment is the same. Carefully reading the boxes and calculating how much of the product is required over the same period of time to manage a chronic ailment, like allergies, a person would need multiple boxes of tea to manage the illness for the same period of time. Further, if one were to select an over-the-counter tea based on a visit to the Center for Eastern Medicine in Ulan-Ude, for example, the office visit would not be covered by state health care, but a visit to a doctor at a state health clinic would be covered. That said, anecdotally, there is evidence that medical doctors in state-run clinics sometimes prescribe Tibetan teas or other herbal treatments rather than pharmaceuticals. If one goes to an *emchi-lama* or to a clinic where the teas are custom-prepared, the cost of the tea can be two to three times the cost of pharmaceuticals. The larger point is that medicinal teas are only cheaper than pharmaceuticals when one personally gathers. Several of my consultants noted that one of the reasons for the preference for medicinal plants was that they were more natural than pharmaceuticals, that they were less processed or 'messed with.'

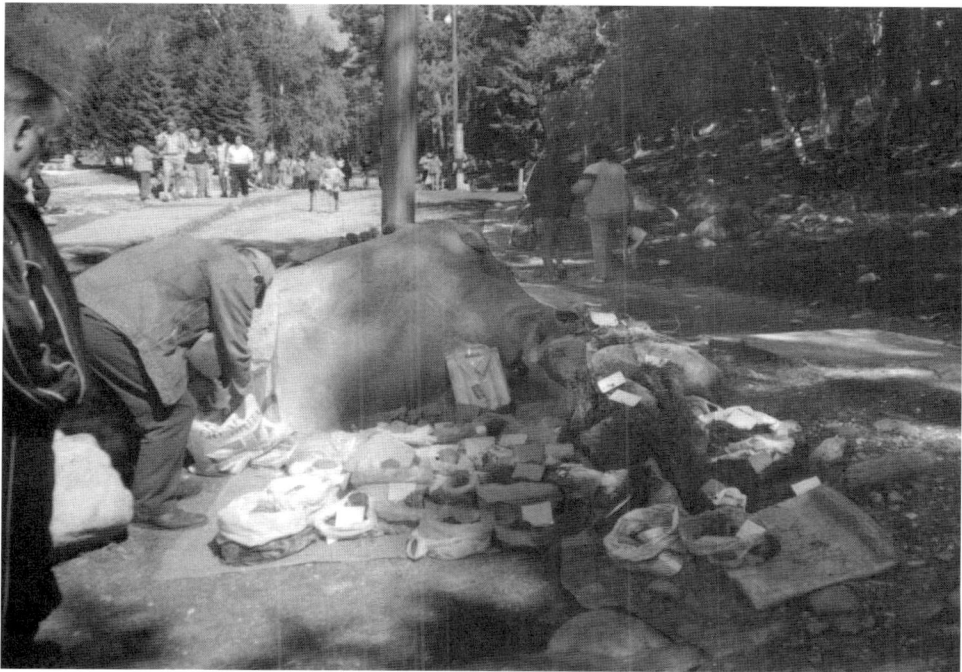

Figure 2.4. *Plant vendor at Arshan, Tunka Valley, 2001.*

Another option that saves money is to purchase individual plants from vendors at open air markets, such as the one in Arshan. On any given day during the summer months, between five and twenty sellers will be set up along the sidewalks that lead to the main set of mineral springs. A typical set up is one or two sellers standing or sitting on chairs or a nearby bench behind a tarp covered with small, open plastic bags. Some of the bags have shot glasses or juice glasses next to them that can be used for measurement. Next to each bag there is a handwritten sign with the common name of the dried plant found within it. Vendors rarely volunteer any information, aside from pointing out indigenous plants, such as *sagaan dali* (*Rhododendron adamsii*), which looks like a dark green, almost brown, thick leaf and is considered a potent treatment for circulatory ailments. If a person has questions about the plants, s/he is invited to read the placards or the vendor hands over a book, typically a field guide to medicinal plants of the Baikal region.

Not all vendors are present everyday and with the help of some of the local vendors, I estimate that there are about fifteen local sellers and the same or a greater number of sellers from outside the region. The ethnic composition of sellers is about 60% ethnic Russian and 40% ethnic Buriat. According to the local sellers who are better able to judge, the overwhelming majority of customers are tourists from outside the region, typically from Irkutsk or Ulan-Ude. One seller set the estimate at 70% tourists. Foreign tourists often stop and look, but (myself excluded) rarely buy. In order to increase their inventory, vendors will trade with one another or buy from forest wardens. The transaction I observed was after the wardens returned from the mountains where they were clearing brush for a fire break. One of the shrubs that they cleared out was a medicinal plant and they had several 20 or 50 kilogram flour sacks stuffed with the branches. While selling plants violates local regulations, the National Park authorities turn a blind eye to selling at these markets.

A question that arises regarding plant harvesting is whether or not the way in which they are collected is sustainable. On a number of occasions, Tunka residents raised concerns that outsiders would not or did not take the same care in gathering medicinal plants and were causing irreparable harm to stands of rare and endemic species. Many guide books, however, have precise instructions or guidelines for sustainable harvesting (*see* Table 2.1). In interviews at the Center for Eastern Medicine in Ulan Ude, I asked about the origin of the plants in their pharmacy.

Table 2.1. Recommendations for sustainable harvesting of medicinal plants

Grasses/plants	Do not pull up by the roots
Leaves	Always leave some leaves on each plant
Flowers	Leave at least one-third for self seeding and plant renewal, especially for those plants that multiply through seed dispersal
'underground parts'	Collect only after the plant has peaked and produced seeds. Leave part of the root, especially for those plants that multiply through shoots
buds and bark	Collect only from felled trees, not living trees

From: Bogdanova and Bichikhanov 1991.

The doctor I interviewed said that, in the past, pharmacists and doctors gathered all the plants themselves. In recent years, however, they have been buying the majority of their plants from other collectors. In the days following my interview, she and a colleague were headed to the Tunka Valley where they would gather some plants, but would also purchase plants, typically those that were out of season, from local vendors. I pressed her on the question of sustainable harvesting. She replied that one couldn't really over-harvest any of the above-ground parts if the leaves and flowers were clipped correctly [Rus. *akuratno*]. She mentioned that the roots are trickier, and that one should not remove them entirely and would need to allow two years to pass before collecting in the same location. In the end, she concluded that even the 'less than attentive collector' could do little harm to plants. The pharmacy at the Center for Eastern Medicine even has a chart on the wall that instructs visitors on the part of the plant and time of year to collect each of the more common plants.

Table 2.2. Medicinal Plants Free-Listed by Informants in the City of Ulan-Ude (listed in rank-order based on salience. starred plants are common to the Tunka Valley).

Common Name (Russian, unless noted)	Scientific Name	Common Name (English)	Salience
*romashka	Matricaria chamomilla sp.	Chamomile	.537
*podorozhnik	Plantago (major)	Common Plantain, White Man's Foot	.396
aloi	Aloe vera	Aloe	.346
*bogoroditskaya trava, chabrets, aia-ganga (Bur.)	Thymus serpyllum	A variety of thyme	.251
*pustyrnik	Leonurus cardiaca L.	Motherwort	.232
*tisiachilistnik	Achillea millefolium	Yarrow	.227
kalendula	Calendula officinalis	Calendula	.214
zveroboi	Hypericum perforatum	St. John's Wort	.162
*malina	Rubus sachalinensis	Raspberry	.155
*brusnika	Vaccinium vitis-idaea	Red Whortleberry	.149
valerian	Valeriana officinalis	Valerian	.149
zolotoi us'	Callisia fragrans	Golden Tendril	.138
shipovnik	Rosa majalis	Rose hip	.124
*krapiva	Urtica dioica	Nettle	.115

Despite the fact that plant collecting is not a common activity in the Tunka Valley, I must note that many locals can recognize a set of medicinal plants quite well. This became obvious from the free-lists of plants I asked people to record.

My research also showed an interesting distribution of common knowledge of plants across Buriatiia. Most people who compiled free lists of plants in the city of Ulan-Ude identified between four and seven items. On these lists there were ten plants that appeared on at least one-third of the 18 lists. Another four showed up on at least five lists (*see* Table 2.2). I found the common plant knowledge of residents in the city of Ulan-Ude surprising since they often cited plants that were commonly available in Russia but not specific to Buriatiia. People in the Tunka Valley, whom I interviewed, frequently listed several other plant species that were rarely listed by their urban counterparts. These plants are compiled in Table 2.3.

The plants that are so widely cited in the city work as general tonics (calendula, raspberry, chamomile) while others are used pervasively in Russian folk medicine as well (common plantain). Plants like aloe, *valerian*, and *zolotoi us* are commonly cited in self-help pamphlets in Ulan-Ude and other major cities in Russia; therefore, it is not surprising that these plants were cited on the list compiled in the urban setting. Interestingly, only *bagulnik* and *sagaan dali* (Table 2.3) were among the 42 species compiled from the urban free-lists.

This exercise in gathering plant knowledge on lists demonstrates that the information needed to effectively collect plants does exist, and that people have a general idea about key medicinal plants and their uses. With rare exceptions, local residents actually have books on Tibetan medicine or medicinal plants in their home libraries, but they are treated as general or cultural knowledge, rather than as a resource for gathering. In fact, people often pulled the books off the shelf for me to read when they learned of my research topic. Nevertheless, my rural consultants still preferred to purchase medicinal teas in pharmacies. Residents were also reluctant to purchase plants from vendors at Arshan. Their distrust of vendors is explained by a sense that the vendors lack the training or knowledge to collect properly—either in a sustainable fashion or identifying the correct plant from among similar looking plants. While no one actually stated this as evidence, I think the fact that vendors, rather than answering questions with authority, tend to hand over a guidebook (perhaps the same guidebook that someone has sitting at home) supports the perception of a lack of knowledge.

Table 2.3. Medicinal Plants commonly cited during interviews with plant sellers and residents of Tory and Arshan, Tunka valley, 2005.

Common Name (Russian, unless noted)	Scientific Name	Common Name (English)
oblepikha	*Hippophae rhamnoides*	Sea Buckthorn
bagulnik, Bur. *sagaan dali*	*Rhododendron adamsii* (endemic) *Rhododendron dauricum* (more widespread)	Rhododendron
bagulnik	*Rhododendron groenlandicum*	Labador tea
rodiola rozovaia	*Rhodiola rosea*	Roseroot, golden root
cheremsha	*Allium victorialis*	Wild leek/onion

According to my consultants, books for popular audiences capture only part of the necessary knowledge for collecting and using medicinal plants. The scope of knowledge needed makes it seem prohibitive to collect. One needs to know not only what the plant looks like and what it is used for, which is available in books, but where to find plants—knowledge that is written about in a very general way as in guidebooks that describe habitat. Knowing where to find plants, especially rare varieties, is something you must be shown by another who already knows. When asked what else one would need to know to collect, people suggested a number of other factors: what part of the plant to collect (flower, leaves, seeds, roots), what stage of its life cycle (before or after it goes to seed, while dormant or flowering, and even on the first day of flowering versus at any stage while it flowers), and even what time of day (morning, evening, midday) or under what climate conditions (before or after rain, during dry period). The fact that most plants, even those dispensed through custom teas prepared at temples or eastern medical clinics, are not collected in this way does not seem to deter people from thinking that they lack sufficient knowledge for proper collection. The irony of this point is not lost on everyone. My colleague, Vera, one of the individuals who collects for household use, said, "We're walking on gold" and lamented that her neighbors were not more entrepreneurial at a time when unemployment in the village was at about 30%.

Chapter Two: *Medical Pluralism and Expert Knowledge in Buriatiia*

Medicinal Plants as Expert Knowledge

Within this chapter, I have examined medicinal plant collection and use in rural Buriatiia based on the example of Tunka Valley, an area regionally known for its high degree of biodiversity, including most varieties of medicinal plants used in Buddhist ayurveda medicine. I began with the paradox of why rural residents do not gather plants, despite the high costs of pharmaceuticals and 'natural' remedies, in contrast to the abundance of these plants in their home region. Tunka residents almost universally use medicinal plants, either as folk remedies, over-the-counter teas and tonics, or prescriptions from medical doctors and emchi-lamas. People prepare teas and topical treatments from single plant species, yet only the rare person gathers these plants him or herself. I have concluded that gathering and preparing or mixing plants is seen as a form of expert knowledge.

In terms of healing traditions in Tunka, and more broadly in the Baikal Region, there is general knowledge that is universal, based on the quotidian lives of households. This body of knowledge is not limited to treating or curing illness, but includes knowledge about maintaining health and balance. In broad strokes, we are talking about the pastoralist traditions of the Baikal Region. Knowledge about caring for animals, pastures and recognizing useful versus harmful plants is deployed on a daily basis. Likewise, people focus on balance in their diets, using both plant and animal products. For the most part, however, this knowledge is connected to being healthy and is not associated in people's mind with illness.

General, universal knowledge about health and balanced living stands in contrast to the expert or specialized knowledge that they seek out when their general knowledge fails. While charismatic legitimacy has a role in healing practices (Metzo 2008b), the traditional legitimacy of ancient healing practices plays a more important role in the use of medicinal plant treatments. Medicinal plants are 'proven' treatments with thousands of years of testing and use. The fact that these substances are also studied easily within laboratory settings adds a layer of scientific legitimacy, which is important in the Buriat case, I would argue, because of the high degree of assimilation in terms of language and education.

Herbal medicines produced in the Baikal Region are by and large connected with Tibetan medicine in the popular imagination, which becomes the expert knowledge required to collect, prepare, and dispense medicinal plants. For Russians and Buriats, Tibetan medicine has much the same attraction that it does in the West. Within the context of modernity, "people may seek healing modalities that do not simply effect a cure, but also bring some kind of meaningful order to the perceived causes, and consequences, of a disease. Tibetan medicine, which links an increasingly popular Buddhist spirituality to herbal-based, holistic therapeutic modalities, may offer an ideal mix of the pragmatic and symbolic in this new epidemiologic context" (Janes 2002:282). Thus, even the one-size-fits-all teas have appeal as tonics and become part of the '*bricolage*' of "particular cultural and therapeutic elements [chosen] from among a number of distinctive traditions" similar to the ways in which Americans, in another modern, scientific state, piece together a package of healing practices (McGuire 2002:410).

While the appeal of more holistic traditional medicines generates demand for medicinal plant treatments, the link between Buddhist *ayurveda* medicine and science creates distance between the lay person and this knowledge that is increasingly specialized. Early efforts to modernize the health care system in the Soviet Union at the turn of the century emphasized bureaucratic efficacy by counting workers and extending their lifetime labor output (Field 1957). Alternative treatments remained present in the network of sanatoria and the ability of doctors and scientists to study Eastern systems of medicine abroad. In the 1970s and 1980s, while the authority of biomedicine was being challenged throughout the Soviet Union, Buriat medical doctors traveled abroad to learn Tibetan medicine and acupuncture. Because Ulan-Ude is home to the leading institution for the study of Buddhism in the former Soviet Union which houses a department dedicated to the study of Tibetan Medicine, the 'experts' are also navigating the relationship between traditional and scientific knowledge. The growing interest in these alternatives and the ease of integrating traditional and scientific knowledge moves medicinal knowledge out of the reach of the lay person. Medicinal plants, unlike surgery or shamanic trance, weave together traditional and scientific knowledge, demanding much more of the practitioner in the eyes of typical rural residents. Plants are something that everyone knows a little about, but just like one would not 'dabble' in surgery or attempt to 'cure' a family member through entering an altered state of consciousness, local residents opt to leave the serious work of medicinal plants—the collection, preparation, mixing—to experts.

Acknowledgements
Research in 2000 and 2001 was supported by an IREX Individual Advanced Research Opportunity Grant, a Wenner–Gren Dissertation Fellowship, and an Indiana University Research-in-Aid Fellowship. Research in 2005 was supported by a Faculty Research Grant from the University of North Carolina-Charlotte. The author would like to thank Zhargal Aiakova for assistance in data collection.

Chapter Three

The Development of Tibetan Medicine in Buriatiia

Vindarya N. Gololobova
Translated by Ol'ga Pak

The Tibetan medical tradition has existed for thousands of years. It is rooted in *ayurveda*, a traditional Indian medical system, but has also been influenced by the medical traditions of Nepal, China and Persia. Today, Tibetan medicine is practiced not only in Tibet, but also in India, Mongolia, China and Russia, among other places. It is also gaining popularity in Western countries, spreading along with Buddhist religious practices and leaders. However, in each context, traditional Tibetan medicine adapts itself differently to the local social, cultural and ethnic circumstances as well as to the natural and climatic conditions. This paper discusses how healers in the Republic of Buriatiia, Russia, have creatively adopted this tradition.

The Republic of Buriatiia occupies an extensive territory within Eastern Siberia. It a mountainous region and encompasses diverse landscapes including forests, forest-steppes, and steppes. Buriatiia has a continental climate, with cold winters and short hot summers. These features create a great diversity of local flora. Today, most Buriats reside in the Republic of Buriatiia, but there are also significant populations in the Ust'-Orda Buriat Okrug of Irkutsk oblast', in the Agin-Buriat, Autonomous Okrug of Chita oblast', and within other counties of the Zabaikal Krai. The main religion of Buriats who live in Pribaikal'e and the Ust-Orda district within Irkutsk oblast' is shamanism, and that of Buriats in the Zabaikal region is Buddhism.

The spread of Tibetan medicine within Buriatiia is closely intertwined with that of Buddhism. According to the results of a sociological survey in the Republic of Buriatiia in 2003, 61.3 per cent of Buriats identify themselves as Buddhists; 15.6 percent practice shamanism; 1.6 percent are Orthodox Christians; 15.4 percent are non-believers, and 6.1 percent cited other religions (Manzanov 2005:125).

Tibetan medicine came to Buriatiia along with the Buddhist school of Gelug-pa from neighbouring Mongolia. Buriats at that time were shamanists. However Buddhism did not suppress shamanism but rather legalized it and incorporated their practices into the Buddhist system. Therefore, the Buddhism of today's Buriats includes many shamanist rituals and traditions. The dissemination and adaptation of Buddhism in Russia was possible thanks to a favourable political period, when the Imperial Russian Government preferred a policy of non-interference in Buriat affairs. These circumstances facilitated the development and consolidation of the Buddhist faith, an increase in the number of monks, and the expansion of Tibetan medicine (Aiusheeva 2007:38).

Buddhism was officially adopted in Mongolia in 1576 and D. B. Dashiev, citing historical chronicles, specifies this as the date when Buriats first became acquainted with Tibetan medicine. Although there were Buriat *emchi-lamas* who studied directly in Tibet, Buriats were exposed to Tibetan medicine mostly through its Mongolian variant. Mongols opened *manba-datsanuud* (medical schools at monasteries), translated medical treatises including Jud-Shi and Lhan-tliabs from Tibetan into Mongolian, and ordered the practices of Mongolian folk medicine (Dashiev 2004:453-454). L.V. Aiusheva suggests that Buriats became familiar with Tibetan medicine slightly later, at the end of the 17th and beginning of the 18th centuries. In 1712, one hundred and fifty Mongolian *lamas* of the highest clerical rank, *gelun*, settled among Buriats and began actively spreading Buddhism and Tibetan medicine. Among them were such experts in Tibetan medicine as the Tibetans Agvan Puntsog and Lubsan Shirap (Aiusheeva 2007:40). Zhimba Akhaldaev, from Selenga, became the first Buriat healer and in 1721 began traveling to Mongolia and Tibet to study. Damba-Dorzhi Zaiaev, a Buriat of the Tsongol clan, became another renowned healer who studied philosophy and medicine in Tibet. After seven years of traveling, he returned home and soon attained fame as a skilful doctor (Badmaev 1991:57) (Fig. 3.1).

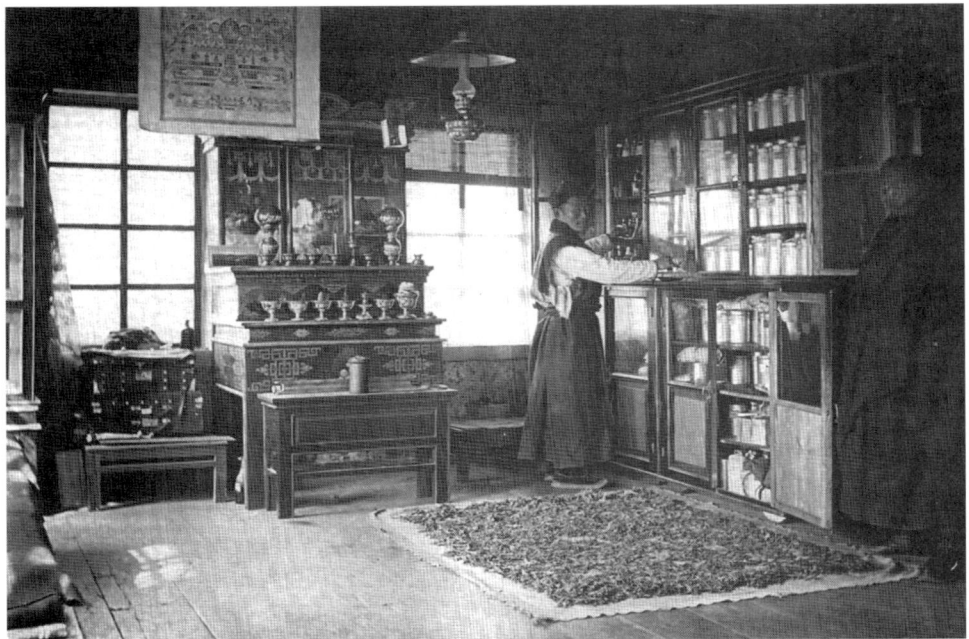

Figure 3.1. *A pharmacy of an* emchi-lami *at the start of the 20th Century (Aseeva* et al. *2008).*

Buddhism was officially adopted in Russia, specifically in Buriatiia, in 1741. *Lamas* organized the first medical school in the Tsugol Datsan [monastery] and Buriat *lamas* invited teachers from Mongolia to Buriatiia in 1869. Then, toward the end of the 18th century, a Buriat named Guru-Darmy Biliktuev started teaching in the Tsugol Datsan (Aseeva *et al.* 2008:33-34). Later, the *emchi-lamas* of various monasteries including those of Atsagaty, Tsongol, Agin and Iangazhin organized medical departments and started printing xylographs on Tibetan medicine. The most renowned school of Tibetan medicine, organized by *emchi-lamas* C.D. Ireltuev and Agvan Dorzhiev, was located in the Atsagat Datsan. The Buriat clergy recognized that Tibetan medicine helped consolidate Buddhism, and therefore they encouraged *lamas*-healers to practice at the monasteries. By the end of the 18th century, Tibetan medical practice had become a significant part of everyday life. Customary law codices even specified tariffs for treatments performed by *emchi-lamas*. From the second part of the 19th century, Russian settlers also began seeking the services of *emchi-lamas* (Aseeva *et al.* 2008:30-34).

An expert in Tibetan medicine and the history of Buriatiia, Galdan Lenkhoboev (1907-1991), states that until the start of the 20th century, there were two schools of Tibetan medicine in Buriatiia: Khori and Selenga. The *emchi-lamas* of the Khori School studied

Tibetan medicine, mostly in Tibet, while those of the Selenga School were educated by the Mongols and in the Mongolian language. Galdan Lenkhoboev (Lenkhoboev and Zhambaldagbaev 2003:13) identified himself with the Selenga School. In general, the Khori School has preserved the theoretical and practical aspects of the original Tibetan traditions, whereas the Selenga School has adapted Tibetan medicine to local conditions in Buriatiia.

Buriat Folk Medicine

Before Tibetan medicine was introduced to Buriatiia, the local population practiced their own form of folk medicine. This knowledge did not rely on any formal theoretical training but was passed down orally from one generation to another. Ethnographers divide Buriat folk medicinal practice into several spheres: shamanic treatments, healing magic, bone-setting, and treatment with herbal, animal and mineral remedies. Each healer employed the different treatments to varying extents. The local population considered those who were able to use both practical techniques and healing magic to be the best healers.

Buriat folk healing methods include wrapping the sick person in the skins of a newly slaughtered animal, laying the patient on warmed-up soil, cauterization, bloodletting, prescribing animal and plant medicines, healing magic, bathing in mineral springs [*arshan*], and dietary cures. A key technique in healing is a type of attention to physical traumas where the *lama* uses his hands to massage or move muscles, veins, and bones, including broken bones [*kostopravstvo*]. Khakasses, Iakuts and other peoples of Siberia and Central Asia use similar methods. Tibetan medicine incorporated some of these folk healing practices and techniques. For example, edible wild plants used in Buriat folk medicine were included in the recipe books of Tibetan medicine under Tibetan names, as local substitutes for imported ingredients (Aseeva *et al.* 2008:15, 26).

Buriats, like many other peoples of the world, conceptualized health as the optimum balance of hot and cold in the human body. Diseases were named after organs and by adding the words 'hot' or 'cold' [in the Buriat language, *khaluun* or *khuiten*, respectively]. Tibetan medicine, as is generally known, also classifies diseases caused by hot and cold, complementing Buriats' long-established notions about health.

If the cause of a disease could not be identified, folk healers blamed evil spirits for the sickness, and in these cases shamans were consulted. They viewed disharmony between the human being and the surrounding world to be the major cause of any sickness. It was believed that such a disharmony could result in the loss of one's soul, consequently hindering the person's own ability to recover. Shamans treated their patients with healing magic and rarely used medication. They used massage, charms and spells [*tarim* in the Buriat language], water [*yhan tarim*], stones [*shuluun tarim*], and wrapping the patient in the hides of newly slaughtered animals [*adaha tarim*]. They also used rituals and ceremonies: for example, the *khurylkha* ceremony was believed to assist in returning an absent soul. Some have identified an element of psychotherapy in the way that sick people recovered due to the shaman's strong suggestions and to self-suggestion (Mikhailov 1987:165-169). Some methods of healing magic were not incorporated into the arsenal of Tibetan medicine due to their obvious discrepancies with the principles of Buddhism. However, *emchi-lamas* often approached the treatment of diseases pragmatically. For example, if a Buriat *emchi-lama* decided that it would be most effective to wrap a patient in the hide of a newly killed animal, he would refer the patient to a shaman or a folk healer for the required ritual. Mongolian *emchi-lamas* also used to perform this type of cure themselves, despite the prohibition on killing animals in Buddhism (Pozdneev 1993:164). Buriats still use this method of treatment today, but only as a last resort.

Buriats of Pribakail'e, who were not influenced by Buddhism, have preserved their traditional folk medicine to a larger extent. However, their shamanic practices are fragmentary and take place mainly within the home. Their most widely-known folk treatment today is the movement and setting of bones and muscles, which Tibetan medicine has not been able to fully supplant. Experienced bone-setters *baryaasha* [from the Buriat verb *barikha* meaning 'to hold'] help people when Tibetan medicine is less effective, for example, in cases of fractures and dislocations, concussions, and repositioning of the foetus in pregnant women.

Information on cauterization and bloodletting is very limited and there are no folk healers practising these methods in Buriatiia today. However, cauterization and bloodletting are employed by *emchi-lamas* within the frameworks of Tibetan medicine and many contemporary *emchi-lamas*, when necessary, supplement oral medication with these types of treatment. For example, the *emchi-lama* Chimit-Dorzhi Dugarov, well known both within and outside of Buriatiia, uses cauterization and bloodletting in his healing practice. *Lamas* of the Ivolga *datsan* are also familiar with these techniques.

Medicinal Raw Materials of Tibetan Medicine in Buriatiia

Many herbal ingredients required in Tibetan recipe-books are unavailable to *emchi-lamas* in Mongolia and Buriatiia; therefore they substituted imported raw materials with local analogues. The Mongols ordered the experience of indigenous Mongolian folk medicine into a coherent system, and identified and classified the medicinal qualities of local flora in accordance with Tibetan examples. Gradually, the Mongols found replacements for many imported raw materials that were hard to obtain. The proportion of local plants in Mongolian traditional medicine amounts to 57 percent, whereas the proportions of Tibetan, Indian and Chinese materials comprise 11.6, 11.3, and 9.6 percent, respectively. Buriat healers replaced imported ingredients with local types to an even greater degree. In their recipes, the flora of the Zabaikal region amounts to 85.06 per cent, whereas Indian and Tibetan ingredients make up 3.64 and 3.46 per cent, respectively. The substitutes used vary between different regions of Buriatiia and because of these differences, researchers describe three distinctive branches of Tibetan medicine: Tibetan medicine proper, Mongolian medicine, and Buriat medicine. Despite considerable differences in the assortment of medicinal raw materials, all the branches share common theoretical ground, the same concept of illness, principles of healing and the like. They are also all characterized by their common religion (Aseeva *et al.* 2008:32).

Buriat *lama*-healers in almost all *manba-datsans* compiled their own *chzhory*—collections of recipes adjusted to the specifics of local flora. The founders of medical schools also collected their own recipes, and their pupils and followers further enriched those collections, organizing and rewriting them. The Buriat *chzhory* were simply lists of tested recipes, listing the ingredients and dosages of a remedy in both the Tibetan and Buriat languages. Instructions for use were either missing or written in the Mongolian script,[1] Buriat *lamas* hardly ever altered the names of recipes, their structures or instructions, but the ingredients could be replaced completely with local equivalents (Dashiev 2004:458). In addition to recipe-books, Buriat *lamas*-healers compiled reference books where they designated local substitutes under the Tibetan names of medicinal raw materials (Aiusheeva 2007:64). Buriat *datsans* published as many medical books from the middle of the 19th century, as did Tibetan and Mongolian monasteries at that time.

---

[1] [Translator's note] The Mongolian script is an ancient Mongolian writing system that was used before the introduction of the Cyrillic type of writing in Mongolia.

What were the principles determining how local medicinal materials were substituted for imported ones? *Emchi-lamas* knew local plants very well and could identify their properties following their knowledge of 'tastes' which, according to Tibetan medicine and philosophy, are the combination of five *mahābhūtas* (the main elements): earth, water, fire, air and space. A taste could be sweet, salty, burning, sour, bitter or astringent. *Lamas* specified seventeen properties of food and medicinal agents to be taken into consideration when finding remedies for certain diseases. In addition, *lamas* always observed how a remedy could affect the inner warmth of the body. *Emchi-lamas* often interpreted the effect of the climate, food and medication on the patient in terms the concept of 'inner warmth.' Inner warmth was viewed as a bile that facilitated digestion, and all processes within the body depend considerably on it. Bile is thought to help keep tissues and inner organs warm, replenish the body's strength, and determine the length of a person's life. A state of inner warmth was achieved by consuming the correct foods and having a good climate and living conditions. Warm and cold were viewed as the essence of all seventeen properties of medicinal agents. The locations where plants grew were also taken into account when identifying the properties of plants: plants growing in dry, stony places were believed to possess warm properties, while plants from humid places with loose black soils had cold properties. Neutral properties were attributed to plants equally influenced by both the sun and the moon (Lenkhoboev and Zhambaldagbaev 2003:35-37).

When selecting substitutes, *lamas* took into account the prescriptions of Buriat folk medicine which fit the Tibetan tradition well. Modern chemical tests have revealed that even when the substitutes were not even phylogenetically close to the original Tibetan raw materials, their effect was analogous. The local substitutes could be even be slightly stronger than the original components. For example, the Altai aster contains more saponins than the alpine aster and therefore is a good substitute for this imported component. Over the long period that Tibetan medicine was practiced in Buriatia, *lamas* were able not only to substitute difficult-to-access ingredients but also to enrich the Tibetan pharmacopoeia considerably with local raw materials. In addition, they broadened the range of use of several component plants (Asseva *et al.* 2008:72-78).

Buriat *lamas* strictly observed specific temporal and spatial rules when collecting medicinal materials. The Tibetan medical canon Jud-Shi [*Chdzud-shi*] stressed that the places where herbs and plants were gathered must be pure and pleasing. If the Jud-Shi stated that certain herbs should grow in stony soil or along riverbanks, *lamas* followed those recommendations. Buriat *lamas* often collected plants and herbs near their *datsanuud*, the locations of which were always carefully chosen. They had to be in pure places, at the tops of hills and not far from *arshanuud* [water springs].

The dry continental climate of Buriatiia created a mosaic of different landscapes, such as mountain forest-steppes, forests and steppes with a mixture of grasses. This varied environment resulted in a diverse ecology and allowed *lamas* to find plants with the required properties. *Lamas* from the Aga and Tsugol Datsans collected herbs in the areas of Urdo-aga, Tsokto-hhangil, Mogoitoye, Zugalae and in the Onon River valley. *Lamas* from the Atsagat Datsan not only gathered, but also transplanted plants that were difficult to access into more convenient places. For example, a large field of yellow Day Lilies still grows near the Atsaga Datsan after having been transplanted decades ago (Fig. 3.2).

The renowned practitioner of Tibetan medicine, Pandido Khambo Lama XII Dashi-Dorzho Etigelov (1852-1927) used to collect medicinal plants near the Iangazhin Datsan (demolished in Soviet times), where he was the chief *lama*. This location, called Barzhagar, is situated near the holy places Olonoy obo and Shunehete and not far from the *arshanuud* Uta Bulag and Sagan Zhalga (*Vstrecha s Khambo Etigelovym* 2003:20).

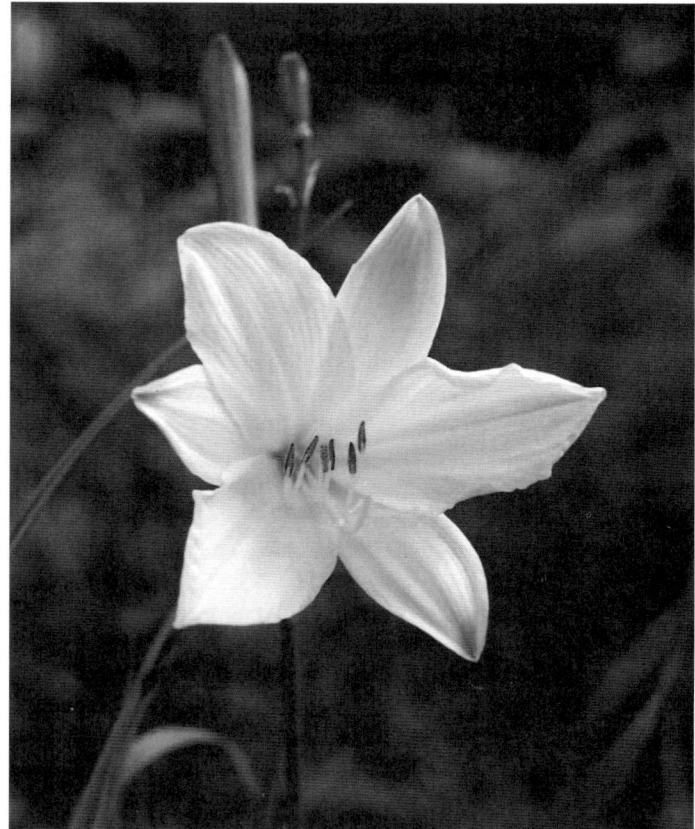

Figure 3.2. Krasodnev zheltyi—*yellow Day lilies*. Photo by V.N. Gololobova.

Buriat *lamas* adhere to the rules established by the Tibetans when collecting medicinal raw materials. Roots, branches and wood are gathered when their juice or sap is dried out; i.e., in the spring or autumn, whereas leaves and sprouts are collected during the growing season (Fig. 3.3). Flowers are taken when they are in bloom, so the timing depends on the flowering period of each plant. Fruits are gathered in autumn when they are ripe. Such rules correspond to scientifically determined recommendations on collecting medicinal raw materials and mean that the plants are collected when they are especially rich with active ingredients. Buriat *lamas* also used Indian, Chinese and other imported materials in the preparation of medications; however, they only imported ingredients that would survive the journey, for instance roots, wood, fruits and bark. Large volumes of myrobalan fruit trees, red and white sandalwood, cinnamon, cloves, peppers, ginger, cardamom, ferula, etc. were imported (Aseeva *et al.* 2008:71-72).

Unfortunately, some plants available within the territory of Buriatiia and previously used as substitutes for imported materials have now become endangered species. For example, the habitat of the redwood buckthorn (*Rhamnus erythroxylon*), a substitute for red sandalwood, is shrinking due to intensive economic development of the region. Ural liquorice is registered as an endangered species in the Republic of Buriatiia. In the 19th and 20th centuries, *lamas* actively looked for substitutes within the local flora of the Zabaikal region. But today they travel to other countries such as India, Tibet, China and others for the required primary materials (Aseeva *et al.* 2008:121).

Chapter Three: *The Development of Tibetan Medicine in Buriatiia*

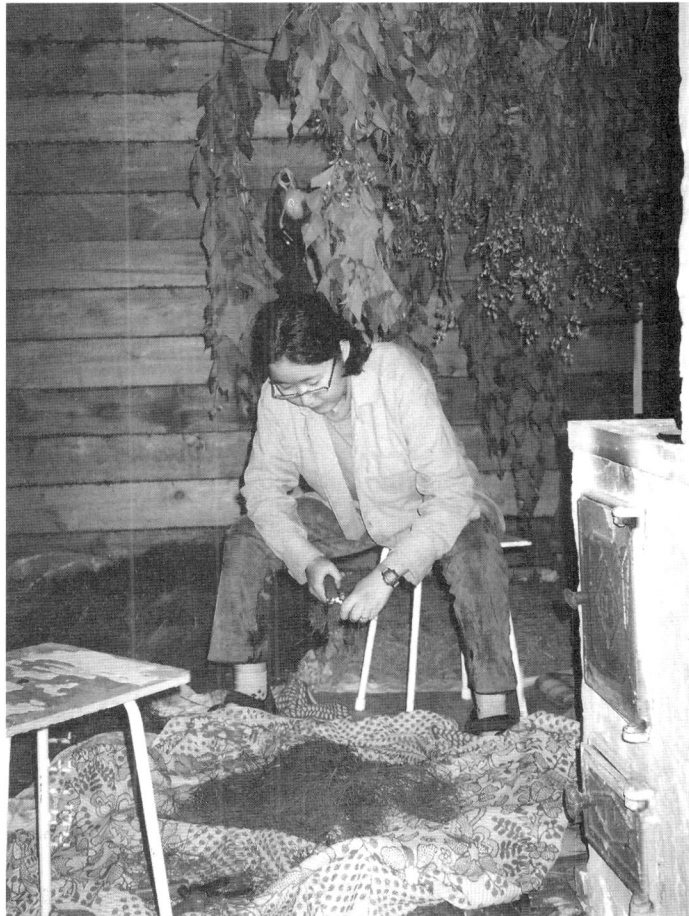

Figure 3.3. *The preparation of medicines.* Photo by V.N. Gololobova.

Tibetan healers also used animal products to produce medication. The Jud-Shi prescribes the use of horns, bones, flesh, liver, tongue, fat and other animal parts. For example, Galdan Lenkhoboev, a practitioner of Tibetan medicine, used to use the heart of a horse to prepare one of his medications. He cut the fresh heart into pieces and dried them in the sun, then reduced the pieces to powder and used this to make remedies for heart diseases. He also used 'stone-oil' [*mumio*], deer tails, antlers, tendons, tortoise flesh, crabs and snakes, shells, etc. Buriat *lamas,* as Buddhists and deep believers, could not kill animals even for the benefit of other people. Killing animals breached the *lama*'s vows and could result in evil outweighing the good. Therefore, *lamas* did not kill animals for the preparation of their medication but obtained animal ingredients in other ways. First, they could substitute vegetable analogues for the required animal materials. Such replacements were possible in many recipes because they were multi-component and often contained several ingredients with the same effect. Second, *lamas* could obtain the required parts of animals that had already been killed by someone else; e.g., from hunters and herdsmen. The fact that recipes in Tibetan medical practice, in Tibet and Buriatiia alike, contain primary materials of animal origin testifies to the antiquity of this tradition, which has preserved fragments of pre-Buddhist medical knowledge.

Emchi-lamas also use inorganic ingredients in their recipes. This group of primary materials includes metals, gems and stones, brimstone, borax, stibium, arsenic, calcites, various oxides and salts as well as medicinal ashes produced by means of burning plants or the organs of animals. Buriat *lamas* often substituted local material for Tibetan inorganic ingredients. For example, there are no recipes in the *Bolshoi Aginskii Chzhor*, the most complete medical recipe-book of Buriatiia, containing gold, silver, diamond or emerald. *Lamas* chose the remedies required by the local population and prepared the recipes with practical logic, picking out those recipes that they could identify and prepare (Aseeva *et al.* 2008:90).

Galdan Lenkhoboev offered prayers and tributes to spirits connected to each place [Bur. *serzhem*] where raw materials were collected. Paying tribute to the spirit of a certain location is a shamanist ritual that has been assimilated by Buddhism. Buriat *lamas* also say prayers and mantras devoted to the Medicine Buddha while preparing medications. These actions are believed to obviate obstacles that would prevent the healer from curing his patient effectively, or the inner obstacles of the patient him/herself (Mikhailov 2006).

The method of consuming a medication determines how finely it is powdered. Decoctions and infusions are prepared with water, which requires that the raw ingredients be reduced to a fine powder. *Lamas* grind all the components into a special mortar and then mix them together (Figs. 3.4 and 3.5). Some preparations are boiled for just 2-3 minutes. Others are boiled until they are reduced to the volume of one-third of a cup. Others are simply sprinkled into boiling water. Pills are made with the addition of honey, water, oil and treacle. Dry extracts and medicinal wines are prepared using technologies similar to contemporary ones. Ash-based medications are prepared by burning the ingredients separately and then mixing them together, or by crushing or grinding all the ingredients and blending them with oil, milk or broth, which is then worked into a stiff mixture and burned in a covered pot with no access to air (Aseeva *et al.* 2008:115-118). Decoctions are the type used most frequently by *lamas*. Pills containing precious stones and ash-based preparations are used less often. Galdan Lenkhoboev used only powders that could be blended with water or milk, or simply taken with water (Fig. 3.6).

Contemporary scholars who have analyzed the complicated recipes of Tibetan medicine conclude that the prescriptions include components designed to:
1. regulate the specificity of a disease (cold and heat);
2. correct imbalances in the body's regulating systems;
3. target damaged organs and tissues directly.

Medicinal mixtures achieve their efficacy due to several factors. First, each component reinforces the pharmacological properties of the others. Second, each medicinal ingredient treats the body as a whole. Third, the medicine takes into account multiple possible causes of a disease (Petrov 2004:30).

Now we will turn to how the raw materials of Tibetan medicine of Buriatiia are collected and processed. Usually, the methods for processing the raw materials are passed on orally from teacher to pupil; the latter masters the process by collecting raw materials himself. *Lamas* gather herbs and flowers in the appropriate season, observing strictly all recommendations of peak harvest time. Then *emchi-lamas* clean the medicinal herbs, chop and dry them in the open air, in the sun or under a tarp. It is important that the plants do not lose their colour during this process (Fig. 3.3). Some of the herbs used are poisonous; for example, Fisher's spurge, and these must be boiled in milk to eliminate the poison. Minerals also require special treatment: the *lamas* often scorch, clean and crush them in a metallic mortar.

Chapter Three: *The Development of Tibetan Medicine in Buriatiia*

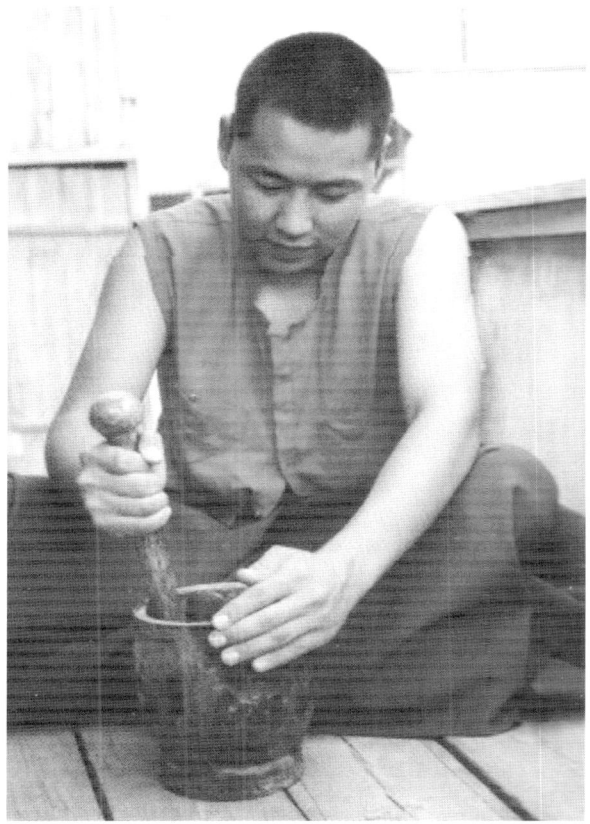

Figure 3.4. *Pulverizing medicinal materials in a mortar (Ochirov 2006).*

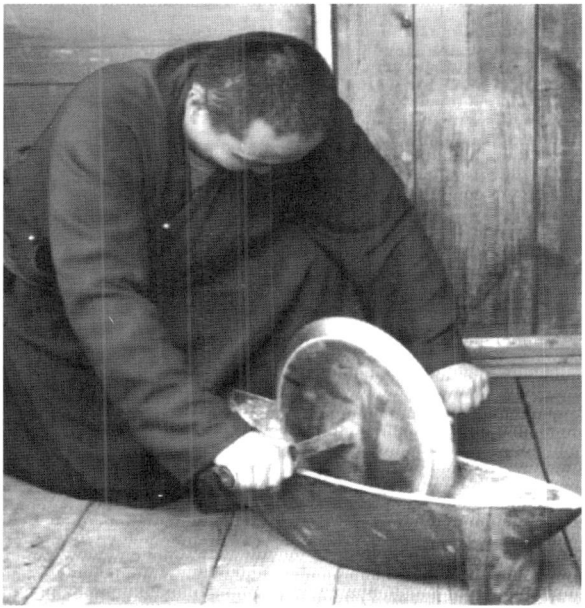

Figure 3.5. *Grinding medicine with a hand-mill (Ochirov 2006).*

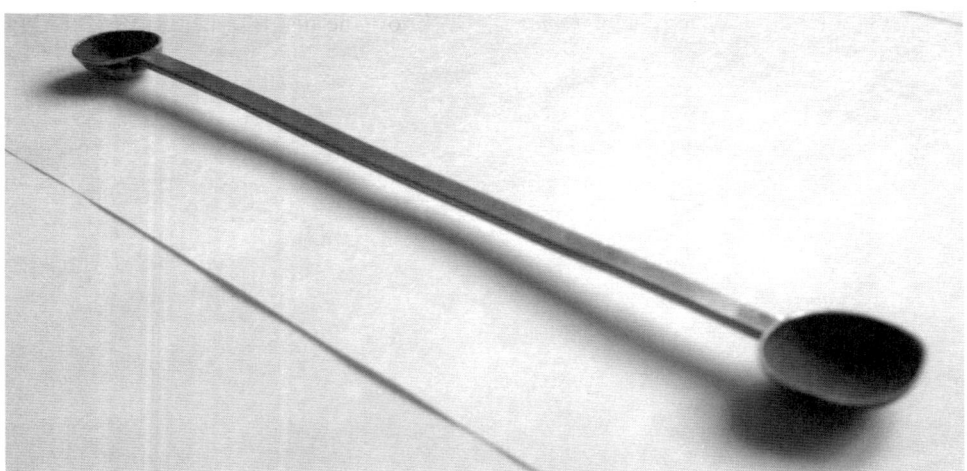

Figure 3.6. *A measuring spoon for medicine.* Photo by V.N. Gololobova.

Today, there are factories in Mongolia and India that specialize in producing Tibetan-style medication and therefore *emchi-lamas* in Buriatiia are able to buy ready-made preparations. Some Buriat *lamas* take advantage of these, while others prefer to make the preparations themselves and to collect the raw materials within Buriatiia. For example, *emchi-lama* Iuri Tsydenov from the Aga Datsan mentioned in his interview to a local newspaper that the primary materials for medications are collected in the Aga Datsan by *lamas* and *khuvaraguud* [novices]. If local components for making medications are scarce, *lamas* buy them from China or Mongolia. However, Tsydenov himself prefers local herbs, considering them to be the most suitable for his preparations (Dashizhapova 2007).

Methods of Diagnosis and Treatment

The main diagnostic techniques of Tibetan medicine include pulse diagnosis, interviewing the patient, and a general visual inspection of the patient. Pulse diagnosis is an important diagnostic method. It allows the *lama* to diagnose the state of the internal organs. Feeling the pulse, *Emchi-lamas* are able to classify the disease (whether it is cold or hot), and to diagnose the state of the body's own regulatory systems (as *shii*, *shara* or *badagan*). The method also allows the *lama* to localize the disease and any accompanying disorders. According to the rules of pulse diagnosis, a doctor determines the state of a patient's internal organs strictly through certain points on the radial artery at the patient's wrist. There are six such points, three points on each wrist, called *tson*, *kan* and *chag*. On the right wrist of a man, the *tson* point reveals the state of the lungs and the large intestine; the *kan* point is related to the liver and gallbladder; and the *chag* point reveals the condition of the right kidney and the bladder. On the left wrist of a man, the *tson* point relates to the heart and small intestine; the *kan* point to the spleen and stomach; and the *chag* point to the left kidney and the genital system. In women, the *tson* point relates to the same internal organs as in men, but in the opposite relation to the left and right wrists. While feeling the pulse, an *emchi-lama* takes into account such characteristics as the rate, strength and pattern of the pulse (Fig. 3.7). In addition, the *emchi-lama* considers the patient's constitution, the time and place of the examination and specifics of the patient's way of life. All these provide complementary information about the condition of a sick person.

Questioning a patient helps *lamas* find out how the disease began and its clinical course, as well as the specifics of the patient's diet and way of life. A general inspection of the body allows *lamas* to identify the patient's type of constitution by observing the skin, tongue, eyes, muscles, etc. Characteristics of the patient's urine, breathing, movement and general appearance are also considered. Palpation is used by *emchi-lamas* to estimate the patient's temperature and muscle tone, as well as the sensitivity of certain points in the body and how painful they are when pressure is applied to them (Nikolaev *et al.* 2004:30). *Lamas* also pay attention to the landscape around the place where a patient lives, seasonal changes and astrological information in order to diagnose the patient and choose a treatment. *Lamas* practicing in different geographic zones say that each location determines certain characteristics of the clinical course of diseases.

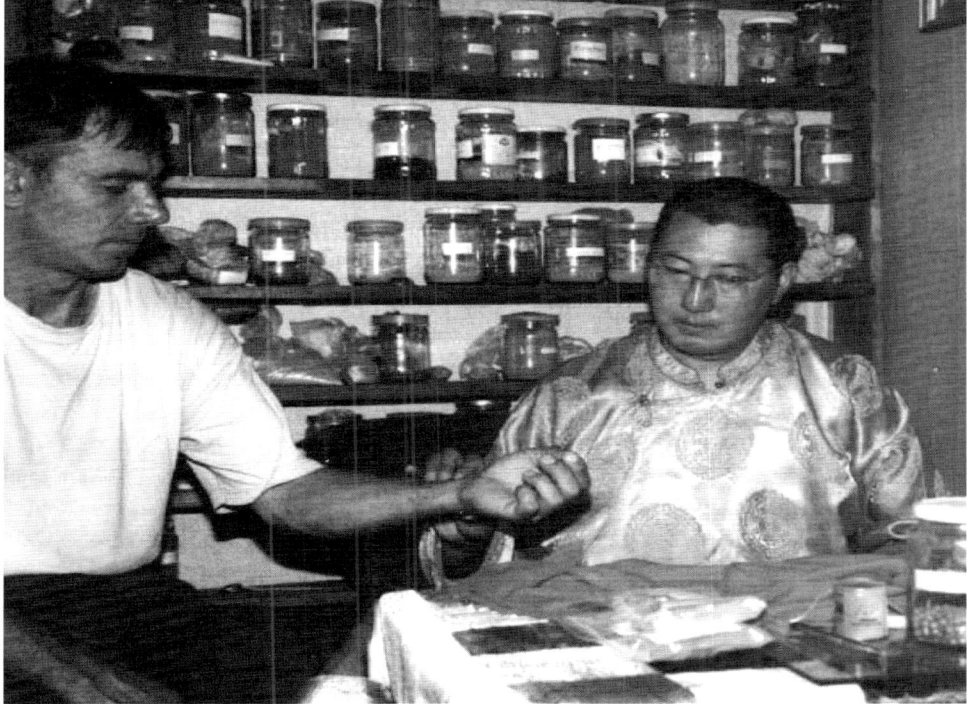

Figure 3.7 *Pulse diagnostics (Ochirov 2006).*

Today many *emchi-lamas* also use the diagnostic tools of biomedicine. Therefore, before beginning their own examination of a patient, they often familiarize themselves with the results of any ultrasound radiography or other types of diagnostics. They also often refer their patients for a contemporary official medical examination in order to obtain a more accurate diagnosis and to control treatment. *Emchi-lamas* deal mostly with chronic diseases and refuse emergency cases and acute infectious diseases (Aiusheeva 2007:136).

Astrology and medicine are interwoven in Tibetan culture, so *lamas* rely heavily on astrologic information for prognoses and to choose a favourable date for beginning the treatment. In Buriatiia, the Mongolian astrology *zurkhai*, which is a Mongolian variant of Tibetan astrology, is widespread. *Zurkhai* has two main functions: warning and prediction. Buriats who believe in *zurkhai* seek assistance from *lamas*-astrologists when experiencing difficult or complicated situations and, having described the situation, are given certain recommendations. Often *lamas*–astrologists have the gift of foresight and can pre-empt a person's misfortunes, diseases, losses and futile efforts. *Zurkhai* can help people specify favourable days to begin a journey, treatment or some other important undertaking; it can provide recommendations on the choice of a life partner, and so on. *Emchi-lamas* actively use *zurkhai* to determine favourable days for a treatment and predicting its outcome.

Doctors of the Tibetan medical tradition can advise patients to correct their way of life and behaviour in order to facilitate their recovery, so *emchi-lamas* also explain the rules of a recommended diet and way of life to their patients. This is important, because health depends mostly on the efforts of the patients themselves. Many people suffer from diseases related to exposure to cold and unsuitable eating habits. Exposure to cold results in diseases of cold, such as rheumatism, nephritis, heart disease, diseases of the legs and feet, etc. *Lamas* advise their patients on the issues of proper clothing (for example, it should be warm, appropriate to the season, etc.) and recommend medication and cures aimed at increasing inner warmth (for example, heating of the body and taking baths).

Unsuitable food and bad eating habits are another problem; *emchi-lamas* assign a diet that complements the patient's constitution. However, there are recommendations common for everyone; for instance overconsumption of fruits and vegetables with cold properties is believed to result in excessive exposure to cold and, as a consequence, in various cold diseases. The traditional Buriat cuisine is well balanced in terms of cold and hot properties and ideally suits people residing in Siberian conditions. However, Buriats have always preferred food with warm properties. The staples of this cuisine include meat, dairy and green tea, and many dishes with healing effects. For example, the soup *khorkhog* used to be cooked for preventing diseases and for replenishing a person's strength after a wasting illness. Its preparation requires the following: bits of each type of a ram's bones and inner organs were to be put into a wooden pot and covered with water. Then nine red-hot stones were to be immersed in the water; they had to be replaced with fresh hot stones till the contents of the pot boiled. This soup was and is considered to be very effective for keeping the inner warmth in the proper state and, therefore, for protecting a patient from illness (Lenkhoboev and Zhambaldagbaev 2003:20). Some researchers state that Buriat cuisine is narrow; however I would disagree with this opinion because the traditional cuisine of Buriats is the most adapted to the climatic conditions of their life and includes all the necessary components to keep the organism fit and healthy. Buriats have always been noted for their good health and diseases have been quite rare among them.

A successful treatment requires contact between doctor and patient. There is a decided lack of contact in contemporary Western medicine, coupled with a lack of trust by the patient in the doctor. Doctors tend to spend more time paying attention to tests rather than communicating with their patients. This situation negatively influences the results of the treatment (Kravchenko 2007:222). In contrast, doctors of the Tibetan medical tradition try to start a dialogue with their patients. They understand that the outcome of treatment depends to a large extent on the patient's own efforts. *Emchi-lamas* believe that trust and compassion are the key factors of a successful treatment. Buddhist ethics and vows do not allow them to pursue their own benefits in their relation to their patients, so if an *emchi-lama* cannot help a person, he will not deceive them with false claims (Mikhailov 2006).

Emchi-lamas always pay attention to the way patients feel. After examining a sick person, a *lama* briefly explains his or her medical condition to the patient, in an accessible way, as well as the chosen method of treatment and the expected results. This is necessary in order that the patient is psychologically prepared for the treatment. For example, some types of migraine are associated in Tibetan medicine with over-excitation of the gall bladder. So, medication aimed at vascular disorders should be complemented with gall bladder treatments. If a medication may provoke exacerbation of a condition, the *emchi-lamas* inform their patients about this beforehand and illustrate it with examples.

Chapter Three: *The Development of Tibetan Medicine in Buriatiia*

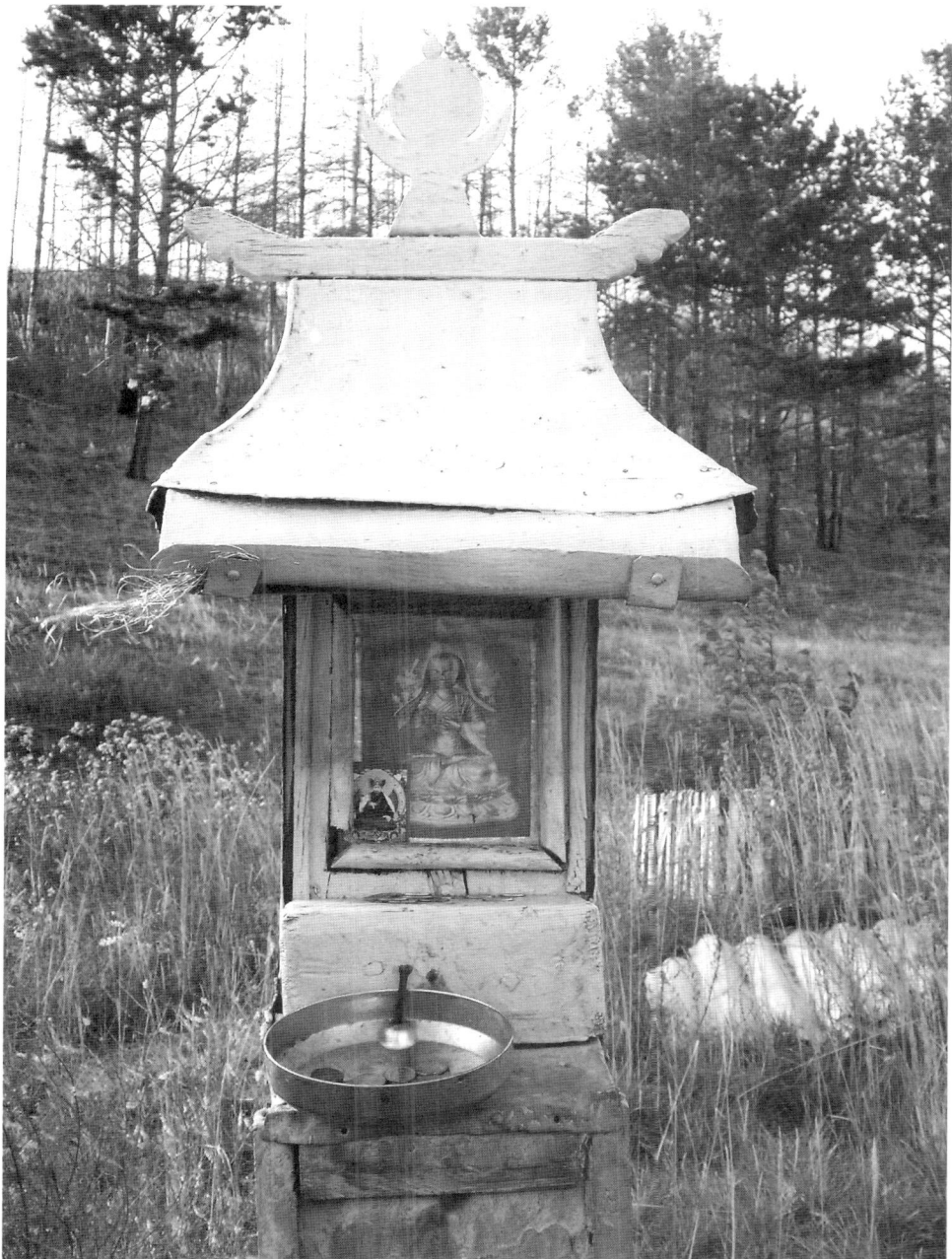

Figure 3.8. *The* arshan *Uta-Bulag*. Photo by V.N. Gololobova.

Tibetan medicine is not limited to the use of medication. When necessary, medication-based treatment can be supplemented with bloodletting, cauterization, acupuncture, medicinal bath-taking, massage, physical exercises and the performing of various rituals.

As in Tibet, *emchi-lamas* resort to rituals when a prolonged treatment with medication is not effective. In such cases, *lamas* associate a disease with the influence of evil spirits or karmic factors. To cure these types of disorders, *lamas* say prayers and read sacred texts. The repetition of mantras and prayers has a psychotherapeutic effect, so a resort to prayer is sometimes exactly what is required for recovery.

Tibetan medicine also adopted and revised various folk methods of healing, such as treatment with water-springs. Taking baths in mineral springs or hot springs [*arshanuud*] was and still is one of the best-known types of cure among Buriats. There are many springs with various medicinal properties in Buriatiia. *Lamas* identify them by the taste of the water, specifics of the soil and vegetation around the springs, the characteristics of a location (for example, whether it is situated at the southern or northern side of a hill, at the top of a hill or on the plain), etc. (Lenkhoboev and Zhambaldagbaev 1983:77). Today, at the exit from a spring, one may see a wooden or stone plate with information on the spring's medicinal properties and use. The choice of spring to use is complex and should take into account both the properties of the spring and the disease to be treated. Therefore, Buriats ask *lamas* or shamans for their advice on where to take medicinal baths. *Lamas*-astrologists estimate, with regard to the year of a person's birth, whether it is recommended to take medicinal baths during a particular year and if so when and how many, whether the baths taken would be effective and which spring is the most suitable (Fig. 3.8).

Passing on Knowledge

Many researchers of Tibetan medicine in the Zabaikal region note that practicing *lamas* often do not have any special medical training. Many *emchi-lamas* had *khuvaraguud* [pupils] who helped them with collecting raw medicinal materials for preparations and assisted at medical checkups of patients. Such an experience allowed the pupils to acquire knowledge about the preparation and prescription of medications. *Lamas* who had not completed the full course of medical training practiced among the non-wealthy population of remote *ulusy* [settlements] and were known as *emtei-lamas* (in the Buriat language, this means 'a *lama* who has medicaments'). The majority of *emchi-lamas* cared about their reputation and were popular among the population. They restricted their practice to a moderate variety of time-tested medications that they prepared according to recipes learned directly from their teachers (Aiusheeva 2007:67).

In Soviet times, when religious practices were banned and government policies threatened the very existence of Buddhism and Tibetan medicine in the country, some healers began to practice Tibetan medicine without a formal Buddhist education. It is mostly thanks to those people that the Tibetan medical tradition in Buriatiia has continued and this unique knowledge has not been lost. The life story of Galdan Lenkhoboev, a practitioner of Tibetan medicine in Soviet Buriatiia, is a good example. His parents wanted him to pursue a Buddhist education and consulted with Dashi-Dorzho Etigelov, the *shiretui* [chief *lama*] of the Iangazha Datsan. Etigelov, however, foresaw the forthcoming hard time for religion and advised Galdan's parents that their son would be better to acquire a Buddhist education outside the *datsanuud*. Lenkhoboev gained knowledge of Tibetan medicine from his maternal uncle (name unknown), who was an *emchi-lama*. In 1923, he began working as a cabinet-maker and worked as a pattern-maker at the 'Mekhanlit' plant for thirty-seven years, during which time he put forward new plans to rationalize production and to improve product quality. Galdan Lenkhoboev was also an activist and served as a deputy for both district and city Soviets. In addition, he was a gifted artist whose wooden and stone crafts used to be exhibited in various museums of the cities of Ulan-Ude, Leningrad, Moscow, and Paris. Lenkhoboev assisted a renowned archaeologist, A.P. Okladnikov, working for him as a guide. Throughout all this time he had been collecting information on the customs and traditions of Buriats. He translated the ancient medical treatises

Chapter Three: *The Development of Tibetan Medicine in Buriatiia*

Jud-shi, *Lhan-tliabs* and *Shel-phreng* into the contemporary Buriat language and compiled a Russian–Tibetan–Buriat reference book of medications used by Buriat *lamas*. He wrote a number of research papers, in which he summarized his observations on the basis of Tibetan medical theory; the first of these comprised information on the cold and warm properties of food and medicaments. He resumed his medical practice in the frameworks of Tibetan medicine after his retirement in the 1960s (Fig. 3.9). For a full bibliography of his works *see* Lenkhobov and Zhambaldagbaev (2003).

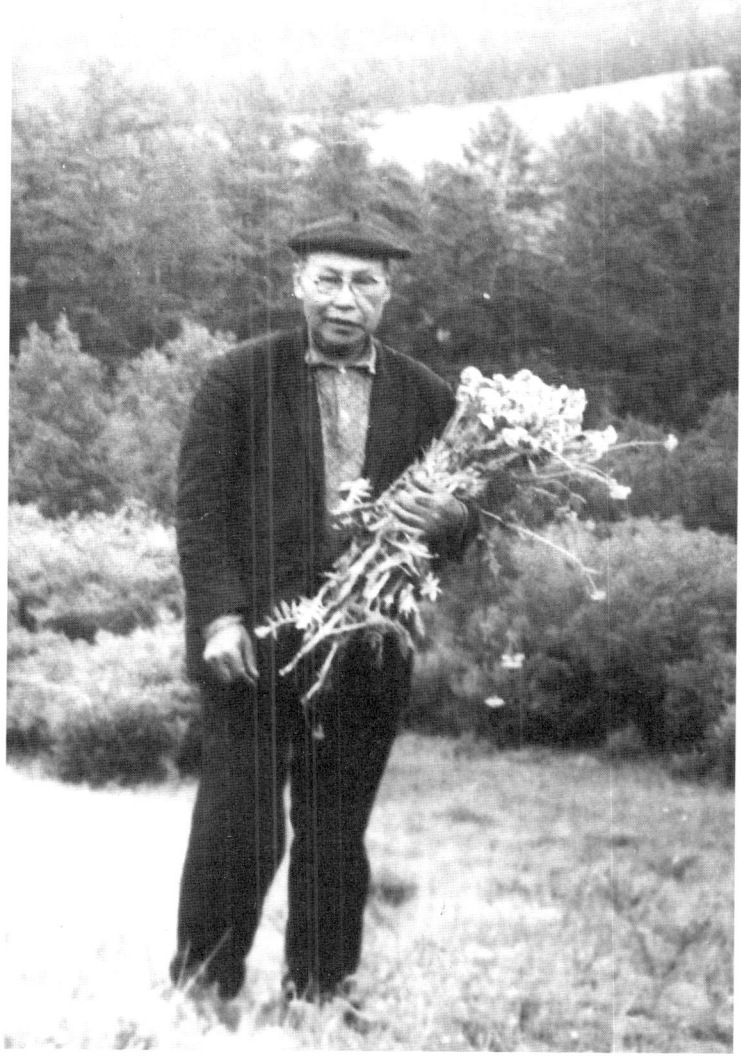

Figure 3.9. *Galdan Lenkhoboev collecting medicinal plants (from the family archive of N.Ts. Zhambaldagbaev).*

Despite the fact that he did not acquire his knowledge of Tibetan medicine from a *manba-datsan*, Galdan Lenkhoboev gained from his uncle all the necessary foundations to practice. Tibetan medicine is considered to be an area of Tantric knowledge, meaning it is not accessible for the uninitiated. One needs to be initiated by their teacher to comprehend and successfully practice this medicine.

Despite various obstacles, Buriats were able to preserve and pass their tradition of Tibetan medicine on to new generations. Today, traditional Tibetan medicine is undergoing a revival along with Buddhism. The Government of the Republic of Buriatiia officially recognizes and supports the Buddhist clergy and Tibetan medicine, as is manifest in the re-establishment of a clerical Buddhist education, including its medical specialization. However, traditional medical education is now somewhat modernized. The duration of training has been reduced from twenty to five or six years and training in Tibetan medicine also requires the study of basic clinical medicine. But, as in the past, *khuvakakuud* learn the secrets of Tibetan medicine under the supervision of their own teachers. Today *manba-datsans* in Buriatiia invite instructors from Tibet, India and Mongolia to contribute to their teaching. Moreover, certified doctors who do not belong to the Buddhist faith also show interest in Tibetan medicine.

Scientific Studies of Tibetan Medicine

The Buriat Scientific Centre of the Siberian Branch of the Russian Academy of Sciences (SB RAS) has been studying the Tibetan medicine of Buriatiia for over forty years. Various specialists take part in these studies: philologists, orientalists, medical workers, pharmacologists, and botanists. In 1975, the Tibetan Medicine Unit of the Buriat Scientific Centre, SB RAS was set up. The Unit collaborated with practising *emchi-lamas* who agreed to share their knowledge of Tibetan medicine for research purposes.

The research fellows of the Tibetan Medicine Unit undertake source studies, and chemical, pharmacological and pharmaceutical research. Philologists from the Buriat Scientific Centre, SB RAS translated the treatises *Jud-shi*, *Vaydurya-onbo*, *Lhan-tliabs*, *Kunsan-nanzod*, *Ontsar-gadon derzod*, *Dzeitskhar Migchzhan*, and the unique *Tibetan Medicine Atlas* from Tibetan into Mongolian and put them to use. They deciphered and specified medical terms and concepts, including names of diseases and medications. The Laboratory for Chemical and Pharmacological Research carries out fieldwork studies of the medicinal plants of Buriatiia, and develops methods of standardization and technologies for preparing medicaments. The Laboratory for Experimental Pharmacology and Pharmacotherapy, under the supervision of Dr. S.M. Nikolaev, explores the pharmacological properties, mechanism of action, and efficacy of new medications. Based on the theoretical ideas of Tibetan medicine, researchers at this laboratory have identified and described the mechanisms of some widespread diseases more accurately. They discovered a previously unknown molecular–biological mechanism of damage to cell membranes in cases of ischemia and hypoxemia of human organs. This discovery stimulated numerous studies both within Russia and abroad and allowed the development of new methods of treatment and prevention of such diseases (Nikolaev *et al.* 2004:49,60).

The Laboratory for Pulse Diagnostics, under the supervision of Doctor of Technical Sciences, Professor V.V. Boronoev, developed an automated pulse-diagnosing complex (known in Russian as APDK). After successful tests, the Ministry of Health Care of the Republic of Buriatiia approved the use of this diagnostic device in medical institutions and research laboratories. In 1989, researchers of the Buriat Scientific Centre, SB RAS and medical workers organized a state medical institution for treatment and prevention of diseases in the city of Ulan-Ude, Russia—the Eastern Medicine Centre. The doctors of this centre use the diagnostic and treatment methods of the Tibetan medical tradition, such as pulse diagnosis, herbal therapy, medicinal bath-taking, bloodletting and moxibustion. For pulse diagnosis, the doctors use the new automated pulse-diagnosing equipment. Dr Ts.D. Turtuev, who operates this apparatus, asserts that, based on his observations, pulse diagnosis is a very useful element in medicine. Pulse diagnosis allows the doctor to obtain complete information about the functional condition of human internal organs in a relatively short time—about 15 to 20 minutes. The automated pulse-diagnosis complex is suitable for mass screening of the population, assessment of the course of disease in the process of a patient's treatment, and for preventive diagnosis of diseases at the earliest stages of their development (Turtuev and Boronoev 2004:38).

In addition to diagnosis and treatment, the Centre also researches Tibetan medicine and licenses traditional medical practice; it produces herbal medications and organizes medical tourism.

Certified doctors who have acquired additional education in traditional medicine practice at the Centre. The Department of Medicine at Buriat State University trains doctors within new framework of integrative medicine. Besides basic medical and biological courses, this approach covers Buddhist philosophy, the Tibetan language and the Mongolian script, homeopathy, herbal therapy and manual diagnostics (Nikolaev et al. 2004:54-55,66). With these developments, it might be possible to conclude that perhaps Tibetan medicine has become secularised.

Unfortunately, Tibetan medicine is not officially approved for medical practice within the Russian Federation. This means that it is practiced in a fragmentary manner and not widespread. Doctors mostly use the herbal preparations of Tibetan medicine because the criteria of clearance for the licensing of herbal therapy practice have already been approved. However, in addition to the herbal preparations of Tibetan medicine, doctors may use other diagnostic and therapeutic techniques that are not a part of classic Tibetan medicine—for example, homeopathy, acupuncture, and the diagnostic method of Reinhold Voll.[2] The complete application of Tibetan medicine requires the questioning of a patient, inspection of the patient's body, pulse diagnosis, urine diagnosis, treatment mostly with medications, and complementary types of cure. This variant has been preserved by *emchi-lamas*. Despite the absence of official approval, Tibetan medicine is widely practiced in Buriatiia, Kalmykiia and Tyva (Aiusheeva 2007:136).

Conclusion

The history of Tibetan medicine in Buriatiia demonstrates the flexibility by which it adapted to natural and climatic circumstances. Based on universal knowledge of the five *mahābhūtas* and the 'taste' qualities of food and plants, Buriat *emchi-lamas* elaborated on the Tibetan medicine theory of the inner warmth of the body. They were able to almost completely replace imported and difficult to access ingredients for their medicinal preparations. Therefore, researchers now identify a Buriat branch of Tibetan medicine. Since the imported products were chosen by the *lamas* using both Tibetan medical theory and their local knowledge Buriat folk medicine, this branch of Tibetan medicine has preserved fragments of Buriat folk practice and saved it from disappearing completely.

The connection between the Buriat–Tibetan medicine and the Buddhist religion has been continuous and invariable. Notions of a healthy organism, unhealthy states, causes of diseases, and principles of treatment are the same in Tibetan medicine in Tibet, Mongolia and Buriatiia. Thus, Tibetan medicine demonstrates a considerable adaptability. The adop-

---

[2] [Translator's note] A method of diagnosis that combines acupuncture and a galvanometer: a device that measures the electric resistance of skin at certain points on the human hands. The method, introduced in 1958 by Reinhold Voll, is also known as Percutaneous Electrical Nerve Stimulation (PENS).

tion of Buddhism among local populations is one of the main influences on the spread of Tibetan medicine.

In general, Buriat *emchi-lamas* do not deviate from the tenants of Tibetan medicine in diagnosis, treatment and communication with patients. Diagnostic techniques almost always include pulse-diagnosis, inspection of a patient's body and interviews. Some *lamas* complement these techniques with palpation of diseased organs and examination of urine, faeces, phlegm, and blood. The dominant treatment is through preparing medicines for the patient to swallow. When needed, *emchi-lama*s can complement such treatment with bloodletting, cauterization, medicinal bath-taking, massage, physical exercises and various rituals. Fragments of folk medical knowledge were incorporated into contemporary practice: for example, taking healing baths in *arshanuud* and prescribing a healing diet. Some of the explanations of the causes of illness come from Buriat folk tradition. Other aspects of the folk tradition were not incorporated, such as shamanic medicine and the tradition of using one's hands to adjust the body [*baryaasha*]. Nevertheless, the *lamas* were aware of a high efficacy of such techniques and, when required, could refer their patients to folk healers.

The political events of the early 20th century influenced the existence of Tibetan medicine in Buriatiia. The anti-religious policy of the Soviet government threatened the existence of Buddhism and Tibetan medicine. A generation of *emchi-lamas* appeared who could not gain a classic Buddhist education in *manba-datsans*. However, the passing on of knowledge from teacher to pupil has not been interrupted. Today, despite the absence of the official approval of Tibetan medicine in the Russian Federation, studies and the practice of Tibetan medicine are undergoing a revival within the frameworks of Buddhism.

The World Health Organization (WHO) encourages the development of traditional medicine and the integration of contemporary official and traditional medical knowledge. Today, traditional and official medicine are seen to be converging in Buriatiia, as evidenced by the example of the Eastern Medicine Centre, where certified specialists employ the methods of Tibetan medicine in their diagnosis and treatment of patients. Such an approach opens the prospects of a wider use of harmless, effective and inexpensive methods of Tibetan medicine for safeguarding the well-being of a person and of society in general.

Over the centuries, practitioners of Tibetan medicine in Buriatiia have replaced almost the entire list of prescribed plant medicines, and adopted the healing practices of the local population. Today, Tibetan medicine has become an important component of the Buriat traditional culture. It remains popular thanks to the high efficacy of its methods of treatment and the absence of side-effects, as well as the positive experience preserved in the collective memory of Buriats.

Acknowledgements

The author would like to thank her supervisor Professor Iurii V. Popkov. Without his assistance it would have been impossible to write this article. I would also like thank my parents N.Ts. Zhamaldagbaev and L.D. Zhamaladagbaeva for their invaluable corrections and for giving me access to manuscripts and photographs. I would like to especially thank the translator and the editor of this volume for creating this text in English and for their advice and comments on the chapter.

Chapter Four

Healing Springs in the Lake Baikal Region

Janice Brummond

Traditional social interactions being revived by Buriat Mongols in the Republic of Buriatiia and in Northern Mongolia include therapies and ritual cures produced from thousands of years of experience with changing ecological and epidemiological circumstances. Based on often reinvented cosmological understandings of self and society, Buriat Mongols are adapting their ancient healing methods to changing institutional contexts and social needs. This chapter describes the water-related therapies and rituals observed at freshwater mineral springs [*arshaanuud* in Buriat language, *rashaanuud* in Mongolian], placing them in the context of evolving physical and cultural landscapes in the Lake Baikal region.[1]

Whether administered officially in conjunction with biomedical clinical practice or independently by friends, family, or local *buu*,[2] healing practices in Buriatiia use ancient ideas about nature. These are expressed through shamanic customs, the seasonal variations in diet and health practices that pastoral nomads developed for survival in harsh conditions with scarce resources, and Buddhist hygienic rituals and therapies based on Indo–Tibetan and Chinese influences. As an integrated body of empirical, paradigmatic and institutional knowledge[3] (Kalland 2000), the Buriat traditional healing system emphasizes the interconnections between the human body and the universe and is interpreted through the five senses. Based on local experience and knowledge derived from Mongolian, Indian, Tibetan and Chinese medical practices, Buriat traditional medicine incorporates the fundamental and integrated principles of balance [*tegsh*]; harmony [*arga-bilig*]; the three energy pulses of wind, bile and phlegm [*khii, shar, badgan*]; and the 'hot and cold' qualities and activities of the core elements of earth, water, fire, air and space (or ether).

The belief that the human is a microcosm of larger worlds—seen and unseen, past and present—and that every living thing needs multiple souls to survive (roughly corresponding to flesh, bone and mind), often requires shamanic knowledge and ritual to keep a balance between humans and nature. All natural and man-made disasters, including epidemics of human or animal disease, are believed to be acts of the *lus* [water] and *savdag* [land] spirits that 'live between the earth and sky.' Shamanic intervention can integrate or 'control' these spirits, but individuals must also 'keep out of their path' and make appropriate offerings to keep the spirits appeased. Therefore, Buriat health is both a personal responsibility and

---

[1] This chapter draws principally from my dissertation field research experiences (2001-2002) and post-doctoral research in 2006 which included extensive interviews and biophysical data collection at mineral spring locations near Lake Baikal and in the Barguzin, Chikoi, Irkut, Kyngarga, Selenga and Uda river basins in Buriatiia.

[2] *Buu* refers to general shamanism, usually practiced by a male shaman. Other terms include *udagan* or *yadgan* for females and *ongon*, or ancient shamanic spirits.

[3] Biomedical knowledge also relies on empirical observations, but is generally interpreted through distinct disciplinary approaches and managed applications. Indigenous healing knowledges are 'perceived' (Ingold 1992) in holistic 'ways of understanding' and distributed or institutionalized through complex social relationships and contexts.

a communal concern, using multiple and overlapping idioms for preventing and healing physical and spiritual illnesses.

The oldest recorded medical treatments in this region include the Mongolian therapies of moxibustion and the bone-setting arts [*Baria zasa*l] of the male *barishi* healers (Hruschka 1998) and the midwifery skills of female *bariashad*, all 'holders' of specialized knowledge and spiritual abilities (Humphrey and Onon 1996). As Buddhism spread throughout the region, monasteries became centers or colleges of medicines [*Manba datsanuud*] and physician-monks [*emchi-lama*] developed theories and therapeutic methods incorporating ancient knowledge of plants, herbs and animal parts as well as the use of mineral waters—alone or in the preparation of medicines.

By the 1700s the fundamentals of Tibetan medicine, based on ancient Tibetan tantras and the practical experiences of the *emchi*[4] were documented in the *Atlas of Tibetan Medicine*. This treatise outlines a philosophical framework and includes the formulations of over 1,300 plant remedies, 114 therapeutic uses of minerals and metals, and 150 medicines derived from animals. At the Center for Tibetan Medicine in Ulan-Ude, all of these medicines are used as well as acupuncture, surgery and other traditional and biomedical treatments. Additional folkloric evidence in *tumbe* [books of traditional remedies], documents numerous *dom* therapies that did not necessarily involve special healers. For example, drinking tea for a headache or treating a sore left eye by touching it with your right knee seven times before breakfast. Some cures evolved directly from the nomadic pastoral lifestyle of the Buriat Mongol people, including the liberal use of fermented mare's milk [*airag*], or venesection [blood-letting], which was first used on animals.

Many Buriat Mongols believe that the interconnected spirit and physical worlds have specific contact points on the landscape where individual and communal health can be maintained or improved (Sarangerel 2000:58). These intersections are important symbolic and ritual sites, spiritually powerful and historically significant. Along with sacred mountains, symbolizing *tengri* [the heavens or most powerful spirits], there are numerous rock formations, caves, canyons and *arshaan* water sources that are marked by ancient petroglyphs or white or bright blue silk scarves called *khadag*. Individuals recognize the power of these sites and may perform their own healing rituals, but many people often turn to the traditional knowledge of shamans or lamas who have special abilities and connections within this 'spirited landscape' to help diagnose and treat specific ailments as well as maintain social harmony. The most important site for Buriat heritage and health is Lake Baikal itself, the home of the 'master' of the water spirits (Uha Loson or Uha Khan), but in addition, there are smaller freshwater sources and mineral springs throughout the region that are important ritual and healing centers.

Water Therapies—*Arshaan*

The Buddhist, shamanic or folkloric origins of Buriat rituals and medical treatments involving water are difficult to differentiate.[5] The term *arshaan* has two meanings: 'consecrated or holy water' and 'mineral springs or mineral water.' The special 'spirited'[6] waters of

---

[4] *Emch* is one word for a respected doctor or healing *lama*. *Bag emch* is a healer's assistant, like a paramedic.

[5] In 1846, the Buriat scholar Dorzhi Banzarov documented local shamanic practices in contrast with Russian influences. Walther Heissig (1970) traced the origins of Buriat and Mongolian 'folk religion' to pre-Buddhist times.

[6] *Ezhin* or *ezen* are 'master' spirits of mountains, rocks, plants, etc. and *lus* or *los* are specific water spirits.

arshaanuud may be collected from different freshwater sources such as mountain summits, streams, springs, lakes, dew, rainwater or snowmelt and kept in different containers for months—even years. Some of these healing waters are boiled, others kept in the sun. Still other waters must be used *in situ* or their powers are degraded and lost. Practices of traditional Buriat and Mongolia shamans include 'eclectically combined altered states of consciousness, drumming, chanting, prayers, healing bioenergies, ritual offerings of sheep, vodka, colored cloth, nature cults, (especially springs and cleansing baths)' (Fridman and Neumann 2003:41). Early Buddhist missionaries tried to eliminate aspects of this ecstatic shamanism and replace the social aspects of ancient folk religion with Buddhist doctrine and organizational control. When both Buddhist and folk traditions were further disrupted under Russian and later Soviet influences, many nature-based rituals were forgotten or camouflaged within nationalistic rhetoric and actions.[7] In field studies throughout Buriatiia and Mongolia, I determined that while many *arshaan* remedies and rituals remain linked to nomadic and Buddhist traditions, other behaviors and healing practices at each mineral spring or *arshaanuud* have been adapted to local environmental and social circumstances as well as to changing medical needs.

Arshanuud **and Social Ritual**

According to early records and my ethnographic interviews, *arshaanuud* were traditionally identified and sanctified by 'extrasensitive' people—shamans and later *lamas*—who perform an annual ceremony of blessing and impart their knowledge and experience about how the *arshaan* can be used for healing. The annual blessing or 'invitation to *arshaan*' became a social celebration, much like how villages in Britain traditionally decorated wells (Hope 1968 [1893]).[8] After the long winter, springs are cleared of debris, worshiped and cherished in special festive ceremonies with *arshaan* waters poured into all available bottles and silver bowls. These social occasions of community healing may be timed to coincide with horse racing, *Suur-kharbaan* festivals or *Maidari-Khutal* rituals.[9]

Midsummer is thought to be when *arshaan* waters become most powerful or 'ripe.' *Arshaanuud* are still places of summer holidays as well as pilgrimages throughout the year.

---

[7] For example, Humphrey quotes T.M. Mikhailov's story about the *tailgan*, shamanic ceremony of ritual and sacrifice to ancestral spirits, dedicated to the Parisian Communards who took refuge in Lake Baikal as *Ukhan-Khaalyuud* (water-otters). It was believed that if these spirits were appeased they would help fulfill the Soviet collective fishing 'plan' (Humphrey 1998:408).

[8] Throughout the spring and summer in rural England, wells, springs and other bodies of water are decorated with often elaborate structures and mosaic-like pictures made of flower petals, mosses and other natural materials such as seeds and cones. The traditional practice of well-dressing or well-flowering may be linked to early Celtic rituals celebrating the powers of fresh water, Christian practices of naming healing waters after saints and blessing wells with flowers on the saint's name day or community thanksgiving for escaping the ravages of the Black Death in 1348-1349. The custom almost disappeared in the 1950s but festivals to 'dress' wells have been revived in some villages, primarily for the tourist industry.

[9] From observation and oral testimonies as well as from information in *Amazing Meeting* by A. Lamajaa as quoted in Arakchaa (1995:2). The *Suur-kharbaan* ('shooting the target') festivities are held in July in Buriatiia as is the *Nadaam* (festival of the manly sports) in Mongolia. Both often entail visits to nearby spring waters or spas. Many annual Buddhist rituals include healing waters taken from local mineral springs or from Lake Baikal.

Usually in August, *Usn Arshaan* and *Usn Taiklagn* include gathering at spring locations, blessing the water, and making sacrifices to the water spirits. Monks and prayer leaders come to chant and bless the waters, and then everyone, including animals, is allowed to drink the waters. The celebration of New Year and *Sagaalgan* [White Month] includes prohibitions on spring water use except for special ritual purposes. Other water rites are directly linked to Buddhist ceremonies. The *90* [fertility ceremony] unites earth and water to create and sustain life. Symbolically, consecutive offerings to the water and the trees ensure the productive union of the daughter of the master of the waters and the son of the master of the rain. Other life-cycle rites of birth, marriage, and death, all incorporate *arshaan* waters with incense and chanting in all stages of the rituals.

The most obvious material evidence of ritual at spring sites is the tying of blue *khadag* or prayer flags [*but*] near the water source (Fig. 4.1). Some springs have nearby *oboo*, ritual rock cairns, or a cleared space for related ceremonies (Fig. 4.2).

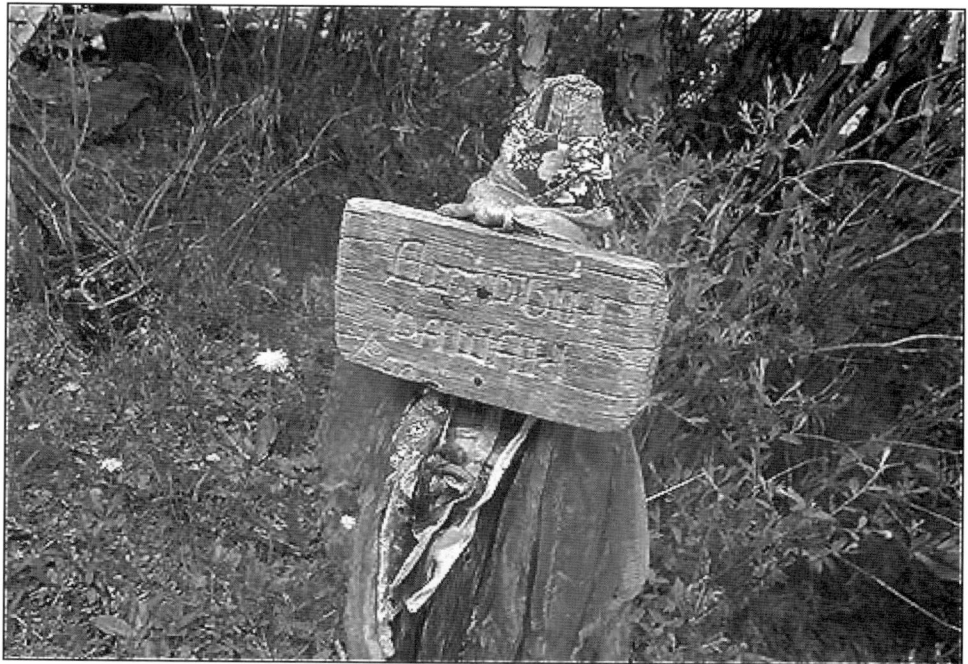

Figure 4.1. *Ceremonial* khadag *marking of a mineral spring.*

Healing Powers of *Arshanuud*

The healing properties of individual *arshaan* in Buriatiia are locally well-known but only sporadically documented.[10] Each water source considered *arshaan* has specific treatment regimes or recommended cures that are implemented in three principal ways: soaking or balneotherapy; drinking; and steam inhalation. Adjunct therapies include mud, acupuncture, massage or exercise regimes.

---

[10] Some data on the medicinal values of Mongolian *rashaanuud* were included in Soviet and Mongolian regional spring studies (Smirnov 1932; Namandorj *et al.*1966). Individual spring systems in Buriatiia have more extensive data (Botoraev 1991).

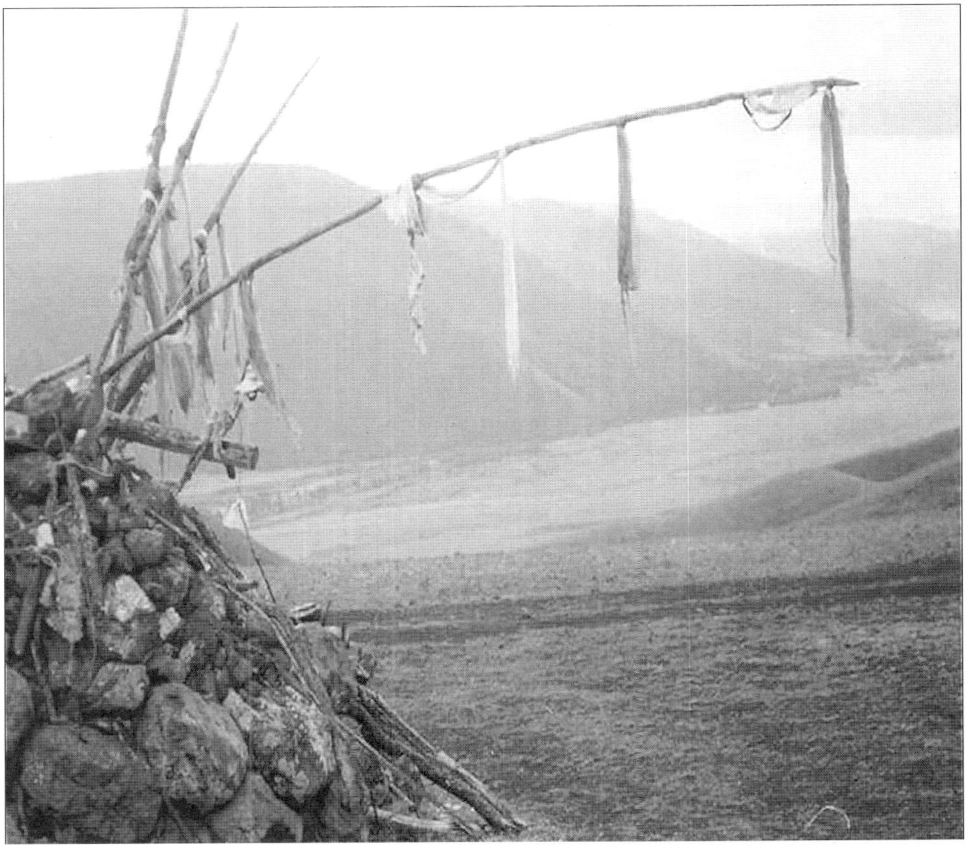

Chapter Four: *Healing Springs in the Lake Baikal Region*

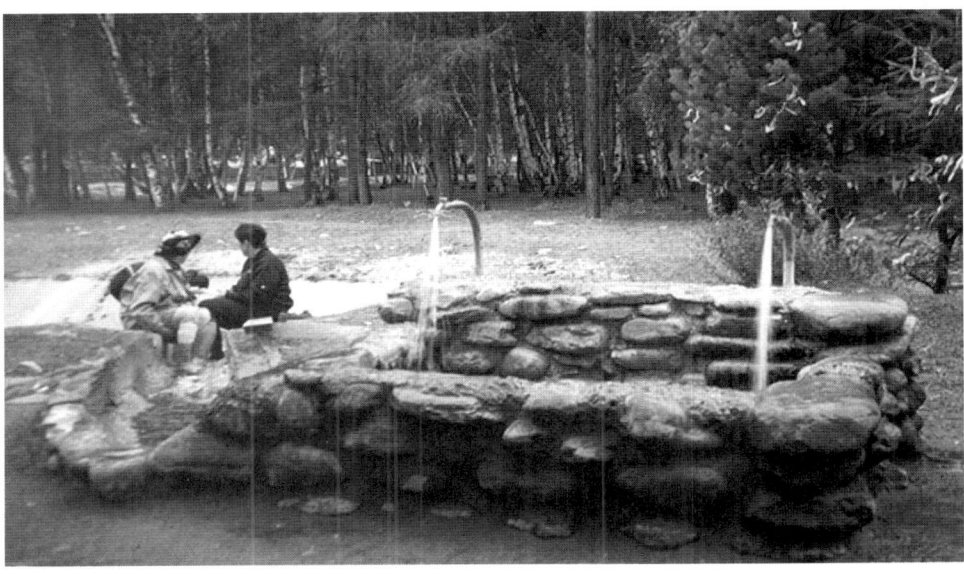

Figure 4.2. *Photo of* oboo—*ritual rock cairn.*

Figure 4.3. *Foot-soaking at Arshaan Saiani, Tunka Valley, Buriatiia.*

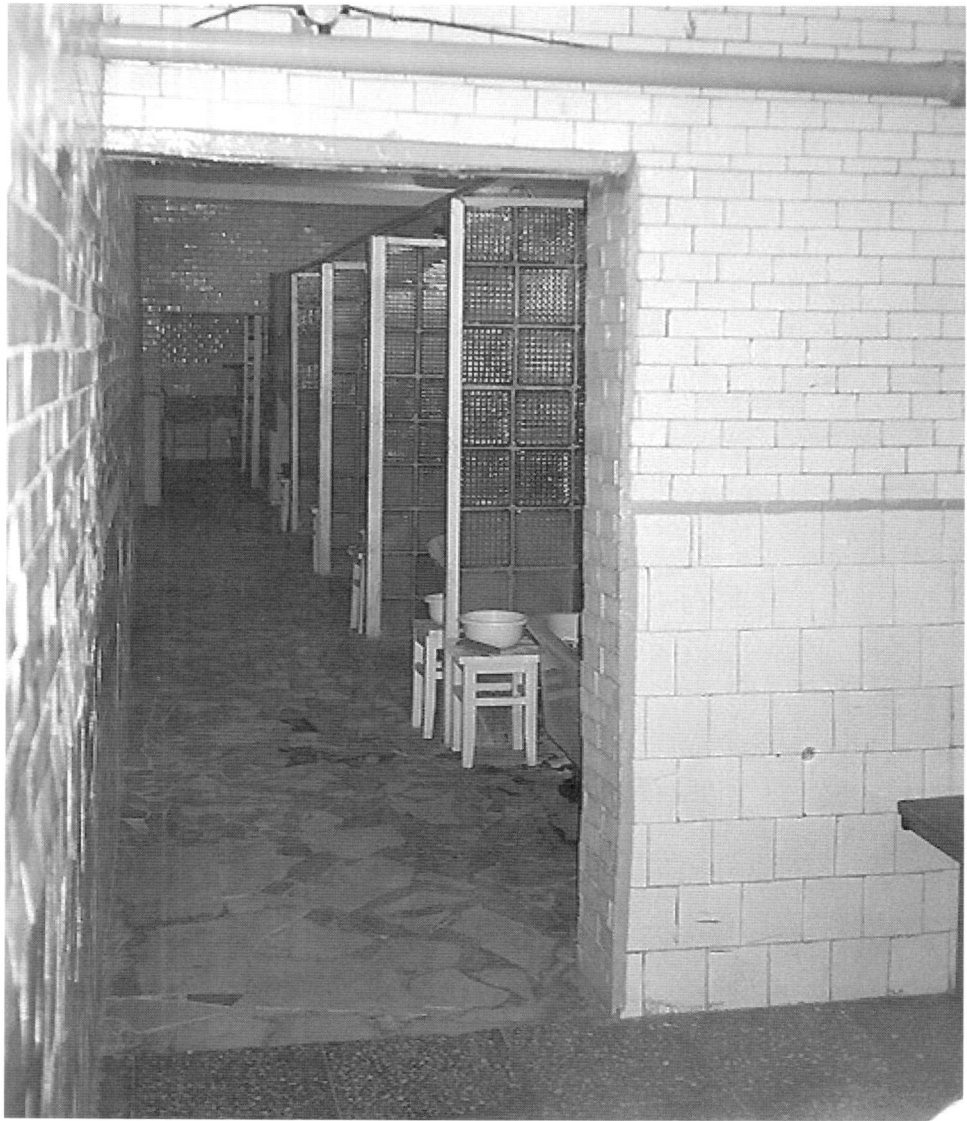

Figure 4.4. *Therapeutic baths at Nilova Pustyn, Tunka Valley, Buriatiia.*

Soaking and Bathing

Soaking therapy in this region developed during the violent conquests of Chinggis Khaan. Victims who were losing huge amounts of blood from wounds were placed in the abdomen of a recently slaughtered animal (cow or camel). The wounds would be soaked in the healing, hot blood of the animal. Animal dung or hot sands were also used. If hot springs were nearby, wounds could be cleansed and soothed in these waters (Bold and Ambaga 2002) (Fig. 4.3).

According to Bold and Ambaga (2002:25; 50) the earliest known treatise on balneology from this region is *Balneotherapy: How it can help you, its applications and hygienic uses* by Tsahra Gevsh Luvsanchultem (1740-1810). Another important work is the Buddhist tantra entitled *Rashanii Tsatsral* [Spa Springs] (1639) by Lamyin Gegeen Luvsandanzanjantsan. A distinctive ancient prescription is to make a soaking bath by adding a decoction of ephedra, juniper, willow, wormwood, and rosemary called the Five Springs of Dandar (Ligaa and Tsembel 2003). To-Wang, a 19th century *khan*, developed mineral springs as spas within his *banner* (administrative district), recording the healing properties of the waters as well as other traditional weather lore and herding advice (Bawden 1968). This traditional knowledge corresponds to modern studies documenting the healing benefits of soaking in mineral waters, especially thermal baths (Lamoreaux and Tanner 2001; Altman 2000) (Fig. 4.4).

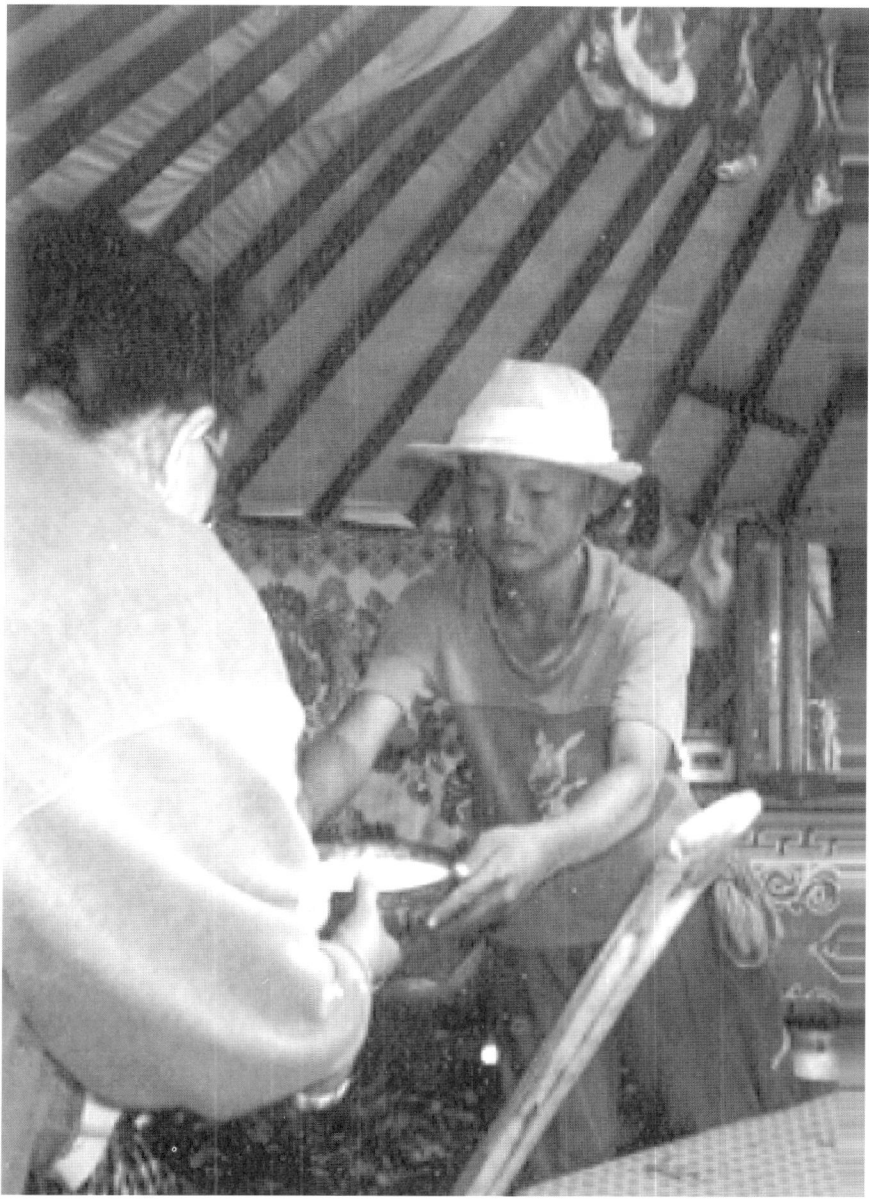

Figure 4.5. *Ritual drinking of* airag *(fermented mares' milk).*

A second traditional Buriat healing treatment is to drink special mineral waters, either alone or in combination with herbal potions. Drinking rituals vary in different locales throughout the region. In Buriatiia, the Eastern Buriats take a small amount of liquid on their fourth finger of the right hand and flick droplets in each of the four directions prior to drinking. Western Buriats either throw a portion of the beverage over their shoulders or touch the earth (or table) with liquid. Taken seriously by people of all ages, these habits are related to the nomadic ritual of throwing milk on the hearth before eating and drinking. Beverages are often combined—with milk, alcohol, and *arshaan* mixed into silver or ceramic bowls [*aiaga*] that are never allowed to remain empty (Figs. 4.5 and 4.6).

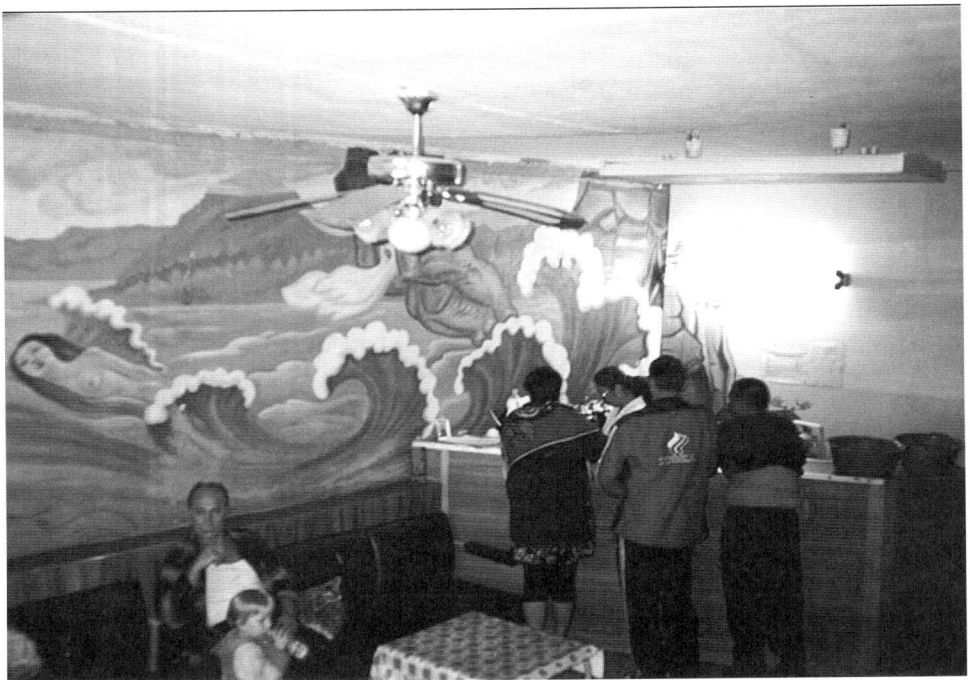

Figure 4.6. *Drinking regime at Nilova Pustyn spa, Buriatiia.*

Drinking Mineral Waters
Some people add small stones to their waters before drinking, believing this to further enhance the powers of *arshaan*. Drinking habits also vary by gender, with cups or bottles of certain *arshaan* reserved and sipped by women and others used exclusively by men.

A third method of using mineral waters involves inhaling a combination of steam from *arshaanuud* and 'smokes' from medicinal plants. Inhalation of hot spring vapors is an especially powerful cure for asthma, sinus problems, allergies and other lung and respiratory disorders. In Buriatiia the traditional *bania* or steam bath is often part of *arshaan* therapies and a shaman's initiation ritual [*ugaalga*] includes steam purification using *arshaan* with wild thyme (*Thymus serpyllum*).

As in other spring locations around the world, coating parts of the body with mud is believed to remove toxins, heal the skin, and relieve arthritic and muscle pain (Altman 2000). The mud pools at Shumak and the bottom sediments of Lake Kyren in Buriatiia and a series of lakes in North Central Mongolia (Toson Nuur, Booruljuut, and Gurvan Nuur) all contain especially soothing ingredients (Fig. 4.7).

Chapter Four: *Healing Springs in the Lake Baikal Region*

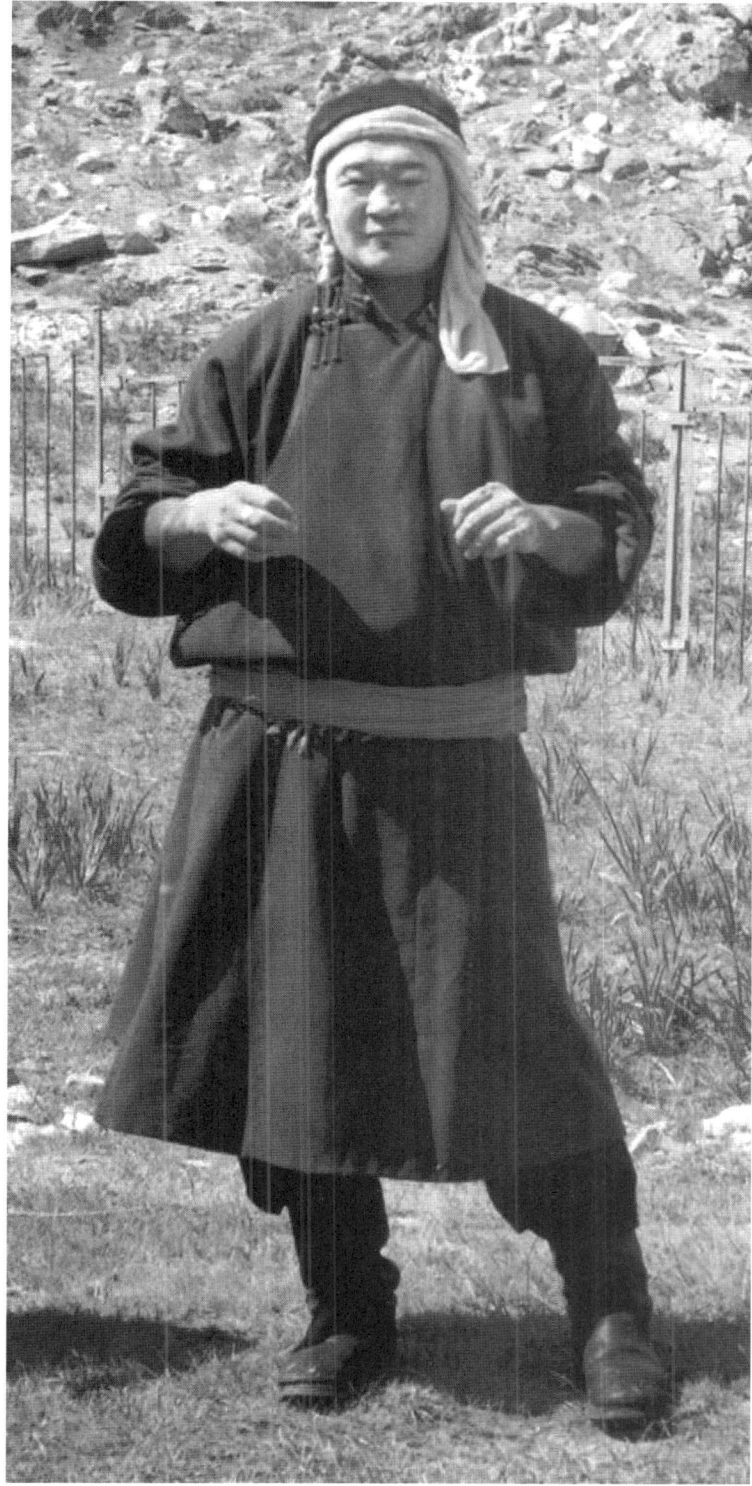

Figure 4.7. *A herder uses mud for skin therapy, Mongolia.*

At some spring locations, hot and cold water treatments are combined and chemically diverse waters are used in complicated sequences of drinking, bathing, and inhalation. Traditional therapies at springs may include a regime of physical exercise and fresh air, or a conserving regime of relaxation therapies including massage and meditation. Acupuncture techniques may be used in both types of regimes, for stimulating certain pressure points or for alleviating pain and reducing tension.

Medicinal Plants and Diet

Critical to traditional treatments at *arshaanuud* are plant and animal-based remedies, and dietary prescriptions (Fig. 4.8). The traditional Buriat Mongol nomadic diet is interrelated with cosmological principles, grounded in centuries of indigenous knowledge related to climatic conditions, grassland resources and animal population dynamics. The most important aspect of a balanced or *tegsh* diet is knowledge about the 'hot and cold'[11] foods which should be consumed in specific combinations, depending on the season. Knowledge of medicinal plants is also localized and specific to most spring locations. No parts of plants are excluded from medicinal use, even those known to be poisonous:

A flower rejected by the butterflies is poisonous, but it can become medicine when it is properly composed. Like a notorious thief who can become a good and useful person when he is properly trained and taught, a poisonous plant can become a very effective medicine. In fact, the *Emchi* use medicines prepared by poisonous plants when the disease is severe (Bold and Ambaga 2002:26).

Historically, mushrooms (fly agaric or *Amanita muscaria*), cannabis, and *datura* were often used as shamanic inebriants, mixed with water or milk and the juice of sweet plants (Schultes and Hoffman 1992). Now this practice seems to be less prevalent, possibly due to the widespread use of *airag*, *arkhi*, and other alcoholic beverages.

Arshanuud in the Landscape

The social significance and medicinal values of *arshaanuud* are further influenced by their place in the regional landscape. The Lake Baikal region has distinct landscape types—biomes—that determine the character and medicinal values of each spring, for example alpine, taiga and steppe biomes. My field data collected in 2002 and 2006 points out diverse medicinal practices and other social traditions at spring systems in each biome.[12]

Arshaanuud in Alpine Areas
At the edge of Lake Khovsgol, in Northern Mongolia near the border with the Buriat and Tuvan Republics is the well-known Khar Us *rashaan* (N 50° 56' 7.8", 100° 14' 48.1", Elevation: 1673 m). It is a fast-flowing spring discharging laterally off the side of a hill in a series of cascades clearly marked with an *oboo*, *khadag* and wooden signs indicating

---

[11] This knowledge is based not on the temperature of foods, but rather their interrelationships with the elements of earth, wind, fire, water, air and 'ether' and the three 'pulses' of wind, bile and phlegm. The complexities of these dietary rules are documented in most Tibetan medical texts such as those translated into English by Ven. Rechung Rinpoche (1973) or in Russian by Petr Badmaev (*cf.* Gusev 2000), Bazaron (1987), Asheeva *et al.* (2008), among others.

[12] I distinguish biomes with the habitat-based WWF ecological land classification which puts Burtiatiia in the Paleoarctic ecoregion.

different medicinal uses. The main source spring is used for drinking and general health, while a secondary flow is for stomach ailments and other smaller cascades are marked for headaches, nerves and muscles, and internal organs.

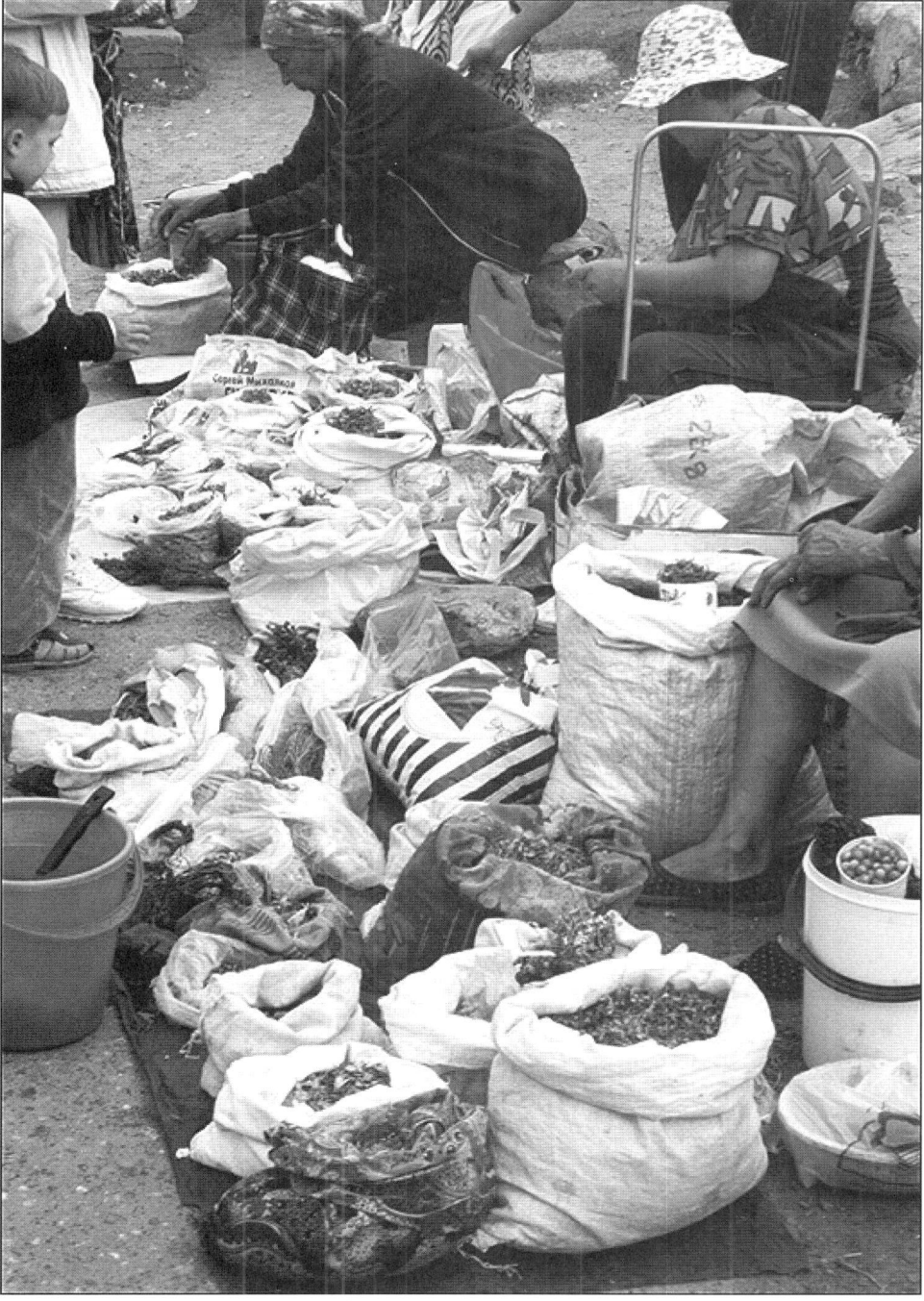

Figure 4.8. *Women selling medicinal herbs at Arshaan Saiani, Buriatiia.*

Combination and Adjunct Therapies

In the spring (late May–early June) this area is extremely busy with '*rashaan*-ers' from all over Mongolia and Buriatiia. Camping above the spring or along the lakeshore, many people time their annual visit to coincide with the spawning of Siberian grayling (*Thymallus arcticus arcticus*). People can scoop up hundreds of fish from the side channels in a matter of minutes. They may smoke or dry some fish, but most of it is used immediately to make a special soup with the *arshaan* waters, believed to increase virility and boost the general immune system.

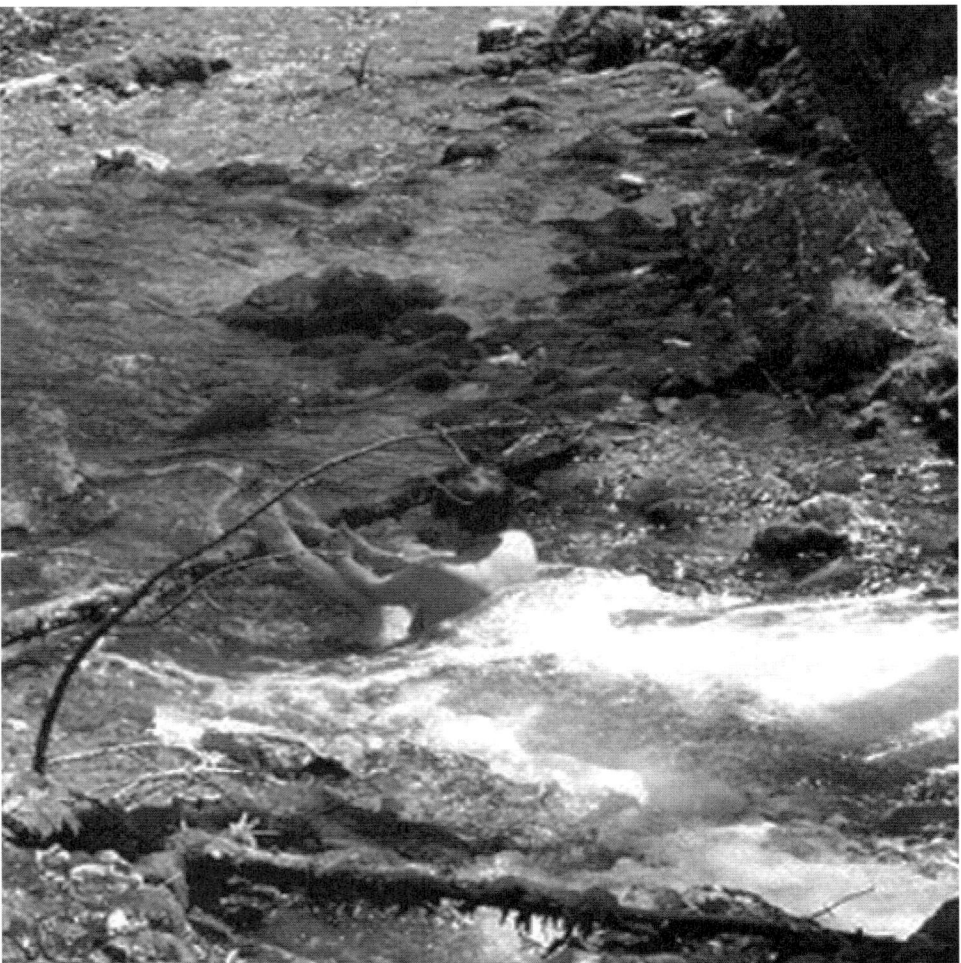

Figure 4.9. *Water massage therapy at Khar Us rashaan near Lake Khovsgol, Mongolia.*

Therapeutic hot springs in this landscape type are infrequent, but those found near the summits of mountains, such as Khoyto-Gol springs and the Choigan *arshaan* where Tuva, Buriatiia and Mongolia meet in the Eastern Saian Mountains have special historical and cosmological connotations for many people, since they are 'closer to Tengri,' or the heavenly spirits (Fig. 4.10).

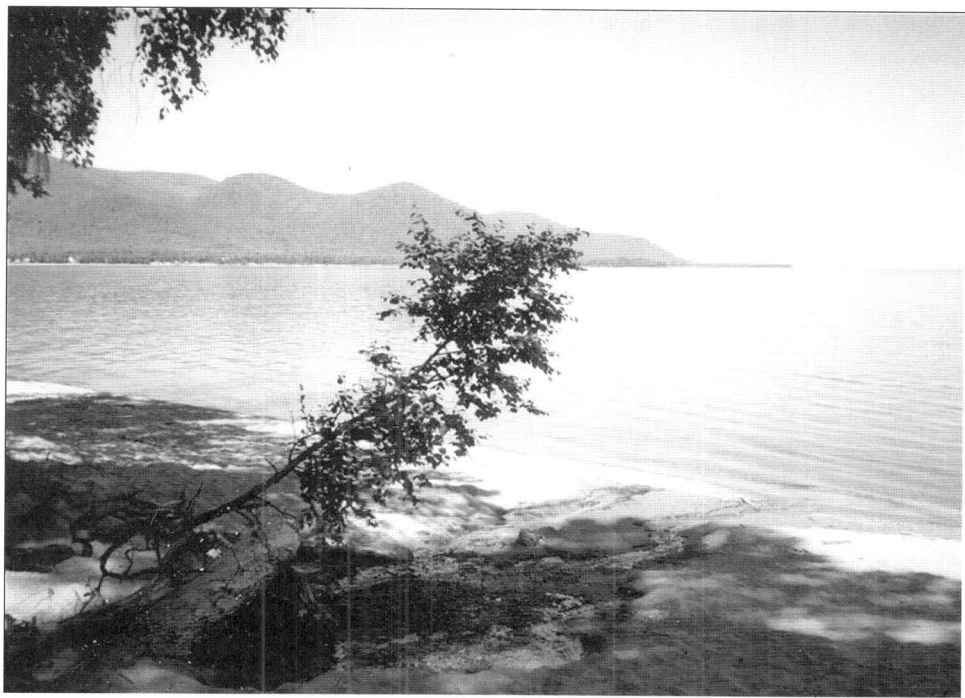

Figure 4.10. Arshaan *for eye treatments flowing into Lake Baikal.*

Taiga Springs

Most of Buriatiia and about 10 percent of Mongolian landscapes are classified as taiga and are part of the largest continuous forest in the world. The Siberian boreal system is coniferous, with mostly Siberian larch (*Larix sibirica*) and Siberian pine (*Pinus sibirica*). Home to important, often endangered wildlife,[13] the taiga also contains various mosses, lichens, rhododendrons, pea trees (*Caragana arborescens*), ginseng, mushrooms, and berries that are important for traditional medicines. Bilberry bushes (*Vaccinium vitis idaea* L.) and smartweed (*Polygonum hydropiper*) often are found near springs and used in infusions with *arshaan* waters. Many springs in the taiga are relied upon for their clear, cold drinking water as well as for medicinal purposes. Developed springs in Buriatiia's taiga zones include those of the Tunka Valley; the famous hot alkaline springs of Khakuses and Dzelindenski in the Severo–Baikalsk district; Garginski kurort in Kurumkan district; and Goryachinsk in Prebaikalsk. There are also many smaller springs that flow directly onto the shores of Lake Baikal, revered by many Buriats, as well as by Mongolians, as the Sacred Sea of their ancestry (Fig. 4.11).

Tunka Valley, Buriatiia

In 1894, the Tunka Valley taiga area of Buriatiia was 'discovered' for its special waters. Extremely popular with local and foreign tourists, Arshaan Saiani was developed as a showcase spa during Soviet times and became an important treatment center for the children of

---

[13] Taiga mammals include musk and roe deer (*Moschus moschiferus, Capreolus pygargus*), European elk or moose (*Alces alces*), brown bear (*Ursus arctos*), wolf (*Canis lupus*), and sable (*Martes zibellina*). The Eurasian River otter (*Lutra lutra*) has been declared an endangered species in Buriatiia. Hot springs in this region contain the endangered Russian ratsnake (*Elaphe dione* Pall.)(Dorzhiev and Namzalov 2001).

Chernobyl—victims of the 1986 nuclear disaster. The chemical and medicinal properties of these waters have been studied extensively for over 70 years (Botoroev 1991). Approximately 40 outflows of hot, cold, and warm carbonate waters have been differentiated and are used in elaborate spa regimes. The main cold spring water comes from the Kyngarga River valley—a steep cascade from the Eastern Saian and Khamar Davan mountain ranges.

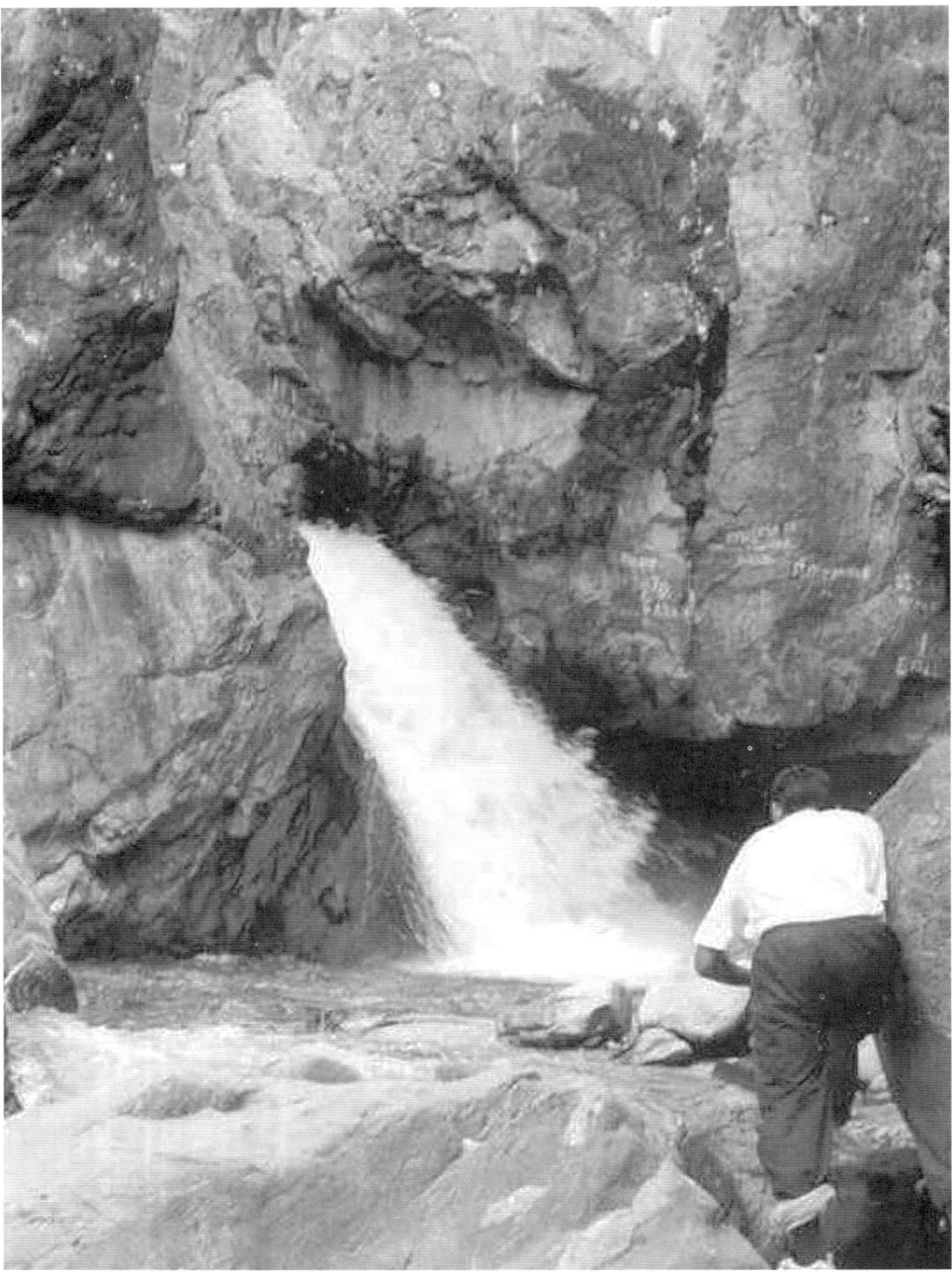

Figure 4.11. *Kyngarga River source—Arshaan Saiani.*

Another Tunka Valley *arshaan*, the Dzemchuk or 'Pearl' tourist complex, is located adjacent to the Irkut River and includes an artesian hot sulfate spring, a mud pool, and hot methane waters flowing from a well. These waters and muds are known for alleviating pains in the joints and nervous disorders. The legend of Dzemchuk is that a rich merchant showered pearls over the area when his son who could not walk was cured by these waters (Fig. 4.12).

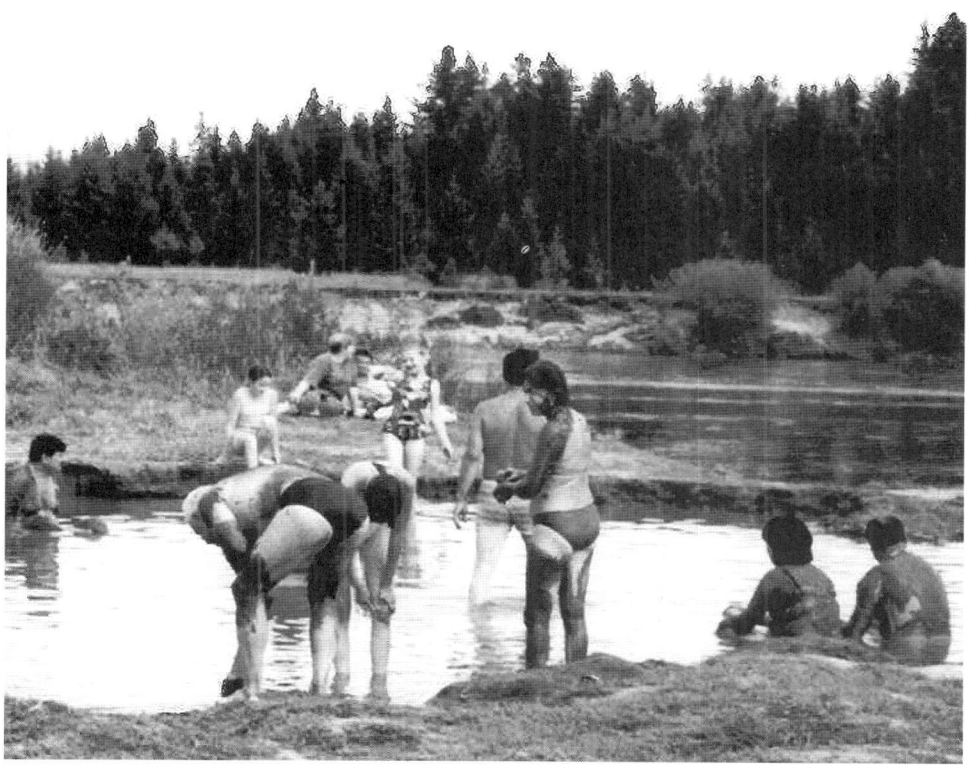

Figure 4.12. *Mudbaths at Dzemchuk hot spring, Tunka Valley.*

Nilova Pustyn is an historic spa area with three separate *arshaan*, hidden in the deep canyon of Ikh Ukhgun River, a tributary to the Irkut. The main two enclosed hot springs reach temperatures from 38 to 43 degrees C. and are used for therapeutic baths to cure skin diseases and arthritis. The medicinal waters are highly mineralized and undrinkable, containing trace elements of fluorine and radon. The third cold alkaline *arshaan* is known to cure eye ailments and is also drunk for general health benefits. There is renewed interest in this site's historic associations with the Russian Orthodox sect of 'Old Believers' [*semeiskie*] in Buriatiia and with the sometimes violent reconciliation of local beliefs with Buddhism. According to oral histories, the *lamas* burned all shamanic evidence and also 'converted' the most powerful shamanic forces that are believed to be based in the Saian Mountains. Thus, many people spoke of the particular healing powers and 'force' of waters from the Tunka Valley as being 'almost as important as Baikal.'

Shumak

Slightly more than a 2,700 meter pass from Nilova Pustyn is the mineral spring of Shumak. The spring area is a 175 meter-long fissure, with over 100 different mineral water flows, 51 of which are hot springs reaching temperatures over 40°C. Local people claim that these waters are 'uniquely purifying' because of their special elements and living organisms in the water. According to Buriat legend, Shumak was discovered when a local hunter followed a wounded bear to the site. After bathing and drinking from the springs the bear was cured and the hunter was convinced of the powers of the *arshaan*.

As in other forested zones of the world, legends and ancient narratives describe how the forest holds both magical and dangerous powers. Several people explained how during the 'dark times' of Soviet oppression, many of the *lama*-ist and shamanic rituals were 'kept alive' by elders at *arshaan* in the forest using secret, carefully crafted ways.[14] These oral traditions and rituals are now often transformed, not only into educational tools for young Buriats interested in restoring their heritage, but also as a cultural attraction for tourists and those interested in the spiritual legacies of indigenous peoples. Recreational and leisure activities are being added to the therapeutic regimes at some previously restricted *kurort* locations to attract more visitors and stimulate economic activities.

Mountain and Forest Steppe Zones

Where the taiga meets the steppe, there is a transition zone of forested mountains, broad river basins, and hilly pastures. Covering much of Mongolia (25%) and the lower elevations east and south of Lake Baikal in Buriatiia, these areas contain the major urban centers of both Buriatiia and Mongolia as well as important historic sites. These mixed zones have a high degree of biodiversity (Finch 1999) but are increasingly vulnerable to political changes in land control and large-scale resource developments. In addition to the mix of plants and animals found in the taiga, these zones have large populations of typical steppe creatures such as *tarbagan*, Siberian marmot (*Marmota sibirica*), and hawks, kites and bustards. A common 'cool' medicinal herb found throughout this biome is the endemic Mongolian Adonis (*Adonis mongolica*) that is a very effective treatment for cardiovascular problems and fevers.

Springs in this type of natural zone vary widely, but many have been developed into sanitoria [*kurort*] using combined Western and traditional techniques. The *kurort* in the Selenga River basin of Buriatiia and Northern Mongolia are often places of pilgrimage for Buriats.

Purportedly where one of Chinggis Khaan's sons, Ogedei Khaan, drank to cure a stomach illness, Avraga *rashaan* (N 47° 5' 41.2", E 109°10' 6.7", Elevation: - 1187m) is a bicarbonate and carbonic gas spring claimed to be useful for curing more than thirteen diseases of the internal organs. The flow is covered by a pump house and access is controlled by the people in a nearby *ger*, to the consternation of some local visitors. Further north and east in the Buriat area of Dadal *soum* in Mongolia is another complex of spring waters with historic connections to Chinggis Khaan. The Khaju Bulag or Chinggis Khaan spring is one of the clearest and coldest (2.9° C) in the region. The nearby three medicinal lakes of Gurvan Nuur are also part of a shrine to Chinggis Khaan. The site was developed as a sanatorium in 1949 with 60 beds. In 1961, it expanded to a year-round facility with 150 beds and received 1,300 patients annually at its zenith in 1963. Now the spa averages 138 patients and the facilities are also open to tourists. The main treatment is *shar*, a clay mud

---

[14] As James C. Scott (1990) describes in his work on social resistance, Buriat social and ethnic traditions were likely carefully camouflaged or 'hidden' in other social actions that either complied with or ignored Soviet restrictions.

used for treating arthritis, heart disease, and nervous disorders. The clear air of the region is also recommended for combined exercise and diet regimes.

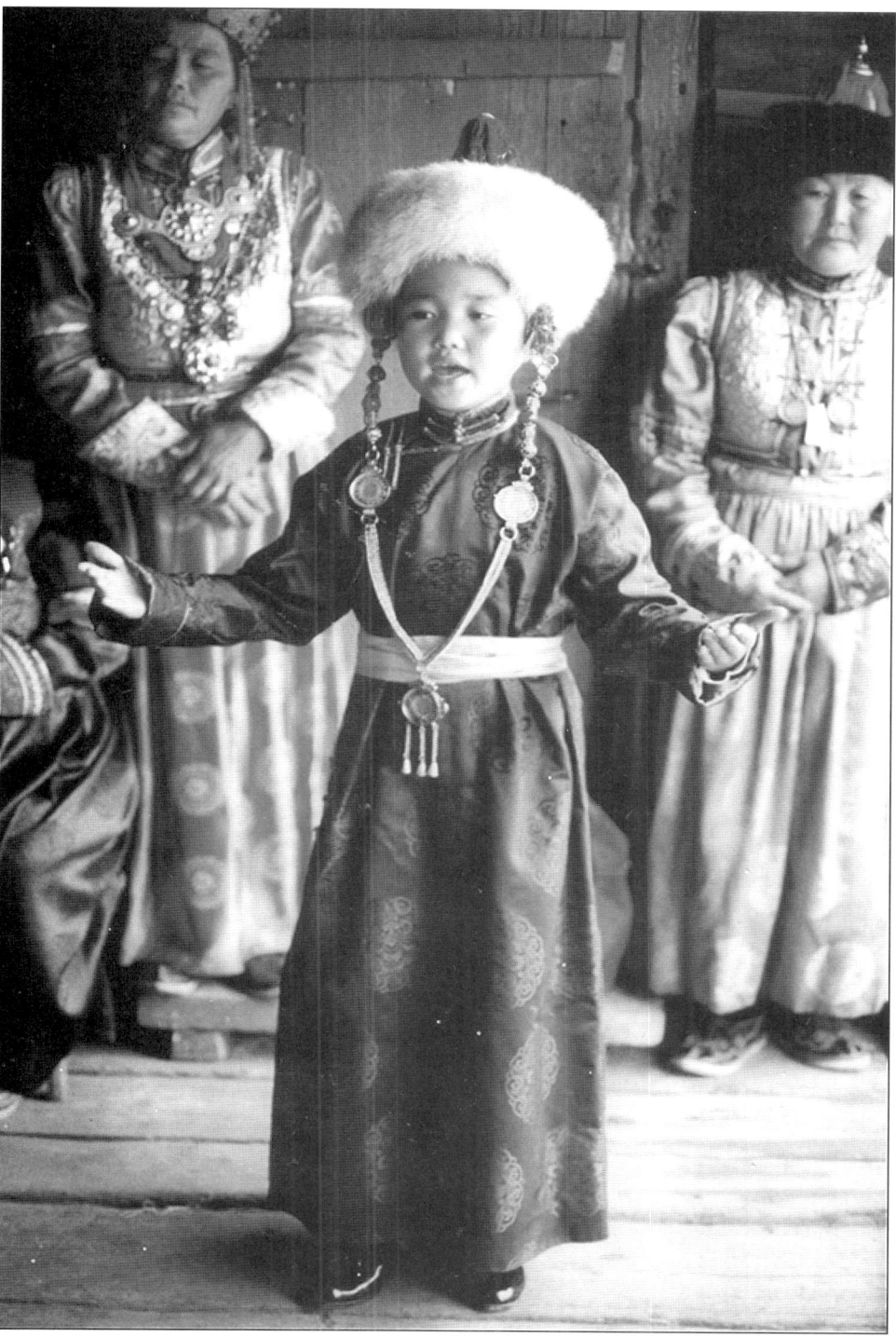

Figure 4.13. *A young Buriat singer at an* arshan *near the Chikoi River.*

The Healing Landscapes of Central and Southeastern Siberia

The Khasurtai *arshaan*, located in the Khorinsk district of Buriatiia off the Kurba River northeast of Ulan Ude, was one of the first *arshaan* documented for its medicinal powers. In 1865, Vanchik Sagin, a local *bag emch*, wrote up his conclusions about the powers of Khasurtai, after several years of 'making various sick people drink it, bathe in it, and make ablutions with it' (Poppe 1957). As part of a chain of small mineral lakes and springs known for being *gudzhir* or briny, Khasurtai waters are used in conjunction with a 'hot' diet to cure a variety of disturbances of vital functions [*khii*].

Springs in Steppe Biomes

The steppes of Buriatiia and Mongolia hold ample evidence of Eurasian paradoxes. Central to nomadic identities and historical events, they are often as isolated and misrepresented as nomadic herders themselves. Seen as vast, empty and unchanging, steppe grasslands are actually ecologically diverse and dynamic systems that have been transformed over centuries by human and animal interactions as well as by changing geological and climatic conditions. Freshwater springs in steppe zones were almost all free-flowing and open, but usually small and difficult to locate. Most of the *arshaanuud* in this region have an extremely sour taste and are recommended in small doses for stomach troubles and to improve digestion. During my fieldwork, the local herders claimed that many springs are flowing lower than usual because 'they have lost their *arshaanuu*' and they whistled to create bubbles and a higher flow (to release the water spirits). They also considered it an insult to the *lus* to let any containers of this special water touch the ground.

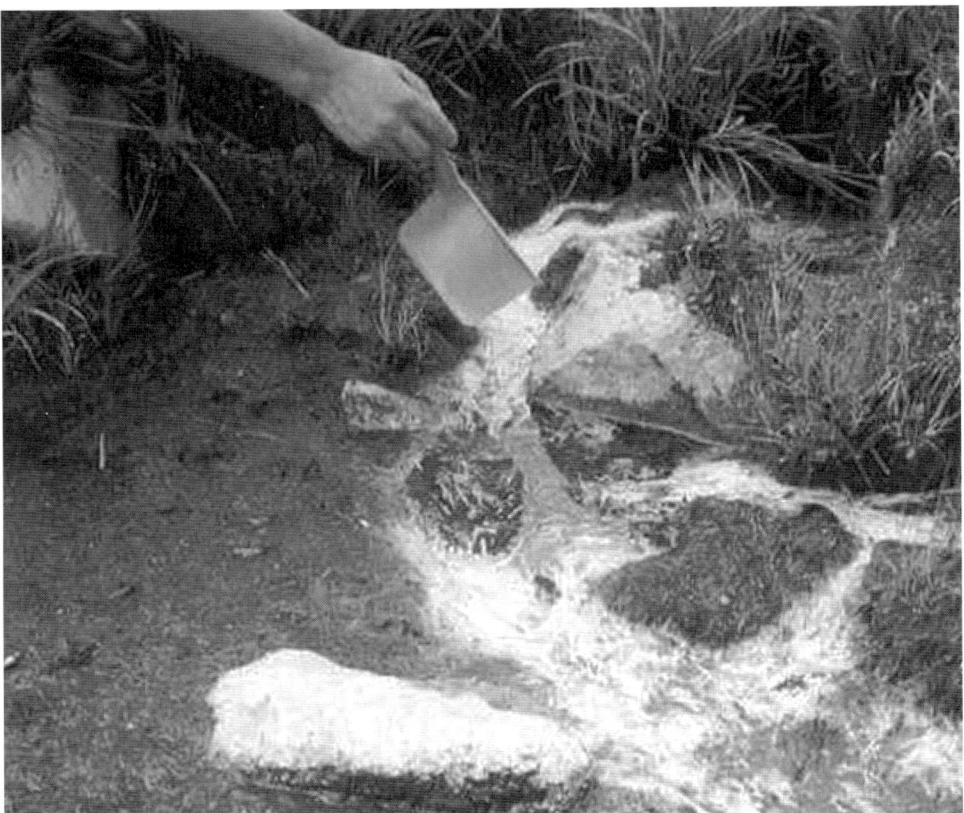

Figure 4.14. *Steppe spring, Dund Baidlag Dood.*

One of the oldest known medicinal springs in Mongolia, Utaat Minj, is a hot spring located near the eastern regional town of Choibalsan, and it is used for treating many ailments including rheumatism, skin irritations, kidney, spinal column and other pains. Some people even claimed that Utaat Minj waters can 'cure' HIV/AIDs. The regime includes sitting in the steam and inhaling three times daily.

In the Selenga River Valley in Buriatiia and Northern Mongolia and the Uldz River valley in Eastern Mongolia, there are many small lakes and marsh muds with curative properties. Buriat herders use these local *arshaanuud* and small medicinal lakes for watering their animals and treating general health problems. Local steppe herders are especially adept at recognizing the quality of pastures by their color and texture.[15] In their own diets, herders use *cheremsha*, wild steppe leeks (*Allium odorum*), for a protein source and knotweed (*Polygonum avicalare*) for its high levels of Vitamin C (150-450 mg%) (Ligaa and Tsembel 2003:128). Characteristic vegetation also includes various grasses and sagebrush (*Artemisia frigida*) as well as steppe lupine (*Termopsis dahurica*) and 750 other flowering plants, many used directly or indirectly for improving the health of either livestock or humans. Medicinal plants include: seabuckthorn (*Hippophae rhamnoides*) which is prescribed for coughs; Sweet sedge (*Acorus calamus*), a bitter nerve stimulant; the fennel-like rue (*Peganum nigellastrum*) used as a purgative; and Ural licorice (*Glycyrrhiza uralensis*). Found in boggy areas around steppe springs this licorice is a treatment for asthma or gastric ulcers when mixed with *arshaan* waters.

Some of the more gaseous, shallow steppe ponds are becoming eutrophic, perhaps due to mining in the region or climate change, but remain important sites for wildlife habitat and for watering livestock.

Healing Waters in Context

The healing practices observed at the *arshaanuud* presented in this chapter are only part of complex and on-going regional discourses about health care, resource conservation and heritage protection for Buriats within the Lake Baikal region. Many Buriats continue to consult *emchi* and shamans informally and rely on the religious ritual and Tibetan medicine practiced under the auspices of the Buddhist *lamas* at *datsanuud*. Others use government or private health services that often incorporate aspects of formal *ayurvedic* or Chinese medicine into standardized diagnostic and treatment regimes.

Many Buriats also use familiar folk remedies that have been passed on through word-of-mouth from their grandparents or other knowledgeable persons who had secretly continued traditional medical practices during the years of repression. Some people now claim that they were initiated into the shamanic arts during these dark days, but others dispute the healers' purported powers. Still others believe that the revival of traditional medicine is crucial as an alternative or supplement to the deteriorating national health care sector and limited access to affordable medicines.

While it is difficult to document all the permutations and circumstances of Buriat uses of *arshaan*, indigenous plant and animal medicines, and manufactured pharmaceuticals (*see* Metzo, this volume), the following therapeutic comparisons can be made (Table 4.1):

---

[15] These observations corroborate studies on Mongolian herder knowledge reported by Maria Fernandez-Gimenez (2000). Further studies conducted through the University of California at Davis document the botanical veterinary medicines used by pastoral nomads to improve the health of their herds.

Table 4.1. Comparative therapeutic uses of plants, medicines, and waters (%)

Diseases	Western Medicines*	Indigenous Medicines*	Healing Waters
Inflammation	7	12	14
Dermatitis	1	15	18
Gastro-intestinal	2	17	25
Ob/Gyn	14	7	4
Cancer	4	1	3
Cardio-vascular	10	2	8
Nerves	29	10	14
Renal-Blood	17	11	7
Anti-microbial	12	9	3
Others	4	16	4

* (Balick and Cox 1996, 56)

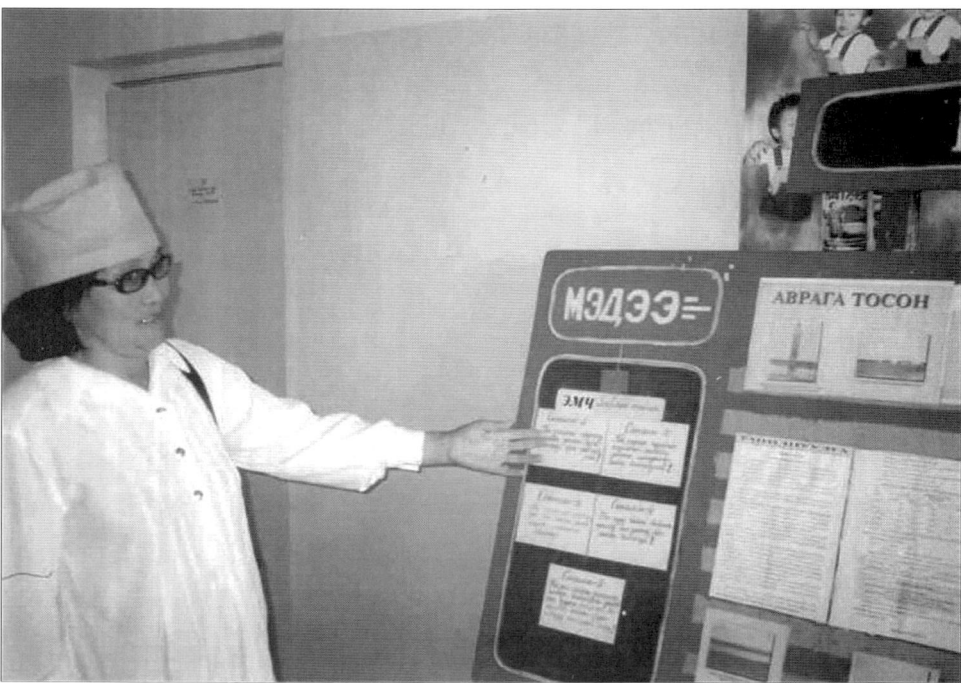

Figure 4.15. *Photo of* Emch *at Avraga Toson Spa, Northern Mongolia.*

In addition to integrating traditional Buriat medicine and the use of *arshaan* with formal healthcare systems, many Buriats are drawing connections between their traditional healing practices and larger concerns about biodiversity protection, historic and cultural preservation and legal protections for cultural and intellectual property. The increased popularity of mineral springs and health resorts in the Lake Baikal region for tourism and recreation has instigated some controversies in both rural and urban areas of Buriatiia.

Chapter Four: *Healing Springs in the Lake Baikal Region*

According to some informants, the overuse or misuse of *arshaan* waters has degraded not only the local ecology, but also 'angered the *lus*—water spirits.' They believe that bottling and otherwise disrupting the *arshaan* waters for economic or personal gain, without 'proper' acknowledgement or compensation to local Buriats and the '*lus*—water masters' will have negative consequences for the 'power' of the *arshaan*.

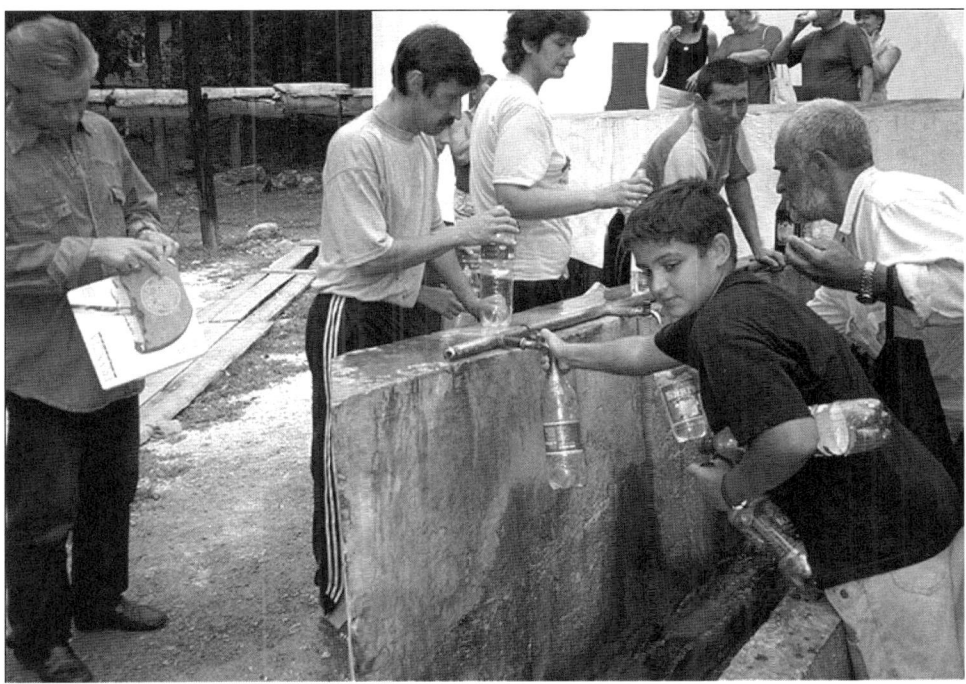

Figure 4.16. *Bottling thermal waters at Arshaan Saiani, Tunka Valley, Buriatiia.*

Others are also worried that the shamanic and Buddhist rituals practiced at *arshaan* locales are being taken out of context and appropriated by tourists, 'new' shamans and other outsiders. As in many other parts of the world, the indigenous knowledge and cultural heritage that is linked to the particular places and natural features of the Lake Baikal region is inextricably linked to changing Buriat individual and social identities. Many Buriats are eager to 'hold onto' and pass along their distinctive traditions to the next generation. Because of Soviet disruptions and currents forces of 'globalization' some people may not be as concerned with misinterpretation of Buriat traditional medicine or practices since they themselves are unclear or confused about the 'proper' methods. They are willing to blend ancient rituals with modern practices and attitudes about medicine and nature in order to meet their personal health and social needs.

The inter-related environmental, ritual, social and medicinal practices I observed at each freshwater site that I visited in the Lake Baikal region demonstrate that many Buriats use a range of integrated healing idioms—physical, spiritual, individual and collective—as well as localized environmental knowledge to maintain their well-being and social identities. Encouraging increased Buriat stewardship, local control and therapeutic uses of *arshaanuud* will be an important strategy for continued natural and cultural heritage protection in the Lake Baikal region.

The Healing Landscapes of Central and Southeastern Siberia

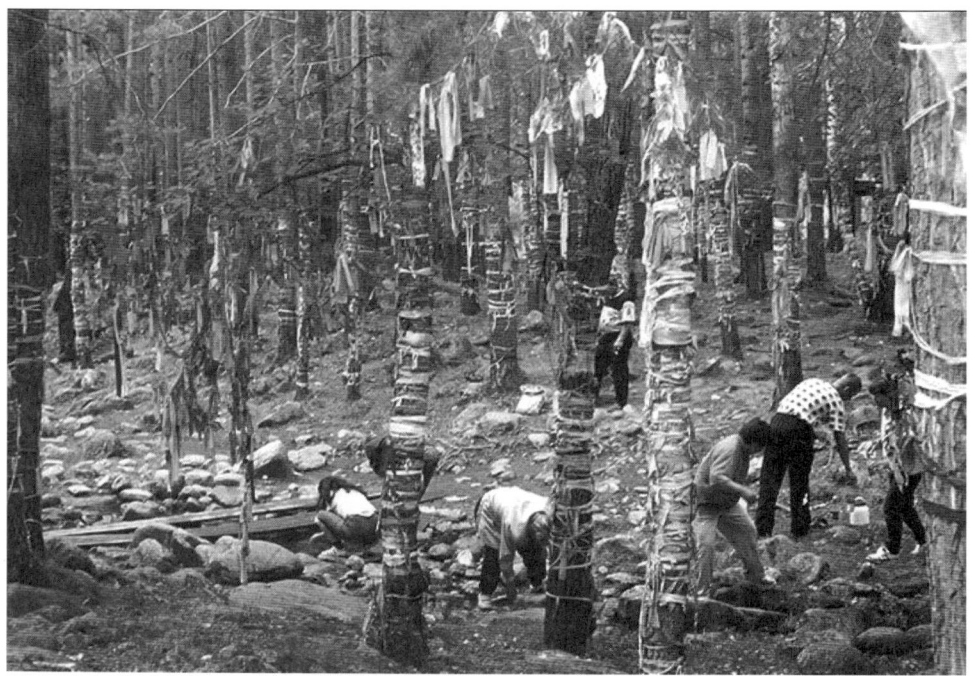

Figure 4.17. *Arshaan Saiani.*

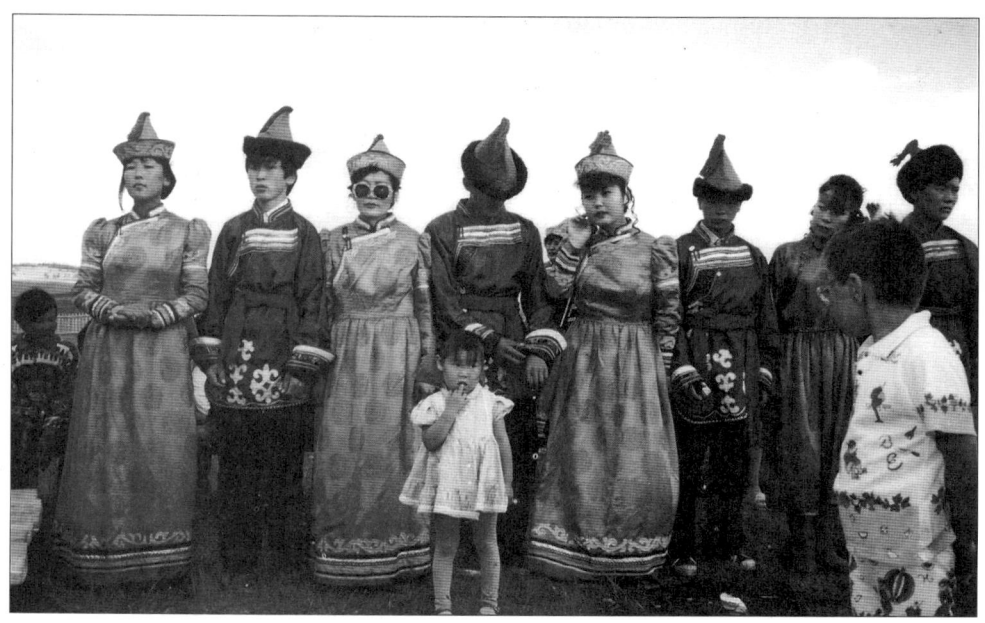

Figure 4.18. *Buriat youths at Suur-kharbaan festival near Khorinsk, Buriatiia.*

Chapter Four: *Healing Sprirgs in the Lake Baikal Region*

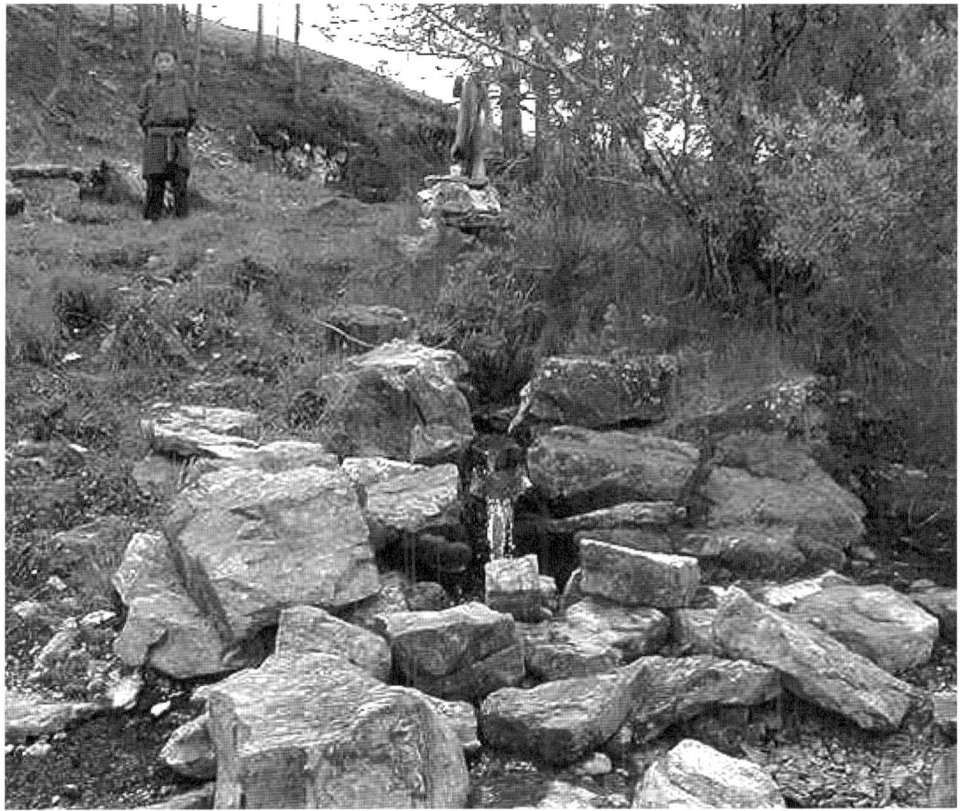

Figure 4.19. *A young Buriat 'guardian' of* arshsan.

Chapter Five

The Paradox of Alcohol in Western Buriat Communities: Vodka and Ritualized Commensality in Ekhirit-Bulagat Raion

Joseph J. Long

Introduction

The decision to include the following ethnography in this collection on health and healing was informed by presenting the material in two particular contexts. First, in the anthropology graduate writing seminar at the University of Aberdeen, a number of important issues centered on alcohol consumption were discussed among students working with indigenous peoples in the circumpolar North. While my own descriptions of rites of commensality were occasionally critiqued for not sufficiently stressing problems that could arise with the obligation to drink, students working with indigenous North Americans felt that to portray commensality surrounding alcohol in any kind of positive light would be highly problematic given the high mortality rates and instances of violence associated with drink in their field-sites. This led to a discussion on the need to present a more nuanced and rounded picture of alcohol consumption in indigenous communities that would account for the fact that consumption practices often lead to violence and illness but also underpin local forms of sociality and commensality, particularly where alcohol consumption is associated with ritual offerings for ancestral spirits.

We had, it turned out, stumbled onto an old debate. In the 1980s, Room (1984) charged anthropologists with 'problem deflation' in overlooking the problems associated with alcohol, while Heath (1987) suggested that research focusing on alcohol as a problem tends to overstate its impact. Since that time anthropologists describing alcohol consumption among indigenous peoples have tried to take greater account of the cultural context of consumption while addressing associated problems (e.g., McKnight 2002; Saggers and Gray 1998). All of us in the Aberdeen seminar felt that sensitive accounts of people's motivation for drinking would provide a sounder basis from which to address the problems associated with alcohol than the blanket condemnation that is occasionally directed at northern indigenous communities. Moreover, nuanced accounts can help counter the stereotypes of drunken indigenes that still persist around the globe. I felt uneasy when, upon hearing that I was working in Buriat communities, Russians in the city of Irkutsk often made derogatory comments about Buriats as heavy drinkers without understanding the centrality of commensality to kinship relations and shamanist practice in the countryside. Despite this, I do not wish to draw a veil over the drunken fights, visible ill-health, and addiction I found there.

With this in mind, a version of this paper was presented at a panel entitled *Alcohol and sociality: Cross-cultural perspectives on drinking and personhood* at the 2008 meeting of the American Anthropological Association. There, a number of presenters working in Latin America and Inner Asia described strikingly similar tensions between ritualized commensality involving alcohol and more harmful or deviant instances of consumption. The panel's convener, Mette High, has pertinently written of 'moral drinking' in Mongolia, to describe the formalized obligations of hospitality surrounding social drinking practices, differentiated from more transgressive practices in which drinking is individualized and the formal rules not followed (High 2008). This local moral reasoning in relation to alcohol resonates with the material that follows. In these cases, it seems paradoxical that drinking practices are morally valued given the fact that excessive consumption often heralds ill-health, violence and social tensions, yet a nuanced understanding of ritualized commensality helps explain why this is so. There are, however, discernible tensions that stem from the obligation to drink and these, too, are described here.

First, a caveat: I cannot claim any expertise on health issues or problems with alcohol in Siberia. I have not, at this point, researched alcohol-related illness or violence in a systematic way. Rather, I hope that in presenting an ethnographic description of ritualized commensality and drinking, I can give a nuanced picture of consumption so that these practices may be better understood. I also account for some nascent local responses to alcohol-related problems.

Tailgan Rites, Kinship and Commensality

In western Buriat communities of southern Siberia, clear analogies of form can be observed between ritualized hospitality practices in everyday life and larger ritual events, namely the clan *tailgan* rites that take place in the summer months each year. Western Buriats each belong to a number of clan groupings, from the lineage group, related within eight generations to a common ancestor, and the 'kin-village' [*ulus*], to broader territorial groupings. Belonging to each is defined through patriliny, but constituted through attendance at ritual events. Central to these rites is the offering, sharing and consumption of vodka, along with milk products and meat at large ritual events. In 2006 and 2007, I spent several months living in the villages of Khuty and Novonikolaevsk in the north of Ekhirit-Bulagat *raion*, located in what was then the Ust'-Orda Buriat Autonomous *okrug*, now unified with Irkutsk *oblast'*. There, I was able to attend several *tailgan* rites and observe ritualized hospitality on many occasions.

Tailgan rites involve the slaughter of sheep, goats and occasionally horses. The meat from these animals is cooked and shared among the members of the clan with portions offered to ancestral spirits. I characterize these rites as a form of communion that includes both corporeal kinsmen and ancestral spirits (Long 2010). While the rites cement kinship relations and obligations of reciprocity between corporeal kinsmen, the spirits are also engaged in reciprocal relations and are fed in return for the protection and well-being of clan members.

Tailgan rites are held at a clan's ancestral homeland, often referred to as the 'clan hearth.' They begin with heads of household [*khoziainy*] making libations of vodka and milk products for the spirits. These libations are known as 'sprinkling'—*bryzgat'* in Russian or *tur'iakha* in the local Ekhirit-Bulagat dialect. As vodka is offered, the names of the spirits are spoken by a clan elder or shaman. Each *khoziain* has a litre bottle of vodka and after continually refilling and drinking a little of each glass, each *khoziain* casts the rest forward into the air as an offering to the spirits named. Further libations are made to a ritual fire while circumambulating it clockwise—*po-solntsu*—the direction in which the sun is said to travel. Historical accounts of Buriat offering rites describe offerings of *tarisun*—a spirit distilled from milk with a lower alcohol content than vodka (Khangalov 2004; Tugutov 1978). Though *tarisun* is occasionally offered today, it has largely been

Chapter Five: *The Paradox of Alcohol in Western Buriat Communities: Vodka and Ritualized Commensality in Ekhirit-Bulagat Raion*

replaced by vodka. The switch to vodka may have reflected its status as a prestige good in the twentieth century, a status it no doubt enjoyed when vodka was in much shorter supply.

After the slaughter of the sheep, goat or horse, the meat is cooked and divided up. Some from each part of the animal is placed on a specially constructed pyre known as a *sheree*—the Buriat term for a table—as an offering to the spirits. The rest is divided into shares for each household and each *khoziain*'s share is known as his *khubi*. After further prayers are made to the spirits receiving the meat, and further vodka is sprinkled, the pyres are set alight and each *khoziain* offers a little meat from his *khubi* to the fire whilst once again circumambulating it clockwise. At the end of the rite, the leftover vodka is shared, each *khoziain* eats a little meat, and pieces of meat are exchanged between kinsmen. The rest of each person's *khubi* is then taken home to be shared among his household.

Tailgan rites not only establish a relationship of reciprocity between clan members and ancestral spirits—for whom meat is offered in return for protection and good fortune—but also re-affirm kinship and obligations of reciprocity between attendees. The obligations of mutual aid constituted through *tailgan* rites have been important in the past, and remain so today. Hamayon (1994) has suggested that the institution of the *tailgan*, and the principle of spirits belonging to a particular genealogical lineage appeared in the pastoral milieu, wherein herds as inheritable property became the norm. In such a milieu, it is easy to see how reciprocal labour was necessary for the collective management of herds and that a clear definition of clan membership was vital. In the Soviet period, Humphrey's (1998) fieldwork, carried out on two collective farms, revealed that kin networks remained important to fulfilling roles such as child-care, and partaking in the cycles of reciprocity surrounding weddings. In revisiting these farms in the 1990s, Humphrey (1998) also records the way rural Buriats helped alleviate food shortages for urban relatives in the immediate post-Soviet years.

In the contemporary context of Ekhirit-Bulagat *raion*, it is possible to see how important kin groups have become once again for the rural economy. The collapse of state-supported collective farming has accelerated the large-scale out-migration from the villages that began in the late Soviet era as local Buriats leave to find work in the cities. Families are becoming distributed over a wider geographic area and many villages are now depopulated. Kin networks have become important in such a context. Buriats who have remained in the villages often rely on each other's help for the small-scale farming that exists today. Help is needed in performing tasks that a century ago may have been carried out within herding groups, and in the Soviet era would have been organized by the collective farm. People I knew relied on the help of kinsmen from the cities who returned in summer to help cut and stack hay and firewood for winter. Local kinsmen supported each other in pooling the use of the few remaining working tractors in the village, obtaining petrol, and helping transport hay home. Children, nieces and nephews were also called upon to assist with the potato harvest in autumn, and most of the large-scale tasks relating to the annual farming cycle were undertaken with the support of kin.

Where the state once organized the slaughter, transport and distribution of meat produced by the *sovkhoz*, personal kin networks are involved in the distribution of produce from small-scale farming in the district today. On one occasion, I returned from Khuty to the city of Irkutsk with meat for the market with two neighbours. My neighbours' elder brother came by car from Ust'-Orda settlement to help slaughter a heifer for market and to take the meat back with him. The next day, the son of his wife's sister, also of the Khuty *ulus*, drove the meat into Irkutsk's Novolenina market for sale. When I accompanied Erzhena (with whom I lived in Novonikolaevsk), on her Friday trips to market in Irkutsk, relatives often turned up for milk, sour-cream and curds, much of it for poorer elderly relatives. In the autumn of 2007, I was in Novonikolaevsk to help with the potato harvest and several sacks were sent to relatives in Ulan-Ude as a bad harvest in Buriatiia had pushed up prices that year.

With accelerated migration to the cities and a lack of employment in the countryside, kinsmen from the city are also being drawn upon for financial help. When the daughter of friends received the opportunity to attend a university course in the USA, various members of their *ulus*, the Khertoi, contributed money so that she could go. Following this, a Khertoi university lecturer from Ulan-Ude decided to found a homeland association (*zemliachestvo*) for Khertoi Buriats with a fund for the purposes of supporting younger members of the clan. In 2009, I heard from Khuty friends that a Khuty *zemliachestvo* has been founded for similar purposes. It would seem, then, that the obligations of reciprocity within the clan, constituted through ritual practice, change and adapt to meet contemporary demands.

Ritualized Reciprocity and Everyday Hospitality

Ritualized reciprocity and communion is replicated across scale in local practice. As well as larger *tailgan* rites, each head of household undertakes the annual rite of 'feeding the mongol' in which offerings of vodka and milk products are made to household mongol spirits on behalf of household members. When undertaking journeys by road, offerings of tobacco or vodka are made at designated places along the road, each known as a *bar'sa*, in return for safe travel. A drop of tea is always dabbed on the table for the spirits when drinking in everyday life, and each morning many people sprinkle their first drops of tea on the household's main hearth—usually a brick stove in the kitchen.

At *tailgan* rites, meat and vodka are not only offered but consumed. Offering rites have been described to me several times as 'hosting the ancestors.' and are a ritualized form of commensality. Commensality is also a salient feature of everyday sociality in which western Buriats follow a strict and highly regimented set of rules for the sharing of vodka that echoes many of the patterns described in the *tailgan*. This constitutes an important medium of cementing and symbolically expressing good relations between kinsmen, neighbours, and friends.

When visiting people in the area, a bottle of vodka is almost always given as a gift by the guest, and is usually presented to the *khoziain*. Drinking always takes place at the table. The host will take charge of pouring and the first glass is always sprinkled onto the hearth for the spirits of the household. A single glass is then refilled and passed to each person at the table in turn by the *khoziain*. The sequence always runs clockwise, again, the direction in which the sun travels. In this context, each person's glass is known as their *khubi*. As each person receives their *khubi* they must sprinkle a little vodka on the table for the spirits. They can then show respect to someone present by offering them their *khubi* after first putting it to their own lips. Respect should be shown by the recipient by consuming some, or preferably all of the vodka in their glass. Before resuming the cycle around the table, the *khoziain* will refill the glass and the person who received the *khubi* will put it to their lips before returning it to the giver, who should also drink the glass to the end, ensuring a symmetrical exchange. Vodka bottles are almost always drunk to the end and if one has been presented as a gift, a *khoziain* should produce a second in return. This will be drunk to the end in the same manner. The last glass is presented to the guest who brought the bottle, and it is then passed clockwise around the table. At this point, anyone present in the household, including children, is called to the table to sip a little, or, in the case of children, dab a little on their foreheads.

Chapter Five: *The Paradox of Alcohol in Western Buriat Communities: Vodka and Ritualized Commensality in Ekhirit-Bulagat Raion*

This ritualized reciprocity is an important means of ensuring good relations with neighbours and kinsmen and the strict code of conduct formalizes and reflects the relations of reciprocity that are important to everyday life in the countryside where help is often required for day-to-day tasks. While kinsmen might be called upon for help with major tasks in the farming cycle, neighbours are often called upon for help with management of the domestic herd or homestead. As well as quick favours such as lifting heavy weights, pushing a car out of the mud or borrowing tools, neighbours are called on for herding cattle home in the evenings when people were away, help with milking, or help finding lost animals. A strictly ordered set of rules for drinking practices not only reinforces the principle of reciprocity in relations between neighbours and kinsmen but, through the inclusion of ancestral spirits, sacralizes them.

There are formal analogies between everyday rituals of hospitality and the offering rites I have observed in Ekhirit-Bulagat *raion*. The clockwise (*po-solntsu*) direction of passing the glass and circumambulating the fire is a notable motif. The importance of the fire or hearth as a place of offering is another. The term for a share of meat or drink as *khubi* is also analogous. The analogy is made explicit in idioms used to describe the rites. One Khuty friend explained offering rites as 'hosting' the ancestors, even as 'laying a table' for them. Reference to the offering pyre as a *sheree*—a term that also means table—underlines the analogy. The occasional description of the ancestral homeland as a 'clan hearth' creates further resonance between everyday hospitality and larger rites.

In his study of Iukaghir hunters in north-eastern Siberia, Rane Willerslev (2007) recounts a distinction, well-established in anthropological literature, between reciprocity, which has an emphasis on exchange, and sharing, in which meat from a hunt is immediately divided. I suggest that in western Buriat practice, both sharing and reciprocity are ritualized and sacralized as moral obligation. The division of meat from an animal or vodka from a bottle into *khubi* is clearly an example of sharing. Humphrey (1998) suggests that, in symbolic terms, this emphasizes the fact that portions, like people, are part of a whole. In the case of the *tailgan*, that whole is the institution of the clan. That a *khubi* is then drawn into ritualized exchange, whether in the form of the glass at the table, or in the exchanges of meat once it has been divided at the *tailgan*, seems to emphasize the moral obligations of reciprocity among kinsmen and neighbours.

In emphasizing commensality as a defining feature of sociality, I wish to stress that it is not only the symbolic acts of reciprocity such as the symmetrical exchange of glasses that constitute social ties, but the collective experience of offering and drinking together. I characterize the *tailgan* as a communion because I propose that kinship is constituted as much through the experience of what Robertson Smith (1889) has termed the 'social fellowship' of communion as through the symbolism of ritual action. Invoking Turner's (1969) famous term, I have suggested that the rites are an act of communitas constituted by making offerings together, by working together on the slaughter and butchery of the meat, and also by consuming meat and vodka together (Long 2010). Moreover, if social relations are cemented through communitas and commensality, the process of becoming intoxicated together constitutes a particular kind of collective experience in which inhibitions are reduced, people talk freely with one-another, and a social bond is created (*cf.* Koester 2003). To see that this is also a kind of communitas is to recognize one of the key reasons that people engage in regular drinking together. In the Buriat context, this communitas is sacralized by the inclusion of spirits through the constant offering of libations.

Paradox and Tensions in Local Drinking Practices

While drinking itself is certainly not emphasized as 'healthy' in the villages where I lived, there is an implicit understanding of well-being attached to having relatives and a strong social network, a principle that is underpinned by reciprocal hospitality and drinking. Herein lies the paradox, then. For while commensality, communion and hospitality are ingrained as desirable in the western Buriat ethos, the occasions, and indeed necessity for engaging in reciprocal exchanges have increased in recent years and, anecdotally at least, the increased availability and consumption of vodka have led to increased drunkenness and associated problems.

Several people to whom I spoke felt that the current levels of consumption in the villages began in the late 1990s. Until 1996, the local collective farm [*sovkhoz*] had organized labour locally and employed everyone in roles ranging from herding, engineering and driving to accounting, cultural work, and education. The collapse of collective farming under Eltsin left most people unemployed. At that time, the Novonikolaevsk *sovkhoz* sold off or slaughtered most of its cattle to traders and local people were left unemployed and at loose ends. The contemporaneous rise in the availability of affordable alcohol met the increased demand. While some people seem to have turned to alcohol from boredom and depression at their lot, greater reliance on neighbours and friends among those now relying on small-scale domestic herds sees the increasing strategic deployment of ritualized commensality. Although it is morally valued, in this context the obligation to consume can be problematic and unwelcome.

The dual obligation of consumption and reciprocity is often manipulated when favours need to be pulled. To give one example, when traveling to the neighbouring village to buy supplies or visit the local administration Vitalii, a man with whom I lived in Khuty, a very isolated spot, always carried a small vodka glass in his jeep. He often purchased a bottle of vodka on arrival and would share it with friends and acquaintances in the ritualized manner described above if he met them on the street, or else called in on them. This was a good way of sealing friendships after which he could more comfortably ask people if he could buy petrol from them, or find spare parts for his vehicle. With petrol being in very short supply in the district, Vitalii often relied on getting petrol in neighbouring villages in order to make it back home. He always had a length of hose ready to siphon off a couple of litres if the opportunity arose. He relied on the bonds of reciprocity consolidated through hospitality customs in this way in order to maintain his mobility. On the other hand, what were intended as short trips often turned into whole-day affairs as unemployed kinsmen and neighbours appeared and wanted to drink, obliging Vitalii to produce bottle upon bottle of vodka.

To refuse to partake in drinking would, however, be highly problematic, and on several occasions people bemoaned to me the fact they were obliged to drink even when they didn't want to. When walking through the village of Novonikolaevsk one day with Kolia, a friend who had given up drinking, we chanced upon someone who told us that another friend was celebrating his birthday. Kolia insisted we turn back immediately for fear of being called upon to drop-in and inevitably drink. I too, often found myself taking circuitous routes around certain houses for fear of being roped into such obligations.

In a study of alcohol consumption in Kamchatka in the Far East of Russia, David Koester (2003) describes the way that the rationale of a special occasion is often manipulated in order to create opportunities to drink—public holidays, graduations, even the birthday of a relative not present are cited as reasons to open a bottle. Moreover, Koester points out that a sense of occasion is often created just by the act of bringing out a bottle.

Chapter Five: *The Paradox of Alcohol in Western Buriat Communities: Vodka and Ritualized Commensality in Ekhirit-Bulagat Raion*

This was evident, too, in Buriat communities. Just seeing someone who hadn't been seen for some weeks, or the fact of visiting someone even for a fairly mundane reason were used as opportunities to open a bottle of vodka. If, in Kamchatka, drinking creates a sense of occasion, in western Buriat communities that occasion is sacralized by the ritualized form of drinking practice—the exchange of the *khubi* and libations for the spirits. Vitalii's unemployed acquaintances seemed to create situations for drinking in this way, often citing the fact that Vitalii had made a rare visit from Khuty as reason in itself to drink.

It is in these circumstances that the tension between desirable commensality and alcoholism is evident. Recalling the distinction between moral and deviant drinking, we could suggest a clear moral distinction locally between being drunk, and always being drunk. Whilst many people I knew got drunk without comment on social occasions, there seems to have been a qualitative and moral difference between drinking in company and drinking alone. I was often told that bachelors are not well respected in Buriat communities, where children and marriage are highly prized, and so bachelors or loners that often appear drunk are often regarded in quite a different way to those that enjoy strong kin networks and engage in social drinking. Yet the kind of experience described above suggests a fuzzy middle ground in which those who are already habitual consumers of alcohol manipulate local mediums of reciprocity to find a reason to drink.

Problems and Solutions

I have suggested some ways in which drinking might be seen positively or negatively in local terms, but have yet to touch on the more universal 'problems' of alcohol such as related illness and violence. These are problematic subjects to write about for several reasons. First, I have not investigated these problems in any substantive way, and second, available statistics are notoriously ambiguous. Anecdotally, there is little doubt that alcoholism is present and visible in the local population, and I knew several people locally who were clearly physically emaciated by drink, and whom I constantly witnessed drunk. What is also clear is that violent deaths occur among the local population, and that these often occur after heavy consumption. Several such deaths have occurred in Novonikolaevsk since I began fieldwork there in 2006. It is difficult to establish whether these problems are more or less marked among the local indigenous population than among the population as whole, however, as state statistics on causes of death are only available by region, not by ethnic group.

Research on alcohol as a whole suggests that related problems are certainly not restricted to indigenous populations. Nemstov's (2005) research on consumption in Russia finds that the increased availability of alcohol and lower life expectancy in the post-Soviet era are related and widespread, fluctuating together with one another. From the late 1990s, he demonstrates that consumption across Russia has indeed increased and life expectancy decreased, with higher consumption in rural areas. Nemtsov (2002:1415) also laments that figures on mortality published by the Russian statistical bureau only relate alcohol consumption to causes of death such as cirrhosis of the liver, and alcohol poisoning, while alcohol consumption has a direct impact on increased mortality related to accidents and violence, an influence made clear by Shkolnikov *et al.* (2001) and also by Brainerd and Cutler (2005). Shkolnikov *et al.* (2001) also note the exacerbation of cardiovascular problems in cases of episodic, heavy alcohol consumption.

In my experience, these problems were certainly evident in the communities in which I worked. We might think of two conceptions of 'problem drinking' here, then— local moral evaluation of moral and deviant drinking, and more widespread problems of health and violence exacerbated by the increased volume of drinking in the socioeconomic context of unemployment and increased interdependence. Whether or not consumption is higher among Buriats than other groups, what I have tried to focus on here is the way in which heavy alcoholic consumption is often carried out according to local cultural practices and justified by local idioms of reciprocity and hospitality.

What must also be noted, however, are some emerging local initiatives that propose Buriat cultural practices as appropriate responses to increased alcohol consumption and the broader socioeconomic situation. In Ekhirit-Bulagat raion in 2006, a number of local activists who had given up drinking organized a festival of the traditional Buriat sports of wrestling, horse-racing and archery in the *raion* centre. The event was organized with the support of the All-Buriat Association for the Development of Culture and the occasion was specifically publicized as promoting a return to a healthy traditional lifestyle. If local sociality is based around communitas, then it seems that the promotion of such events, rooted in traditional sociality and with an emphasis on physical health, are an encouraging sign. Likewise, local Buriat cultural associations and activists have made a point of publicly emphasizing the need for socioeconomic regeneration of the region rooted in traditional cattle herding. Irkutsk's Centre for the Preservation and Development of the Buriat Ethnos held a public forum on the theme in 2007, and one local activist from Khuty is attempting to launch a scheme bringing large numbers of cattle bred in Mongolia to the district.

Figures from across Russia suggest that the problem of alcoholism is, of course, much broader than the indigenous population, and socioeconomic regeneration will require a more broad-based effort than that of local activists, but if heavy consumption is often manifested through local idioms of commensality, it seems that local idioms of communitas and an emphasis on traditional herding practice may also be usefully mobilized to combat some of the reasons for reliance upon consumption.

Closing Remarks

The collapse of collectivized herding in Ekhirit-Bulagat *raion* has renewed the necessity for reciprocal relations with kinsmen and neighbours, but the means for securing them often creates a compulsion to drink the vodka that is now in plentiful supply, along with the time to drink it. Practices of commensality, common to clan rites and everyday hospitality, have consumption at their core. These practices are mobilized creatively by Buriats to cement networks of reciprocity and economic support. But these practices can also be fraught with tension and the obligation to indulge in intoxication on a more regular basis than ever before. There is a paradox, then, in a notion of well-being understood as enjoying strong social networks, but the medium of cementing those networks being the consumption of strong alcohol, with potentially serious implications for related health problems and social tensions.

Acknowledgements
My field research in Siberia was made possible by a studentship from the College of Arts and Social Sciences at the University of Aberdeen and a fieldwork grant from the ethnochronology module of the Baikal Archaeology Project (SSHRCC MCRI 412-2005-1004).

I was fortunate to spend 2005-2007 as a visiting researcher at Irtkutsk State Technical University where Artur Kharinskii and his colleagues provided a great deal of practical support and assistance.

Chapter Six

Idioms of Health and Healing in Central Siberia

David G. Anderson

The ways in which we describe 'health' or prescribe 'healing' are one of the more intimate arenas of cultural difference. By definition, each is only understandable if we have a clear picture of what makes a person whole and vibrant. Given this complexity, it is ironic that the 20th century has given us forms of state governance, both capitalist and socialist, which have gone to such lengths to standardize the meaning of both health and healing such that we often lack the words to describe the things we observe or feel. Sociologists have given us very strong explanations of why this should be (Illich 1977; Foucault 2004) but this does not help us recover our words or our powers of observation. This chapter is an attempt to recover idioms of health and healing from Russian, Evenki and Dolgan peoples in Central Siberia and to show how these tease apart some of the central assumptions of hospital-based medical practice.

This ethnographic chapter is doubly comparative. On the one hand, it examines how biomedical practitioners distinguish themselves from local healers in two contexts: Russia and Canada. For the purposes of this volume, it is interesting that the boundary between the two is different in both places, even if the health concerns of the local communities are similar. On the other hand, it also examines a series of structured meetings between Russian, Evenki, and Dolgan nurse-practitioners [*fel'dshery*] and a group of Cree and Tlicho (Dogrib) Dene community health workers under the auspices of a state-funded development assistance programme in 1999 and 2000. To borrow the terms of historians of science, these meetings generated 'friction' or 'messiness' due to the fact that they were structured by very powerful assumptions not always shared by all participants (Tsing 2005; Law 2004). The 'round-tables' and educational materials produced by the project were motivated by very strong doses of prescriptive and paternalistic 'assistance.' However, mediating this top-down structure was the fact that the project was founded on the silent assumption that people deemed indigenous would necessarily find something to discuss. The project did generate useful dialogue, and long-lasting friendships, but it also provided an opportunity to reflect on what words might be lacking in medical discourse (not to mention development discourse). This chapter sets these misunderstandings centre stage. Within the terms of this volume, this case demonstrates that medical pluralism is an unstable compromise built out of concrete discussions and concrete needs. Nevertheless, it does demonstrate that even biomedical systems in the North can be open to local input.

The chapter summarizes several overlapping themes. The first is a frustration and a worry about the misleading meanings contained in very simple words such as 'medicine' and 'shamanism'—words that one might think carry very distinct meanings but that turned out in these meetings to have elastic meanings. The second is a worry about the way in which political exigencies make it possible or impossible to speak about certain practices in certain places—the way in which institutions, by the weight of their presence or the evocativeness of their architecture, predetermine what can be said. The third is a concern about the proper idiom by which to understand health—captured here as a concern over the over-representation of cures that can be swallowed (i.e., plant medicine). These three themes—vocabulary, emplacement, and application—suggest the need for new attention and new dialogues on how health and healing is perceived both outside of medical institutions but also in interaction with them.

In order to understand the context of the ethnography, it is important to summarize briefly the structure of the development project and the players involved. The Canada–Evenki Health Programme was a three-year initiative of the University of Alberta funded by the Canadian International Development Agency (CIDA) from 1998-2001. The project was funded under a memorandum of agreement between Canada and the Russian Federation designed to help Russia's transition to a market-economy and to offset some of the worst side-effects of the collapse of centrally funded public institutions. This project was one of the first attempts by CIDA to send aid to post-Soviet Russia, and undoubtedly one of the first world-wide employing 'front-line' aboriginal medical personnel (rather than urban consultants) in order to alleviate health problems in several indigenous communities in what was then the Evenki Autonomous District.[1] It was also styled as an 'indigenous-to-indigenous' exchange, whereby the consultants were practicing nurse-practitioners in Evenkiia or community health workers in the Northwest Territories or Northern Alberta. The Russian recipient of this assistance was the Tura Medical College—an institution offering mainly indigenous Evenki and Iakut students a formal qualification of 'nurse practitioner–mid-wife' [*fel'dsher-akusher*][2] (Fig. 6.1). In rural communities, located closer to major cities, this qualification allowed these nurse practitioners to work in clinics under the supervision of a doctor. In the relatively remote nursing stations of this sub-Arctic district, these junior practitioners more often than not were forced to take a more independent role if radio communication was shut down or an emergency air evacuation flight cancelled. These conditions led many to develop a unique approach to healing, mixing their formal medical training with locally available solutions. Aside from the obligatory 'round-table' and management meetings the project had the concrete 'outputs' of producing three educational textbooks for use in the Tura Medical College on northern health practice in Canada and supporting the College with appropriate equipment ranging from a computer and Xerox machine to samples of various diagnostic sets for water quality to tuberculosis (Anderson 2001; Anderson and Popkov 2001; Popkov and Anderson 2002). An undocumented result of the meetings was the sense of respect generated in the minds of the visiting Canadian community health workers who wished that such a medical college for aboriginal peoples could be established in Canada (reverse development assistance, I was told by the CIDA project officer, was not welcome in Ottawa). Perhaps the most long-lasting 'impact' of the project was the international attention focused upon a small regional medical college,

---

[1] The Evenki Autonomous District was, at this time, an independent region within 89 equal regions of the Russian Federation. In 2007 the district was merged with Krasnoiarsk Territory to become a municipal county known as the Evenki Municipal District.

[2] The *feldsher-akusher* is a formal educational qualification at the college level [*srednyi*] offered all over Russia and aimed at providing specialized assistants to doctors in urban areas and more autonomous health care workers in rural areas. The qualification takes two years of training in a medical college following a centralized, standard programme. The programme allows only a few hours per week for local content (and the CIDA project was aimed at developing curriculum materials for that part of the curriculum). Nurse-practitioners learned basic skills in administering medication, applying first aid, and assisting in deliveries. In urban areas they work under the direct supervision of doctors. In rural areas, they are permitted to act independently to give 'pre-doctoral' [*dovrachebnaia*] help to stabilize a patient, and to work with community members in preventive medicine and to control infectious diseases.

perhaps helping it avoid being closed in the savage round of budget cutbacks which categorized that period of Russia's history. The Canadian community health workers came from Cree and Tlicho Dene backgrounds. I was the author of the project and the person who organized the face-to-face meetings and translated some of the discussions. The ethnography in this paper comes from the experience of translating these meetings, a set of formal interviews on traditional forms of medicine conducted by Craig Campbell and Anatolii Amel'kin, as well as from my own long-term fieldwork as an anthropologist in this region.

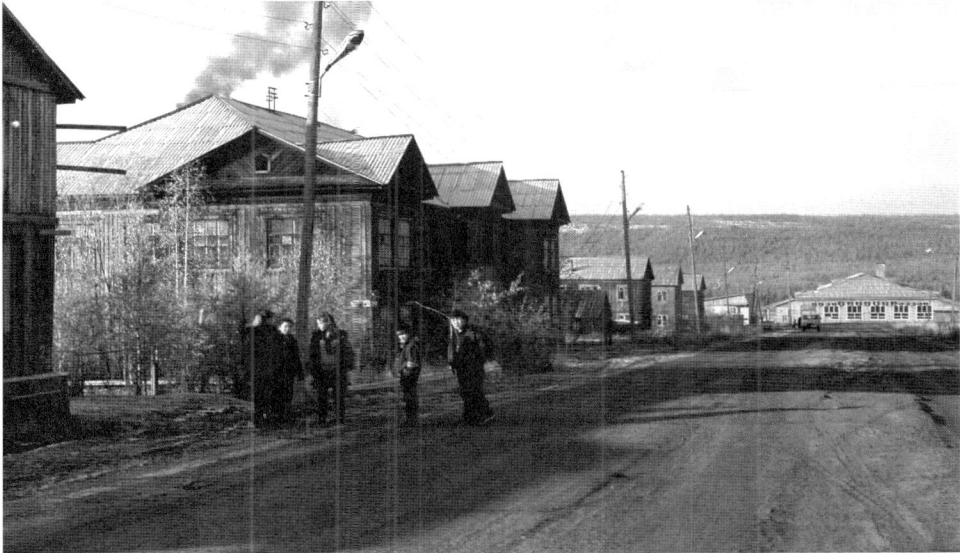

Figure 6.1. *The Tura Medical College, Evenki Autonomous District.*

Vocabularies of Health and Healing

In thinking back over the meetings held under the Canada–Evenki Health Programme, I realized that some of the most profound observations arose out of the simplest problems. From the outset of our discussions, one of the most difficult words to use and to translate was the concept of 'medicine' itself. In both Russian and standard English, medicine and 'medicinal' are often used to denote scientifically standard procedures for healing illness. More often than not, the words immediately imply the use of highly refined and carefully controlled pills. In the minds of many, they may bring forth the image of a sterile building with doctors and nurses dressed in white. Most importantly, they are words which imply that the source of wellness is outside the body of the patient. To be healed, the patient must approach a properly recognized medic in order to bring health into his or her body. In the English used by Cree and Dene people from northern Canada, 'medicine' often means something beyond the standard definition of the term. Medicine refers to a type of powerful knowledge that a person or people may use to make an unhealthy person better (Lux 2001:73; Waldram 2000:607-8). Although there are stark differences between how hospital personal work and the way local Dene or Cree healers might work, this local definition of 'medicine' also contains an important insight that knowledge might be used to strengthen the person rather than attacking the condition.

In Russian, this specific definition of 'medicine' can be most closely linked to practices of 'shamanism.' The Russian word shaman is thought to be derived from the Evenki word *saman* [*khaman*]—meaning 'someone who holds powerful knowledge.' The Evenki term is very similar to the term for knowledge itself *sa-mi* (*kha-mi*). Recognizing the similarities in the central role of knowledge, one sometimes finds in English popular literature that the word shamanism is also used to describe the traditional powerful knowledge of aboriginal people in Canada.

There is a lot written about whether or not it is appropriate to unite all of these knowledge practices under one word, and even more that can be written on whether this knowledge tradition can be can be codified as an '-ism.' Most authors identify a plurality of traditions that can only be unified by their difference from an image of a monolithic type of Western medicine (Humphrey and Onon 1996; Hutton 2001; Sundstrom 2007).

To emphasize the pragmatic quality of their knowledge, Cree and Dene healers have an interesting way of using the word 'medicine.' They tend to use the phrase of 'having medicine' (which we translated into Russian as 'wielding medicine' *vladenie lekarstvom*). This is a possessive idea of a local person temporarily grasping or holding knowledge that could be applied locally. In both standard English and in Russian the same idea cannot exist for medical science. Granted, one can study or learn medicine, but one can never have it or hold it. The most that a community could hope for would be to have a medic—who might in turn have these skills or ideas. Thus in Russian, as in standard English, to talk about a local community having a certain power to heal itself is, in some sense, a different discussion than to talk about medical science.

This cross-over of meanings between 'medicine' as a type of knowledge which comes from outside oneself and outside one's community, and the idea of 'medicine' as a type of intimate knowledge which empowers local people, underscored the main difference of opinion that underlay most of our discussions. The need to have this discussion was forced by a situation where a powerful, centralized state made a decision not to continue subsidizing an expensive but relatively well-developed system of hospitals and nursing stations, not to mention the costly aviation links tying them together. Given this background, the words people used highlighted the way that knowledge was held; whether or not it was held within a system of credentials and subsidies or held pragmatically by individual, community members. Those holding centralized knowledge often protested in the meetings that local, pragmatic solutions could not replace the benefits of participating in a national medical system with the division of labour and the access to specialists that this implied. However, those protests, in that striven period of post-Soviet history, could not replace the fact that communities also should hold local and more sustainable forms of healing knowledge. In the opinion of many, holding or having medicine is very closely related to issues of entitlement within a hierarchical social welfare state where access is often determined by how close one lives to a major city.

Emplaced Medicine and Rituals of Respect

When comparing circumpolar cultures, one of the most common themes is the important value placed on cultures of respect in Siberia, Canada, Scandinavia and Alaska. If in European cultures or American urban culture there is an overt value placed on success, authority, or prestige, in almost every northern culture there is a strong value placed on respect for both people as for living things in the taiga. What we might call this 'culture of respect' is clearly evident within the models of healing that formed the basis of our discussions—and the idea that healing should be done in special places.

In Evenki tradition, for instance, respect is symbolized by 'placements' or the offerings of animal fat or of vodka to the fire before an important meal or when guests first arrive in a home. This is a sign of respect to the invisible master who cares for a family. In a manuscript collection of stories assembled by the Evenki folklorist Lidia Udygyr, there is a nice illustration of this ritual in the words of G.N Udygir:

> When I remember my childhood, when my father returned from hunting to our tent, he first gave a gift to the fire—usually a piece of meat, fat or salted meat. He did this so that he would always have luck. The fire for Evenkis was holy. It gave heat. You could cook food on it after travelling or hunting. According to Evenkis the fire drove away evil spirits from the tent, and illness when someone was ill.

Similar stories were told by Tlicho Dene explaining how coins or shotgun shells were given to the land as a sign that this medicine is of value. These rules of balance and respect between living forms are remarkably common all across the circumpolar North.

Those who value efficiency might be tempted to doubt whether giving gifts of fat to the home-fire or a few coins to the land are bound to improve the quality of the cure. The importance of ritual of this type, however, is quite subtle. Let us take the example of leaving a few matches behind on the land in exchange for a branch of juniper [*khenkere*] (*Juniperus communis*).[3] Evenkis and Dolgans often dried this plant and then used it to produce a smoke which can be used to purify a dwelling, a harness reindeer, or a patient. One elderly woman, Agrafina Bezrukhikh, in Ust'-Avam, once compared *khenkere* to the type of incense used in churches in order to make a place 'holy.' The act of ritually smoking a room with this sweet-smelling smoke leaves a 'clean' smell not unlike the smell of disinfectant that pervades hospitals. The act of leaving gifts on the land shows the type of respect and deference that one shows when consulting a doctor for a prescription. In either case, neither the clean smell nor the fact that one has a properly signed prescription does much to improve the chemical power of the procedure. However, in both cases the fact that a proper respectful procedure was followed sets a context for healing which, in itself, is powerful.

One unexpected and otherwise undocumented event which occurred before the start of lectures of Cree healers at the Tura Medical Institute in 1999 and 2000 was a blessing, or as it was called in English, a moment when we 'paid our respects.' In Cree communities before any important discussion occurs in a political or a healing sense, all those gathered stand up, form a circle, and a prayer is read. The prayer asks the ancestors and the Creator for wisdom and guidance for the event in question whether it be a discussion on land rights or a discussion on how to heal communities of alcoholism. The leader who gives the prayer first 'cleans' himself or herself with the spoke of a dried and braided sprig of sweetgrass (*Hierochloe odorata*). The cleaning procedure is done in a very beautiful way. The person 'washes' their head, eyes, ears, mouth and heart with the smoke so that they can think, see, hear, speak and feel in clear and true way. Then each person in the room repeats the procedure. In the case of our seminars, this important moment, repeated at the beginning of each day, immediately signalled to the assembled staff and students at the Medical Institute that they were about to hear a very different approach to health in healing. The prayer and procedure itself took a significant amount of time—about 15 minutes. For the listeners, who initially sat at their desks properly and politely expecting a rather formal lecture, the

---

[3] Evenkis and Dolgans along the Enisei River often use juniper for smudging. They use the word *khenkere* to identify this plant. A word of the same derivation—*senkere*—is used by Evenkis and Orochens in Zabaikal'e to describe Labrador Tea (*see* Chapters 7 and 8). A more accurate translation of *kherkere* might be 'smudging plant' rather than a botanical term..

fact that they were asked to stand and participate in a ritual from a different place in the circumpolar North immediately unsettled the formal atmosphere at the College.

Although the lectures following the procedure had a fairly standard format in terms of content and length, the initial prayer stayed in the mind of the listeners and prompted questions about the similarities of traditions and outlooks on traditional medicine. When our group was invited to visit the outlying taiga community Ekonda, our Evenki hosts decided to reciprocate with what they saw as an equivalent tradition from their culture. At our welcoming dinner, which took place in the school, an elder took the dried fat of a wild reindeer, ignited it on coals, and passed it around the room in a clockwise circle in order to 'clean' the room and prepare the place for a harmonious meeting (Fig. 6.2). We were told that the old and young people present all 'knew' the ritual but that it had fallen into disuse. The occasion of the visit and the lectures of the Cree healers became an occasion for people in this village to make a strong ritual statement about their tradition and identity as Evenkis, and at the same time to signal their kinship to Crees who had, in their view, a similar ritual. This event was a small one, but often small gestures of contact and reciprocity run very deep. At the end of the visit, I asked our Evenki partners in Tura if it would be proper to begin lessons every day at the Tura Medical College with a ritual of cleansing with the smoke of wild deer fat just as Cree 'community health workers' conduct their sweetgrass ritual before their lessons at similar institutions in Canada. The question immediately brought a smile to the face of the director of the College since obviously it was thought to be somewhat naïve. I imagine that in their minds they were making a distinction between proper day-to-day medical training and the theatre of ritual which our visit had represented.

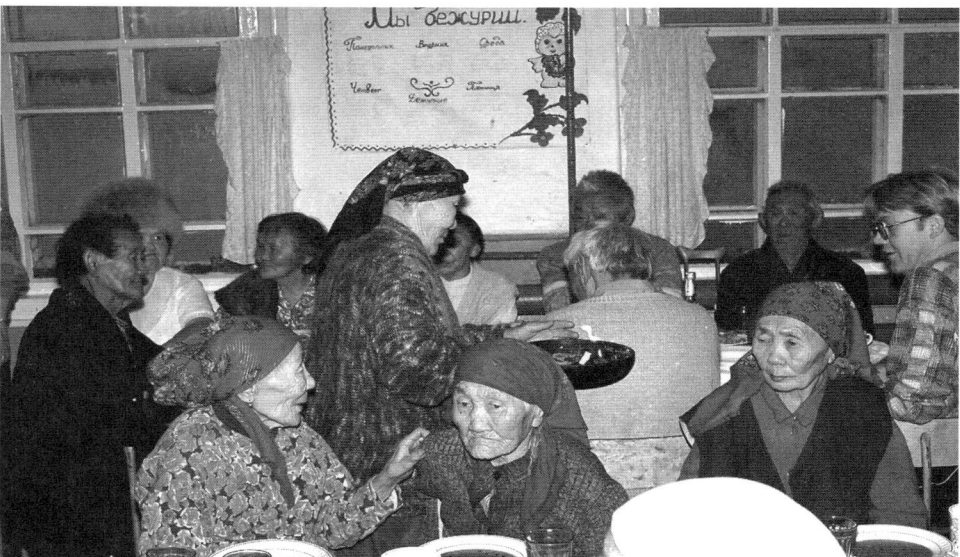

Figure 6.2. *An improvised smudging ceremony in the primary school, village of Ekonda, involving smudging with wild reindeer fat to welcome guests from Canada (Oct. 1999).*

At the most overt level, as symbolized by the smile of the director, the question of power seemed to hang over these meetings—and this power was expressed through a feeling of what was appropriate for one to say or do within a particular space. At the global level, the project officer in Ottawa was becoming increasingly nervous over phrases in each quarterly report that documented aspects of Soviet medical practice that Canadian community health workers felt should be implemented in the Canadian North. The intention of the memorandum of agreement between Canada and Russia was to disseminate best practice on how to anchor a welfare state within a market economy. The message that instead seemed to be coming back was that local communities desired and could make use of healing skills in their own right and they hoped that the welfare state could be embedded instead in their needs. It was clear that it was felt that we should keep these thoughts to ourselves and out of the formal reports on the milestones we had achieved.

At a local level, it seemed that in Russia there were strict lines drawn around the places where medical practice should dominate and the spaces where traditional practice should be allowed to continue. Certainly, it seemed that many felt it was inappropriate for traditional practice to be performed within the architecture of a biomedical setting. By contrast, Canadian biomedical practitioners had become comfortable with small rituals of respect and empowerment within formal settings (as long as the hierarchies of medical education remained unchallenged). This left open the question about which system was more 'pluralistic.' While preferring a crisp biomedical setting when at work, both Evenki and Russian doctors invested a significant amount of their free time collecting and drying medicinal plants, or ensuring they had a container with rendered bear fat at home. Thus we had the impression that in central Siberia these different ways of knowing—clinical medical knowledge and local healing practice—to a great extent ran parallel to each other. In Canada, the different traditions seemed to intersect during certain formal rituals, like the sweetgrass ceremony, but to many it seemed that Canadian doctors did not invest quite as much time exploring alternative therapies as did their colleagues in Russia.

The difference between these independent spheres of knowledge was also captured linguistically. When we spoke about 'medicine' or 'health care' in Russian we were also involuntarily talking about certain official biomedical standards and procedures. However, when we spoke about health [*zdorov'e*] or about folk healers [*'seliteli*] or 'doctoral practice' [*vrachivanie*], then it seemed permissible to speak about purely local traditions such as making offerings to the taiga in exchange for medicinal plants, or about ways of healing the spirit of a patient. When these terms were used, then the words for hospitals, medical colleges, or nursing stations did not appear.

One of the Tlicho Dene participants, Rosa Mantla, captured the mood of these discussions with a story of how an early Tlicho Chief had decided to invite the Government of Canada to build a school in their community. He had a vision of his descendents being 'strong like two people'—that is, of holding and relying upon two types of knowledge simultaneous (and yet keeping them separate and independent).[4] This image of medical pluralism was immediately understood by everyone in the room, whether they be Cree, Dene or Evenki or Iakut. However, it seemed to be understood as a goal that both peoples were lacking. The Canadian First Nations delegates craved an institutional structure for their young students wherein they could begin the work of dressing it with local ritual. The imaginations of the Siberian participants were captured by the sense of strength and confidence by which local traditions could be seemingly successfully placed within the walls of a biomedical facility.

This ethnographic snapshot of what can be said or what can be performed within the walls of a 'medical' institution only captures one side of the controversy of what constitutes

---

[4] An ironic mistranslation of this phrase by a Russian colleague illustrates nicely the sometimes profound cultural difference between local practitioners of medical pluralism and those working in formal institutions. He translated the phrase as making a person 'twice as strong' (*dva raza syl'nee*).

a proper atmosphere for healing. This particular exchange also generated conflicts over what could be made public and what should be silent.

Dene and Cree healers often say that healing knowledge is powerful only when we respect it and when we fear it. Thus, it is not considered proper in many Canadian First Nations communities to talk publicly about the details of certain healing procedures or ailments, since these necessarily involve all of the details of the past relationships of patients with the spirits of the land or with people who might still be present. It would be incorrect to assume that when certain healing rituals were placed in formal medical settings that they were exported without reflections. Both the healers, and the managers of these hospitals, made choices about what was acceptable—much like the smiling doctors and nurses in Tura indicated that they also wanted to make choices.

To illustrate the clumsiness that might accompany the inappropriate staging of a particular practice, I distinctly recall the tangible feeling of embarrassment when one of the Tlicho Dene guests was quizzed by an elderly Evenki teacher on how Tlicho 'shamans' used their drums or which spirits they appealed to in order to heal a person. The Tlicho woman redirected her eyes and refused to answer the question. Perhaps she felt that the question exoticised a type of ritual that this woman felt to be powerful and which deserved respect. The teacher's question was not naïve but was undoubtedly generated by a kind of intellectualized interest in material and ritual culture. She would have known from written ethnography, and perhaps from the stories of her parents, that Evenki healers also used drums. She would have seen some of these drums in the local museum. However, there would have been a three-generation gap between her intellectualized book-knowledge of the practice and the visceral sense of awe and fear that such rituals may have inspired at the turn of the 20th century. Perhaps she was asking since she was interested in reviving such traditions today.

I like to think of this embarrassed encounter as the mirror-image of the smiling embarrassment of the Evenki doctors and nurses who thought it inappropriate to perform smudging rituals in formal medicalized settings. In both examples, there is an important ethnographic lesson to be learned. Healing rituals, like packs of pills, can often be interpreted as being efficient in their own right and independent of the context in which they are taken. Similarly, the healing rituals of loosely defined 'indigenous' people might be thought to be equally evocative in any setting. Although the rituals of smudging, and the use of drums, are crudely common across the circumpolar North, their incorporation into formal institutional contexts must be a product of negotiation to avoid the problem of misplacing rituals. By contrast, biomedical rituals, as efficient as they may be in laboratory experiments, may also be out of place in certain cultural settings—in which case laboratory efficacy and authority might be undermined.

Alternate Healing Applications

Our discussion of inappropriate metaphors was not limited to smudging ceremonies and the use of drums; it also rested on certain categories of healing. When asked to compare traditional remedies, more often than not our Evenki and Iakut hosts were asked to speak about plant medicine. The use of plants to heal is one of the most successful examples of collaboration between indigenous peoples and Euro-American medics. However, in Evenkiia the consumption of plant medicine is just one aspect of the way people heal themselves, and arguably not the most important. What was interesting in these discussions was the difficulty with which alternate healing applications could be understood, since many of them (such as the use of live domestic animal breath for healing) seemed so far away from the biomedical compromise that the Canadian participants were comfortable with.

In this section, I wish to catalogue the different varieties of healing applications among Northern Evenkis before returning to the question of how best to speak about health. These ideas are documented more fully, in Russian, in a book (Anderson 2001).[5]

If we take plant knowledge as a starting point, we find that in Evenki and Dolgan healing practice at least, there are alternative ways of using plants that depart from the European standard of swallowing healing substances as teas or as concentrates. These 'unfamiliar' methods tend to center around the use of dry or desiccating substances, or the use of smoke.

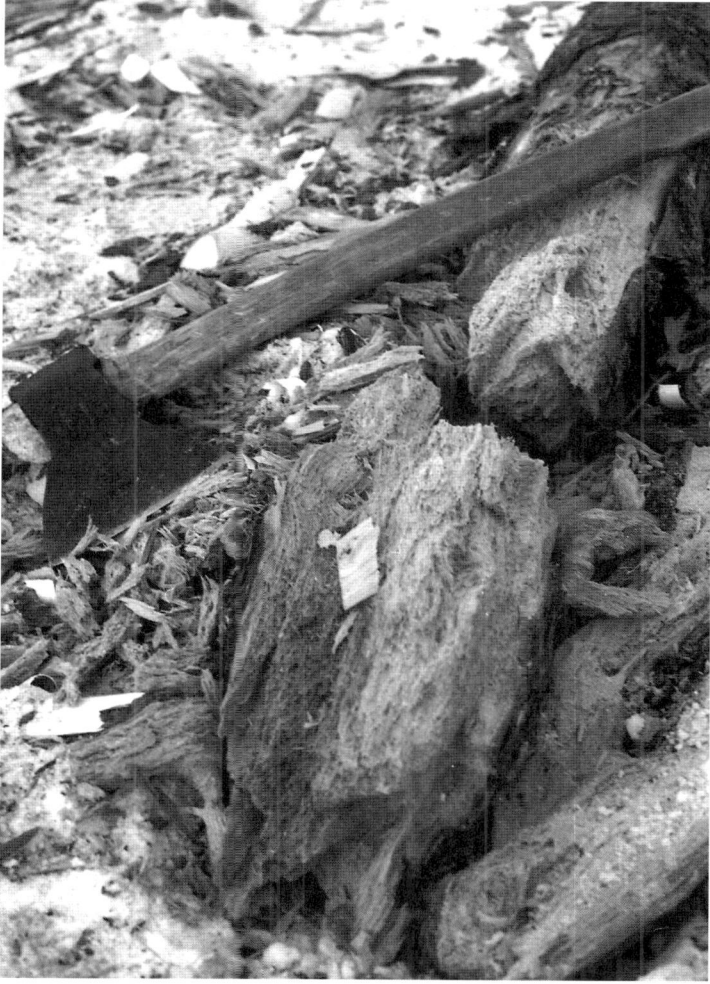

Figure 6.3. *Powdered, rotted larch* kuso *used to dry the skin, from the Kiumbe River Valley, Taimyr.*

---

[5] This volume was a collaborative effort combining interviews conducted by a Canadian masters student from the University of Alberta, Craig Campbell, and several locally-printed sets of interviews prepared by Lidia Udygir and Anatolii Amel'kin. The local publications which were prepared as a curriculum handout for the local language component of a teacher upgrading course by the Tura Centre for Teacher Upgrading.

During the exchange, one of the most widespread references to this idiom was the use of the powder that can be made from dry, rotted wood [*kuso*] of the willow or larch (Fig. 6.3). This powder was used instead of diapers for children when they were carried in special cradles on reindeer from camp to camp. The powder could generally be used to remove moisture from one's hands when working with skins or with lassos, or for women to remove unwanted body products. All elders who spoke about this powder emphasized how much better it was for the skin than the types of artificial towels or diapers which are now used on both the young and old in institutions such as hospitals and nurseries. There was a wide use for bark and for sap in healing infections and wounds. Bark taken from the birch or the larch could be used instead of bandages to heal infected areas.

There are a number of interesting uses of dried, powdered or even digested plant substances in the North of Evenkiia within the Putoran Mountains that, to my knowledge, are unique to the area. Kim P. Mongo (recorded by A. Amel'kin) spoke of the important use of powdered willow for ridding children of worms. In the worst cases, the powder of a dried capercaille stomach could be applied. It is tempting to speculate that in the latter case, the stomach of these birds would contain highly concentrated residues of plant resins.

Dried powders or dusts in the Ilimpei region are more commonly used to heal wounds of all kinds, as in this example from N.I. Sologon:

> If one gets wounded, if one can dust the wound with powder from birch buds [*luba beriozy*] the wound will heal quickly. This also helps for dermatitis. If this doesn't help you can use clay. You rub the clay on the skin until the condition gets better.

In our research, Craig Campbell found examples of using dried tobacco to heal open wounds (as told by N.I. Cheronchina). A similar paradigm was given to us by Evgeniia A. Kureiskaia who spoke of her grandmother sprinkling wood ashes on open wounds to disinfect them. Akseni'ia Bezrukikh, in the community of Ust'Avam, Taimyr spoke about the value of wood splinters [*shepki*] that are produced when lightning strikes trees. These could be powdered and sprinkled on wounds of both reindeer and people. Similarly, the dark 'thunder tobacco' [*eting temperashka*] made by a special type of mushroom [*dozhdevii grib*] that appears after a thunder storm could be used to the same effect. Amongst Evenkis in Tura, the powder of this same mushroom—'lightening mushroom' [*agdyrin*] was also recognized by Galina Ivanovna Khutogoir as often used by elders for congealing blood in cuts.

The use of plants that had been touched by thunder and lightning makes reference to an important aspect of Northern Evenki cosmology. The phenomenon of lightening–thunder, known by the same word *adyl*—is thought to be caused by a living creature that takes the form of a large bird. The thunder is produced by the sound of the bird's wings and the lightening is shot from its eyes (Fig. 6.4). In this case, the healing power of these substances comes from their relationship to this powerful, primal creature.

Similar properties are also associated with bones, teeth or other solid material objects of powerful creatures. Akseni'ia Bezrukikh also remembered how, when she punctured her foot as a little girl, her father removed a bear molar from his knife sheath (he apparently always carried this tooth with him) and scrapped off a fine white powder onto the wound. Her father also carried a special white stone 'the heart of the thunder' [*eteng kherigde*], which he could powder to heal wounds. He would find such stones high up in the Putoran Mountains (Mount Michangda) "where there was often lightening [*groza*]." This narrow, pointed rock, shaped like a pick, could also be pointed toward a part on the body where

Chapter Six: *Idioms of Health and Healing in Central Siberia*

there was a sharp pain. By pressing the stone to the place, the pain could be removed. We also heard of very intriguing remedies involving the use of various rock powders described by some as 'sugar dust' and by others as something similar to diamond dust gathered from cliffs. Such powders could be used to heal sore eyes or stomach discomforts.

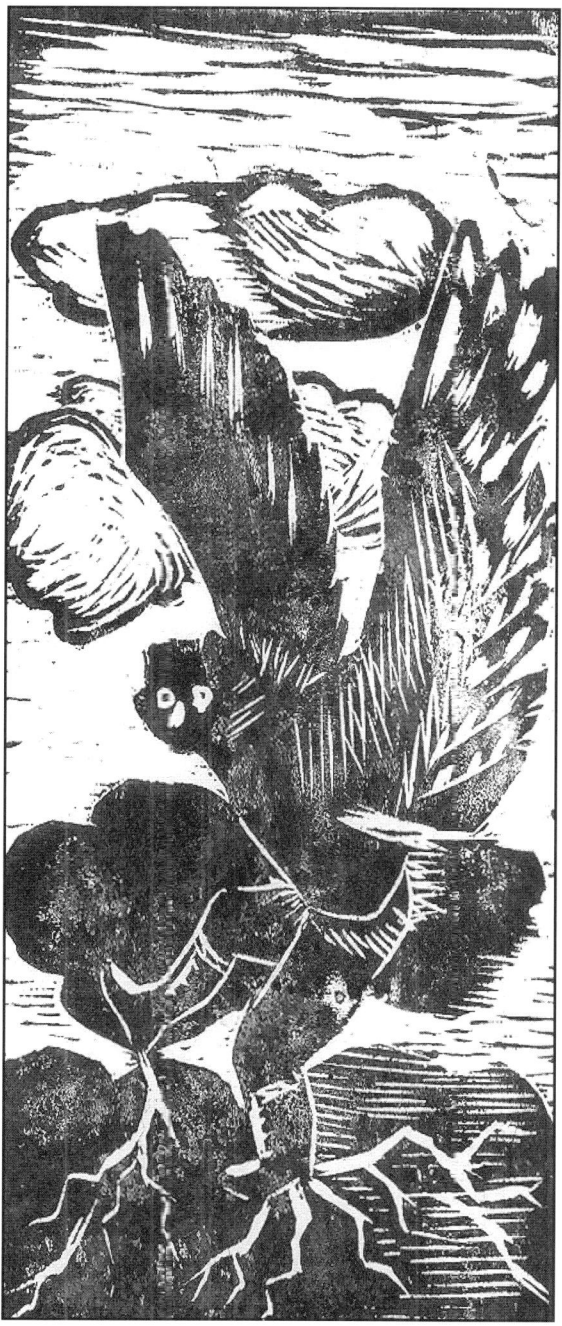

Figure 6.4. *A wood etching 'Thunder bird' produced by students at the Art Department, Tura Boarding School, Evenkiia.*

Plant medicine might also be used as a smoke. We have already mentioned the use of juniper smoke [*mozhzhevelnik*] or dried reindeer fat to 'cleanse.' Here Nina I. Cheronchina (as recorded by C.Campbell) gives more detail on the quieting aspects of this ritual:

> When a man or woman caught an illness, they gather hot embers into a bowl. The embers would be taken directly from the stove. On top [of the embers] they would then place reindeer fat. Then they did like this—they took the bowl in circles around the head in the opposite direction that the sun travels. They did this three times. And [the patient] breathed in this smoke [and exhaled] away from you. You have to breathe in the fat as a smoke into yourself. You start to breathe out and all of it goes out—the sickness goes away.

In this particular situation, Cheronchina is describing the use of smoke to heal a type of psychological or spiritual ailment called *tarymte* which manifests itself as a type of anxiety or spirit-possession.

During our discussions, both L. Udygir and A. Amel'kin have recorded examples of the use of smoke to heal various ailments. In the story told by M.P. Ydygir, her young brother is healed by her mother after falling into a lake:

> They stoked the stove until it glowed red. Mother undressed him and dried his skin until the blood came to the surface. She dressed him in dry clothes. She boiled the tea kettle and gave him tea. Then, she got her [medicinal] grasses from her pouch and steeped them. In the pouch she has a few of these grasses [sic]: cranberries, cranberry leaves, birch fungus, Labrador tea, and mat'-machekha. She gave them to him with a ladle. When any of us got sick we would lie together to warm each other up. Mother would smudge us with Labrador tea and said some words [*prigovarivaia*]. She would feed the fire. My brother started to sweat profusely. He didn't stand up for three days. Mother would change his clothes several times at night. For those days she almost didn't sleep since she kept the fire going. For these three days she barely ate. Slowly, my brother started to get up and walk outside. People came to visit us rarely. We lived alone most of the time.

An interesting related method is a passive manner of inhaling juniper:

> My uncle suffered from asthma. Sometimes it was difficult for him to breathe. He suffered so much the poor man [*bediaga*]. He could no longer hike long distance[s] and he couldn't ski. He could go down a hill but he would go up a hill in tears. He gathered together juniper branches from which he made beads [*busy*]. He made three beads. The 'beads' were made by breaking the branches into short portions and then wrapping them with sinews. My uncle wore these around his neck and breathed in the juniper with the air. That is how he got better. (Karp I. Kombagir as recorded by A. Amel'kin).

A further alternate paradigm of healing is the use of specially-chosen domestic animals as healing agents. Many elders from the north of the Evenki district (Ekonda, Chirinda, Essei) and through Taimyr (Khantaikskoe Ozero, Volochanka, Ust' Avam) have spoken to me and other members of our group about the use of live reindeer for healing. Specifically, knowledgeable shamans would select reindeer which had some sort of special link to a sick person for use in a healing ritual where the reindeer would be tied-up, carried into a tent, and then placed beside the sick person so that the reindeer would breathe on the infected area. Akseni'ia Bezrukikh from Ust' Avam had a particularly colourful rendition of how her eyes were healed as a young girl:

> When my eyes were hurting, my parents contacted a shaman to heal me. The shaman would negotiate with the spirits [*algyr*] to seek their advice. The spirits would indicate a special reindeer which could be used to heal. The shaman showed my parents which deer. They caught the deer and dressed it up in beautiful harnesses with beads. The deer would be 'cleaned' by smoking it with juniper [*khenkere*]. Then the deer would be held for a long time to breath[e] on the one spot. After the procedure, no one would harness or use that deer again.

Other elders commented on the use of reindeer breath to heal sore hands, toothaches, or the above-mentioned psychological ailment *tarymte*. The key aspect stressed in all renditions of the procedure is the use of 'private' deer, 'personal' deer, or very special coloured or extremely white reindeer. This 'medicine' reflects the belief of many Evenkis, Iakuts and Dolgans that certain domestic animals can share the fate of their masters and can be encouraged to take away illness.

A more usual way of using animals in medicine, is to consume different animal parts. In terms of our interviews, these stories of the consumption of fats, or various dried parts of animals were very common from elders in the northern part of Ilimpei district as well as in Taimyr. As listed below in this section, the use of various animal fats was very common. This ranged from the ritual use (smoking) of wild reindeer fat mentioned above, to drinking 'dark' reindeer blood to help one's general health, to the very common use of bear fat to heal skin infections or chest colds. Among more uncommon uses of fat, we heard of the use of wolf fat and wolverine fat for skin and chest colds from Dina Pavlovna Khutukogir. As is well known amongst all circumpolar peoples, bear parts are very important in medicine. The bear's dried gall bladder can be used in various remedies from curing infections in cuts to stomach ailments. The bear's tongue and paws are both thought to be powerful remedies, although the precise treatment procedures remained unclear. M.P. Udygir told of soft reindeer skin used as bandages, and blood taken from the ear of a dog is used to disinfect the region. A different story, from E.F. Udygir, stressed the use of bear fat and reindeer blood to heal cuts and wounds. For all of these procedures it seemed very difficult to get a clear picture of the cure from the general words of the elders. It would help to observe how fat was taken from wolves or bears, or in what way other animal parts would be used for healing. However, in all interviews, the importance of animal part medicine was stressed and deserves further research and discussion.

Each of these 'alternate' or 'unfamiliar' healing applications suggest a unique approach to healing. Whether smoke, or powder, or animal breath is used, the person is healed through exposure to the environment rather than consuming a concentrate into his or her person. This openness to the ecology around suggests a model of the person which looks out or is extended into the landscape, rather than one that moves autonomously through space or through institutions. It is, of course, striking that such methods of healing would be very hard to accomplish logistically in a medical environment of a hospital or medical station—perhaps one of the reasons why these forms of 'taiga medicine' are, in turn, not very well documented. The inconvenience of practicing these cures is transformed into a pathology when practices such as these become invisible due to their exoticness.

Although the knowledge of plant medicine among taiga peoples is important, it is equally important that it does not dominate the entire repertoire of alternative therapies.

Since these meetings have taken place, there is some evidence that 'zootherapies' are gaining some prestige within the cosmopolitan biomedical community. The leading examples, as was the case with plant medicine, come from Latin America (Alves and Rosa 2005; Souto *et al.* 2009; Alves and Oliveriva *et al.* 2010). Each of these authors frame zootherapy as a type of new frontier that is open for research and eventual commoditisation. A similar interest in marketing animal products has also caught on all over Siberia. As Brandišauskas documents in his contribution to this volume, the sale of animal parts to China provides an important income to Evenki hunters today.

Looking beyond these 'alternate applications' of healing knowledge, it is important not to forget that Evenki, Iakut and Dolgan people, much like their First Nations counterparts in Canada, first and foremost speak about healthy ways of living rather than the interventions that one can swallow or inhale in order to feel well again. As Borre (1991) documented long ago amongst Canadian Inuit, eating well and 'living on the land' is an important part of being healthy. The landscape itself can often be understood as a therapy (Wilson 2003).

This emphasis on a healthy lifestyle can also be illustrated linguistically. In contrast to biomedicine, which excels in the classification of sickness and disorder, most northern languages have concepts instead for talking about strength or robustness. A typical idea that one might hear from people who have spent a great part of their lives in the taiga is that they do not remember people being sick (or, alternately, that people were stronger when they were on the land) (*cf.* Metzo, this volume). In general, affliction was thought about in Evenki culture as coming from outside as the result of the power of evil spirits or the action of 'bad places.' The way to avoid affliction would be to avoid afflicted places (such as the old camping places where infection occurred) or to have a certain strength or power that would avoid illness. For example, in the voluminous works of Sergei Mikhailovich Shirokogoroff (1919, 1924, 1935) who wrote about Zabaikal Evenki culture at the time of the Civil War, there are dozens, if not hundreds, of pages of text about spirits and ways of negotiating with them. However, one can only find a handful of examples of medicinal treatments (1935:95-97,181-182) classified as 'technical adaptations' and a very curt but authoritative classification of illness which requires intervention:

> The Tungus distinguish different groups of [medical] cases which are usually treated in a different manner—surgical intervention required by the injury of the bones, skin and of parts of the body are considered as cases of 'breaking' and 'repairing' as natural as any other 'breaking' which may be 'repaired,' surgical intervention for giving an outlet for the accumulated products of a local pathological process (various abscesses); individual slight physiological and pathological disorders; infectious diseases; the obstetrical cases; and the psychomental disturbances (Shirkogoroff 1935:95).

In my own work and indeed own experiences living with Evenki hunters and herders on Khantaiskoe Ozero, one would rarely hear of hunters or herders complaining about the flu or colds. Indeed, there was so much to do when living on the land that there did not seem to be time for being sick. In my own field notes, I often wrote about a very cursory feeling that I had that the work of hauling wood, moving camp, tending to reindeer itself lent a kind of strength. By far the majority of the remedies recited are either for cuts or breaks, or are applied to children. The words of Evgenia Anufrievna Udygir (recorded by L. Udygir) make a clear link between healthy labour and the absence of illness:

> When my parents traveled in the taiga, we did not know illness. At that time, all Evenkis had their own reindeer. As I remember, my parents never stayed for a long time in one place. Usually we traveled all of the time from place to place. Each time we traveled it was interesting. We children were overjoyed with the change of the camp. I never remember anyone being ill for long. We had cuts and burns. We never knew [about illness] before we started to live with Russians. Now I think it was the taiga that saved us and healed us. Now for a long time no one has any reindeer. I would like to travel again to those places where I traveled with my parents. Now medicines are expensive and you can't afford them on your pension.

In the case of more serious ailments, such as tuberculosis, Oktiabrina Chapogir (recorded by A.A. Amel'kin) spoke with great beauty about a shamanistic cure involving tying a sick young girl to a pine which then 'took' the illness (I have heard very similar stories involving the use of spruce among Dene peoples). No doubt medically trained doctors would find this treatment to be absolutely wrong, but there is an important symbolic element in the treatment that is relevant to understanding how illness is understood. In this example illness is seen as coming from outside the person and it is removed through a ritual of transference to another living thing. Building on our earlier observation that formal medical training and knowledge is often felt to be 'outside' of the community and being 'outside' of the body of the patient, this example brings an ironic contrast by instead defining illness itself as being foreign to a healthy, working life.

Conclusion—Placing Healing Practice

In this chapter I have given an overview of the types of healing strategies used by native peoples in Central Siberia, with a focus on trying to understand the philosophy of healing. I have emphasized that successful healing strategies are placed in particular settings. In order to understand the healing landscape in Siberia, these examples suggest that biomedical settings are just one possible place where healing can occur. While Cree and Dene people feel comfortable bringing some rituals of respect into hospitals and nursing stations, it would seem that Evenki doctors are most comfortable performing traditional cures when they take off their white jackets at home.

My intention has been to 'place' traditional medicines within a larger set of activities which preserve a healthy life, such as respect for the environment and other living things, a healthy diet, and a certain vision of strength. In the English language ethnographic literature, the idea of 'placing' is also used to refer to the offerings of food or coins which are given to the land and its invisible masters as a sign of respect. This image, taken from the traditions of northern people worldwide, nicely captures my intention in this chapter. In my view, it is not so important to judge the healing strategies of elders as being more efficient or less efficient than the pills and injections of clinical medicines. Instead, to use the words of the Tlicho guests, it seems best to strive to be 'strong like two people' and combine both sets of ideas to build a healthy context for healing.

The first step to doing this is to be sensitive to alternate ways of speaking about medicine, applying medicine, and holding it. To do this, we have to let go of some of the narrow ways formal clinical traditions label and describe disease, and focus on how medicine can build strength. Since this particular exchange programme demonstrated that the setting within which one spoke to people strongly influenced what could be said, this chapter suggests that ethnography can be used productively to break down the architectural boundaries which may seem to divide different healing traditions. I have also suggested that it would be unfair to listen only to stories on the use of plant medicines, but instead we should also listen to stories of animal and other 'magical' or 'religious' forms of healing.

There is still much work to be done as this and other chapters in this volume suggest. One unexpected result of this preliminary ethnographic survey is that indigenous healers in different regions stress different 'idioms' of healing. In the ethnography presented here, there seems to be a certain shift in healing strategy when one crosses the Nizhnaia Tunguska River and moves north into the Putoran Mountains. Elders who come from Southern Evenkiia or from the Katanga district tend to elaborate on the complex use of plants and plant powders in healing. By contrast, it seems that elders from the North—Ilimpei district and Taimyr—tend to talk more about the healing effects of stones, lightening-altered plants and stones, animal fats, animal parts, or of the breath of live domestic animals themselves. The difference between these models suggests a different position on whether healing is best conducted by bringing elements into one's body or by strengthening one's relationships with independent animate entities present in the environment.

The examples in this chapter suggest a starker view of medical pluralism than is evident in other chapters in this collection. Whether this is due to the difficult remote conditions of Evenkiia, as compared to Buriatiia, or the common homologies between Tibetan–Buriat medical traditions and formal Russian medical training, healers in Evenkiia tend to keep their local traditions separated in different spaces and in different contexts. Here, we see a parallelism within pluralism that is not as evident in the North Baikal region or the Tunka valley. Nevertheless, the material that Evenki and Dolgan healers shared with us underscore the importance of pluralism and certain, unexpected idioms of health and healing.

Acknowledgements
This chapter was the product of many conversations going back over a period of nearly ten years. The heart of the research was sponsored by the Canadian Government in different forms—first as a doctoral scholarship by the Social Sciences and Humanities Research Council of Canada, and later as a development assistance grant from the Canadian International Development Agency. The work on the Canada–Evenki Health Programme involved a team of more than fifty people. For the work on traditional medicine, I would like to thank my friend and colleague Professor Iurii Popkov of the Institute of Philosophy and Law in the Siberian Section of the Russian Academy of Sciences in Novobsibirsk, Dr. Craig Campbell, now of the University of Texas, Austin, and Galina Khutokogir, Federal Inspector for Evenkiia. Iurii Popkov organized many of the meetings and was responsible for the three publications which resulted from the project. Craig Campbell bravely agreed to live in Tura for a half year with his young family during a time of great social upheaval, providing an important element of continuity between the many meetings. Galina Khutokogir, at this time, was the Assistant Governor in charge of Health for this still autonomous district. It was her energy and insistence that gave birth to the project and her hospitality which made it a success. I would especially like to thank the group of scholars featured in this volume who commented on this paper. Special thanks goes to Justine Buck Quijada who commented on the final draft of the chapter and helped me to see it from a fresh perspective.

Chapter Seven

Spirits, Taiga Medicine, and the Practical Engagement of the Landscape among Orochen-Evenkis

Donatas Brandišauskas

The popularity and influence of a variety of healers, locally referred to as shamans [Rus. *shamany*], *lamas* [Rus. *lamy*] or *zaakhari* (also called *sheptuny*), is growing in the northern part of Zabaikal'e and throughout Siberia (Znamenski 2003). Orochens, Buriats, Russians, people of Cossack descent, and horse herders of Tungus origin living in remote northern villages travel for hundreds of kilometres throughout Zabaikal'e to search for healers who might be able to help treat their diseases. Indigenous Orochen–Evenkis, who call themselves 'reindeer people' and are members of the Tungus–Manchu language group, often invite shamans to perform healing rituals and to lead public festivals. They establish new ritual sites near villages, with the shamans' help, that also become important places for the Orochen minority living in those villages. Today, ritual specialists are asked to help in fighting alcoholism, the 'evil eye,' bad dreams, misfortune and a variety of other complaints such as constant pain in the joints. All of this is happening as the quality of institutional medical care declines in remote villages. For example, the local hospital of Tungokochen Village (Tungokochen County) has recently cut its staff despite the fact that the hospital serves 1,500 people in the village as well as those living in several remote villages. The only other option for receiving clinical medical care is to travel long distances to visit hospitals in large villages or even cities. People predict that Tungokochen hospital will close in the near future. Local people perceive that medical doctors are servants of a formal bureaucracy which has no willingness to help. The decline of trust in medical institutions is also shaped by a general belief that anything made in Russia or China is a *potdelka* [fake]. As one hunter stated, 'there is no benefit left from hospitals' [*R. bol'nitsa paria stala bezpoleznaia*].

During my fieldwork in May 2010 I tried to help one prosperous hunter get a simple blood test so that I could help him access special western-made medicines to treat his arthritis. However, due to the indifference of medical doctors, the absence of certain doctors from their work place, and the lack of the simple equipment required, we had no success. This outcome came about despite traveling for hundreds of kilometres and visiting hospitals three times, making agreements with relatives working in hospitals and negotiating for the test. After this, I was told that it is best to visit a hospital when you are almost dead. Others added that one must be able to walk to a hospital since nobody will take you there. This kind of Orochen mistrust of professional medical care and the popularity of healers is reminiscent of the view taken of the first medical doctors who came to the newly established Tungokochen Village in the late 1930s (Kolednev 2009), as well as the way Paladimov (1929) records Orochens based in Buriatiia describing their medical treatment.

Today, as in the early Soviet period, even though Orochens go to hospitals, they also rely on a variety of healers and use their own taiga medicines and strategies to treat disease. With the growing dependence on taiga resources and economic self-reliance, a knowledge of healing, and of how to harvest and use taiga medicine (animal parts, minerals, plants and healing places) have become increasingly important. Similarly, as in the days described by Shirokogoroff (1929:291), people living in the taiga also suffer injuries caused by falls, freezing, burning, accidental cuts, or from animal attacks. People who continue to follow a subsistence lifestyle, or who have newly turned to this lifestyle, have also become interested in the ways in which one can secure their own luck and well-being through rituals, and by interacting with non-human beings dwelling in the local landscape. Hence, good health is seen as being linked to the social relationships of humans with each other, as well as with other beings, that can be maintained through respect and gift obligations. Successful hunting of animals or herding of reindeer also requires a certain respect to be shown to non-humans. Failing to observe certain moral obligations while interacting with master-spirits[1] can potentially threaten a hunter's life.[2] In this context, the knowledge of elders has become important for solving problems linked to illness or clan curses [Rus. *rodovoe prokliatie*], or for finding appropriate answers or taiga medicines. People believe that spirits of masters that have been neglected for decades influence clan life today, both negatively and positively, as well as the lives of those who continue to use different taiga places (Mazin 1984; Alekhin 1999).

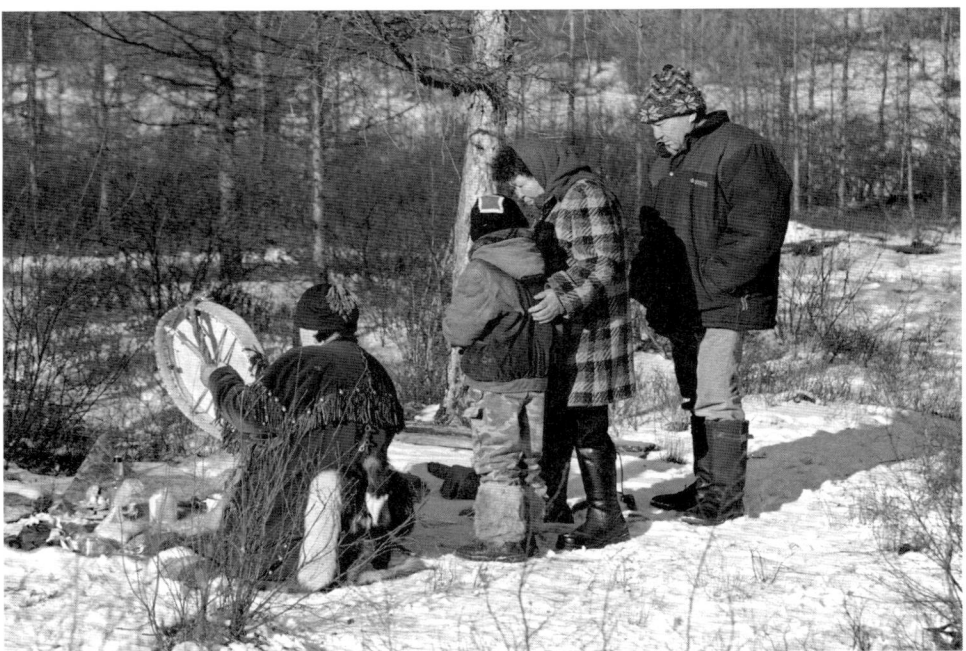

Figure 7.1. *Public healing ritual performed for the Orochen community of Tungokochen County by shamaness Svetlana Voronina from Baunt region (Buriatiia) in autumn 2005.*

---

[1] Most Soviet Siberian ethnographers employ the Russian word *khoziain* [master] to refer to a spirit [Rus. *dukh*] or animal which dwells in different places, or to a spirit placed in objects. In these accounts, the master-spirit [Rus. *dukh khoziain*] commands different landscape features such as a watershed, a hill, a lake, or a celestial object such as the sun or the moon. The master spirit is thought to influence wild and domesticated animals and the destinies of people (*see* the comparative studies by Alekseev 1992:28-59, 76-101; Zelenin 1929; Gurvich 1977; Mikhailov 1987; Petri 1930).

[2] For soul recycling among Oroks in Sakhalin, *see* Kwon (1998:119) and for Siberia, *see* Hamayon (1990:365-72).

Chapter Seven: *Spirits, Taiga Medicine, and the Practical Engagement of the Landscape among Orochen-Evenkis*

Reflecting the increase in importance of subsistence practices, Orochens have started to associate reindeer herding and the consumption of hunted wild animals with bringing 'strength' to the individual as well as the community. Eating the meat of wild animals is seen as being capable of 'cleaning one's body' as well as helping one access taiga medicine. One who lives in the taiga for long periods and knows how to harvest resources successfully is also seen as having 'special knowledge' linked to their interactions with non-human beings, enabling him to predict misfortune or illness, or to help with healing. Outspoken members of the Orochen community refer to the domesticated reindeer used by Orochens as 'cargo animals,' and they are seen as the herders' source of health. It is said that Orochens who still own reindeer live longer lives. The idea that one shares one's strength with the reindeer is a widespread belief among Orochen reindeer herders and hunters.[3]

Visiting shamans have become much more involved in the performance of public rituals in indigenous communities over the last five years, and also in influencing individual strategies and ideas linked to illness and healing (Fig. 7.1). However, most shamans are based in large villages or even cities, and have no knowledge of life in the taiga; therefore, they are visited by hunters or herders only when they have serious health problems that they are unable to solve on their own (Humphrey 2002). Nevertheless, these shamans recommend that Orochen herders visit their ancestor's ritual sites or clan territories [*rodovye zemli*] in the taiga and leave offerings near the mortuary scaffolds of old shamans. With the collapse of the Soviet system, hunters and herders have become more interested in visiting these sites to ask for help with subsistence as well as to maintain well-being. The reindeer herders of Tungokochen have even established many monumental ritual sites re-enacting rituals of reindeer sacrifice (Anderson 2010). People also consciously interact with spirits during public celebrations such as Aboriginal Day (*Den' Aborigena*), inviting knowledgeable reindeer herders there to lead ceremonies. The importance of these revived rituals is outlined in the words of the former leader of the Evenki indigenous association, Mariia Fedorovna Grigoreva: 'there are many unexplained tragic deaths, suicides, illnesses—even young people die. We need rituals very much.'

Hence, in this chapter, I examine Orochen hunters' and herders' perception of health and illness as being linked to their self-reliance, and practices of subsistence crucial for dwelling in northern villages and remote hunting or herding grounds. I also show how these notions are intermingled with ideas of exchange with non-human beings, as well as adaptations to the post-Soviet socio-economic environment and contested life in the taiga and villages. My main focus is on perceptions of Orochen hunters and herders, since I spent most of my 16 months of field research among several Orochen communities based in villages and the taiga in 2004, 2005 and 2010 in Zabaikal Province (former Chita Province) and the Buriat Republic. However, in most cases these perceptions do not differ much from other hunters and villagers of different ethnic origins (*see also* Basharov 2003).

Discourses and Policies Concerning Orochen Health

Various early ethnographical reports document how Siberian indigenous people perceive illness and their ways of healing, describing the rituals of the little-explored 'aliens' of

---

[3] Orochen elder and craft maker Tamara Naikanchina from Tungokochen village told me about her brother who suffered from epilepsy in his childhood, and after a bad seizure, her father performed a special rite. He killed a young reindeer, cut out its heart, and placed the beating heart on the boy's breast. Only this helped the boy recover.

the Russian Empire (Fisher 1774; Lindenau 1983 [1742]). These descriptions, as well as the works of several generations of Siberian ethnographers (Zelenin 1935, 1936; Shirokogoroff 1935; Mikhailov 1987), examined healing mainly as part of the shaman's specialized role in indigenous societies. Ethnographer Zelenin (1935), in his comparative works, even argued that the shaman's main role was to serve as a medical specialist, rather than to ensure success in hunting or to perform divinations for the clan people. These ethnographies aimed to reveal the main features and evolution of Siberian religions, by elaborating on the activities, worldviews and psychology of shamans.[4] In his comprehensive monograph dedicated to shamanism, Russian refugee ethnographer Sergei Shirokogoroff (1935) describes the 'psychomental complex' of the Tungus[5] people. Here, shamanism was a basis for determining the complex actions of individuals, groups and even whole indigenous societies. Although Shirokogoroff (1935) focussed on the 'shaman's art to control spirits,' his rich monograph also contained information on the Tungus perception of different spirits, and on the manifestation and causes of a variety of diseases and symptoms with descriptions of how these illnesses could be cured. Soviet ethnographer Anisimov (1963) also underlined the importance of the Evenki shaman's role as a 'fighter' against alien spirits that caused illness among the clan people. Anisimov (1963) vividly described a shaman leading a dramatic fight and surrounding the clan's territory with a fence [Oro. *marilia*] consisting of his guardian spirits.

Countless statements in early Soviet ethnographical publications reveal the opinion that there was no proper medical treatment among Orochen–Evenki of Zabaikal'e [Rus. *meditsinskaia pomoshch'*] before Soviet rule (*see* Paladimov 1929; Neupokoev 1928; Samokhin 1929). These reports, written for the Soviet authorities, also stated that nomadic life was very 'unhealthy and created many diseases for Orochens' (Samokhin 1929).[6] The pejorative term 'wandering Tungus' [Rus. *brodiashchie*], referring to the most mobile group of indigenous people and seen as the least advanced, is widely used in the literature of the Tsarist and the early Soviet periods. Nomadic lifestyles were depicted as being 'without any order' and without any 'sense of place' (Sakharov 2000 [1869]:2; Orlov 1857, 1858). The nomadic Orochen lived in *chumy* [conical tents]; Samokhin (1929); Paladimov (1929) and Neupokoev (1928) reported that the living conditions were unhygienic since the *chum* was rarely cleaned. They also underlined the unsanitary habits of Orochens, maintaining that they only dared to wash their faces (Paladimov 1929). These accounts also referred to the common idea of extraordinary Orochen spirit-drinking habits, relating it to an idea about the forthcoming extinction of native peoples (Neupokoev 1928; Titov 1926).

The Soviet authorities aimed to change the material aspects of Orochen culture, their beliefs and their identity through projects that included sedentarization, professional medical care and hygiene (*see also* Leete 2004), based on statements such as Paladimov (1929): 'There is no other way as to sedentarize Orochens, since their hunting lifeways and constant movements, life in the *chum* and even the cold cause them to die out [R. *vymiraniiu*]' (*see also* Zolotarev 1938).

In the early Soviet years, professional medical doctors often competed with shamans and other specialists for patients. The prominent Evenki ethnographer Vasilevich (1971:58) stated that shamans have a monopoly on healing people since they "created [their] own

---

[4] The shaman, in Siberian ethnographies, was said to be a spiritual leader and to be a characteristic of 'primitive societies' (Hutton 2001).

[5] *Tungus* is an older colonial name for Zabaikal'e hunter-gatherer and reindeer herding people, who call themselves Orochen (pl. Orochar) or Evenki (pl. Evenkil).

[6] The ethnographer Titov (1926:8) stated the opposite, saying that settled life brought many negative outcomes for Orochen, including poor health.

explanations of the cause of disease, this way influencing people's beliefs that one's spirit can leave the body." Ethnographers often proclaimed shamans to be mentally ill (*see* Zelenin 1935) and because of this, shamans [Oro. *nimnanivkil*] were soon accused of 'cheating' and 'exploiting' people. They came to be called 'enemies of [the] people' [Rus. *vragi naroda*] and were drastically repressed all over the region in the 1930s (*see* Suslov 1936).[7] However, there was still indigenous resistance against the coercive introduction of professional medicine and the removal of shamans from communities in the early Soviet years, and conflicts ensued between these two different traditions and views of healing (Koledneva 2009; Paladimov 1929).

Shamans were not the only knowledgeable people who continued the traditional ways of healing in taiga camps and remote villages. A variety of other healing specialists knew how to use medicinal plants in healing, could set broken bones, administer head massages, stop bleeding, or perform divinations linked to health issues (*see* the case of Gilton Aruniev in Koledneva 2009). Shirokogoroff (1935:133) also mentions specialist 'painters,' able to neutralize spirits causing a disease through the production of 'placings.'[8] Tungus (i.e., horse herding Evenki) acknowledged that shamans were unable to cure many diseases, and that 'experienced people must pray or had to give a sacrifice before the placing' in order to cure these (Shirokogoroff 1935:134-135). Ethnographer Pu (1983:109) also described respected specialists among Orochens in Manchuria, such as *wutuoginil* who cured smallpox or measles, and *agagin*, who used divination to solve health problems. Finally, in Zabaikal'e a variety of healers [*sheptunil*] and people knowledgeable in healing curses, setting bones, or using medicinal plants are also part of the Russian old settlers and Buriat traditions. The state authorities often showed no interest in these specialists, who continued to practice in villages inhabited by Orochens throughout the Soviet years. Villagers consulted any available healer, including so-called *lama*, shaman or *sheptun*, in the early Soviet years (*see* Basharov 2003; Paladimov 1929).

An Environment of Contested Healing

Zabaikal'e, which covers both Buriatiia and Zabaikal Province, lies at the junction of Siberia, the Far East and Inner Asia. A continental climate characterizes the region, with seasonal extremes of temperature from -60 degrees Celsius in winter and 40 degrees in summer. The northern part of Zabaikal'e is homeland to around 2,500 Orochens. Coniferous taiga, with trees covering the hills and ridges, forms their hunting and herding grounds. The highest rocky peaks of these hills lie above the tree line and are covered with lichen and Siberian dwarf pine (*Pinus pumila*). Permafrost is close to the surface and water is not easily absorbed into the earth, creating a wetland environment. Soviet officials and scientists stated that some northern areas of Zabaikal'e were unsuitable for human habitation [Rus. *kraine dikomfortnoi dlia zhizni liudei*], maintaining that the harsh continental climate, permafrost, shortage of ultraviolet radiation, and temperature and pressure fluc-

---

[7] The people of Zabaikal'e suffered particularly harsh Soviet repressions. Many more shamans survived in remote camps of other Orochen communities in the Amur region and Southern Buriatiia as well as Evenkiia (Turaev 2008; Zabianko *et al.* 2002; Troshev 2002).

[8] Shirokogoroff (1935:149-150) writes that some spirits can enter and exit different 'placings' independently, as well as being invited or enticed by humans to enter specific objects which are then kept for their own needs. This type of 'placing' can be described as an emplaced form of spirit. Therefore, any geographical location, tree, animal, human, crafted item, or part of an organ can become such a 'placing.'

tuations caused great discomfort to the human body (Mikheev 1995). 'Specialist' Soviet land-use policy-makers decided that only certain sites, located in river valleys, were appropriate for permanent settlement because of the difficult 'medico-geographical features' of the region (Mikheev 1995), and villages for Orochens were established in these sites. However, these sites had their own problems. For instance, the former centre of Tungokochen County, Tungokochen Village, is constantly flooded by the Karenga River. Orochen elders used to say that the site was a very bad place to camp; therefore, today people talk about a 'bad energy' in Tungokochen Village that can be felt with the whole body as soon as one enters the village.

Most Orochens live in villages in Baunt County (Buriatiia) and Tungokochen County (Zabaikal Province), which were established in the 1930s by the Soviet state to sedentarize Orochen nomads. The majority of the villagers are of Russian, Cossack and horse herder (Tungus) origin. Many Orochens are now based in the villages; however most men and some women spend almost half of the year hunting in the taiga for fur and game animals. Some Orochens privatized reindeer from liquidated state farms and established clan hunting and herding enterprises after the collapse of the Soviet system. They still travel the taiga throughout the year with their relatively small reindeer herds (up to 500 head), and have a mixed economy, hunting wild animals and using the reindeer to transport carcasses, gear and supplies for their mobile camps.

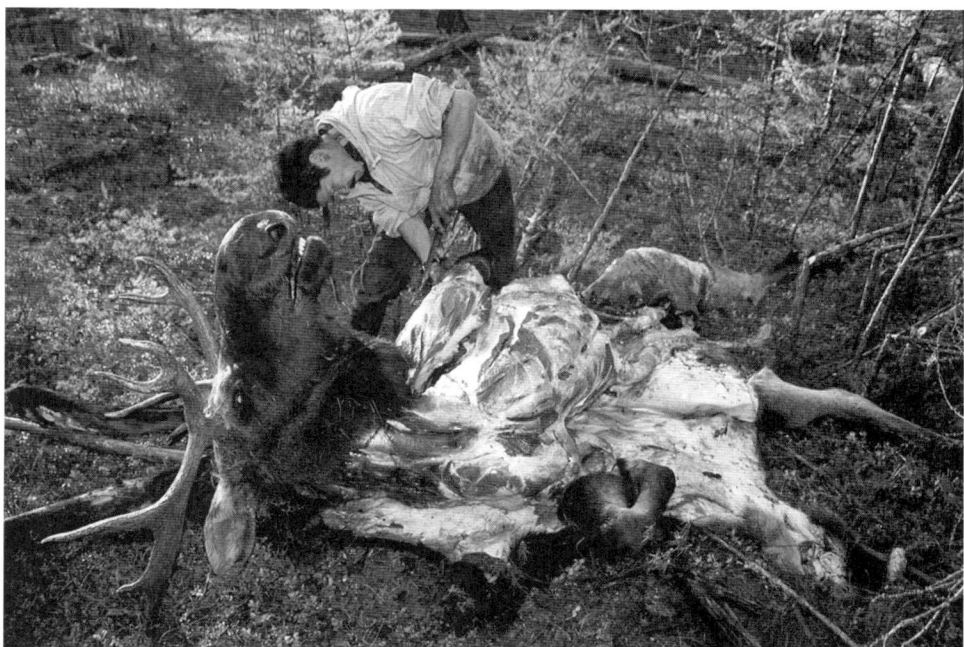

Figure 7.2. *Aleksei Aruneev from the Tungokochen village, butchering the most highly prized hunted animal—the moose.*

The centralized system of resource redistribution and centrally funded economic activities collapsed in the post-Soviet period, and collective property in the villages was privatized. This made the taiga, with its abundance of wild animals, the main source of income and food for many families. People responded to the economic collapse by appropriating taiga territories for subsistence activities (hunting) and increasing their reliance on taiga resources (Fig. 7.2). Villagers rushed to the taiga searching for anything that could be sold, exchanged, or used for their own needs. Consequently, many people visit the taiga frequently and learn new skills by joining organized hunting expeditions. Hunted animals include moose (*Alces alces*), elk (*Cervus elaphus*), grizzly bear (*Ursus arctos*), wild boar (*Sus scrofa*), wild reindeer (*Rangifer tarandus*), roe deer (*Capreolus capreolus*), Siberian musk deer (*Moschus moschiferus*), sable (*Martes zibelina*), Eurasian red squirrel (*Sciurus vulgaris*), Siberian weasel (*Mustela sibirica*), stoat or ermine (*Mustela erminea*), lynx (*Lynx lynx*) and wolverine (*Gulo gulo*). Today, the meat, parts of carcasses and the hides of hunted animals are thought to have special efficacy in the healing of both humans and domesticated animals. Various animal parts have also become an important currency, in the context of a cash shortage and the 'wild market' [Rus. *dikii rynok*] (Anderson 2000a).

Land and resources are scarce and competition for them fierce; therefore, it is quite common for hunting and herding grounds to be plundered. In earlier times, 'the law of the taiga' required salt or sugar to be left in exchange if one took something from a storage platform or cabin, but today 'everyone takes what is left unattended.' The contents of storage platforms, cabins, trap lines and snares are at constant risk of being misappropriated, abused or stolen, and freely grazing reindeer and horses may also be killed for meat, if left unattended. This lawlessness has often reached more drastic levels such as burning the hunting cabins and grounds of rivals, armed skirmishes that result in a high number of 'disappeared people' in the taiga, and even open murders.

Stealing, fighting and murder are, however, not the only methods used in the post-Soviet villages when competing for resources. It is said that villagers also now employ 'black activities' [Rus. *chernota*], for instance to spoil another's success, and *porcha* [damage, spoil] and *zglaz* [evil eye] have become very widespread practices in the post-Soviet villages. These notions are not unique to Zabaikal'e and are known to be used by many old settler communities in Siberia and North-eastern Europe (for old-settlers of Chukotka *see* Khakarainen 2007; for Komi *see* Il'ina 2008). *Porcha* is a conscious magical attack on another person that aims to make him ill. One woman taught me how to give *porcha* to another person, wishing him illness: The simplest way is to write a negative wish on a piece of paper and wrap it in salt, leaving it for a few days so that the 'negative energy' of the written wish would be absorbed into the salt. The salt thus imbued with negative energy is thrown into the targeted person's path, or at least around his house, and it is said that his person will certainly be damaged. *Zglaz* [evil eye] is a negative influence on human activities, when one has 'bad energy' and misfortune and passes it to another unconsciously. It is said that one should not praise items, animals, children or human activities in order to avoid harm.

Today, healers always try to find out whether their patient has *porcha*. As an example, I met an Orochen hunter named Vova, who was very successful. He had good dogs and often came back from the taiga to the village where he was based with full bags of hunted meat. His household was full of different cattle and horses, and he had a good hunting territory, from which he would bring many pelts after the winter hunting season. In addition, his health was good and he had no problems with alcohol abuse. However, he became sick and was unable to walk because of severe pain in his joints. He saw several healers, as detailed below, and all told him that he was suffering from *porcha*, because many people were jealous of his prosperous life and success in subsistence.

When he first became ill, Vova visited a healer who was very popular among the people of Tungokochen, known as 'Khamnigan' (the name of another Tungus Manchu speaking group). She was a shamaness living about 800 km away in Zagulai (Aga Buriat County), and could only be reached by traversing bad roads from Tungokochen. The shamaness, who was in her 60s, used a bottle of vodka without labels as a 'clean source' for predicting illness and future events. She used a variety of methods common to the healers of Zabaikal'e to perform healing rituals for individuals. Typically, she used to feed spirits near her house with candies, cookies, milk and butter in order to lift a *porcha* from her patient, and would give patients suffering from certain illnesses a black tea [Rus. *nasheptanyi chai*] charged with a specific energy, delivered through words mouthed silently while holding a knife above the tea.

However, Vova did not feel well after that visit and could hardly walk or even hold a spoon for the next two months. He decided to visit the local hospital in Tungokochen, where he was prescribed pills and given various injections. However, he had no trust in the local medical doctor, who he referred to as a poacher. Therefore, he moved to the capital of Tungokochen County (Usugli), where he spent some weeks in the hospital there undergoing the same treatment.

Vova was then told that a famous shamaness of Orochen origin from Baunt region was visiting the Orochen community of Usugli village at that time, so Vova took advantage of the opportunity to visit her. He did not feel well after her healing rituals, but he said that the lack of success was probably because he saw her very late at night and he was not well-prepared, bringing only one bottle of vodka bought for healing two patients.

After Usugli, Vova went to Chita city, in the centre of Zabaikal Region, where he visited a Buriat healer who tried to heal him by beating all his joints with a hammer. This procedure did not help either, and only resulted in more pain. Vova also visited a local professional medical centre in Chita, where he was examined and received many papers afterward. However, his health did not improve and he therefore visited Usugli again a few weeks later. People advised him to see a local Russian healer who had a habit of performing healings only at night, but this did not help and left Vova feeling sceptical.

He soon returned to Tungokochen, where he spent several weeks in hospital taking pills and having more injections. After several more months, Vova was advised to visit a Buriat *lama*, who reduced the pain by using massages. Vova was also told to use different charms bought in a Buddhist *datsan* as a protection against evil spirits, and to perform some rituals involving the sprinkling of vodka. This healer, like the others, tried to reduce the power of the *porcha*. Vova was told not to travel in the eastern taiga since five illnesses were located there, while he was told he could meet an evil spirit in the north-eastern taiga. He was also prohibited from attending large gatherings of people, in order to avoid being cursed. Vova started to feel much better after visiting the *lama* several times and drew the conclusion that 'there is no benefit from hospitals at all' [Rus. *bol'nitsa bezpoleznaia*]. He also used a variety of taiga medicines for strengthening his body, learned from his relatives and neighbours, and became interested in massage, minerals and medicinal plants used for healing. The elders started to talk about his long-lasting illness as a sign that could be interpreted as a call to become a certain ritual specialist.

Predictions and Escaping Illness

Porcha and *zglaz* are seen as a kind of 'bad energy' that can be introduced to items such as salt, kettles or coins and directed [Rus. *navesti porchu*] onto another person to cause illness. There are a variety ways to do this, such as throwing the 'cursed' salt or coins into the target's path, spitting into their back yard or house, or through gifting a 'cursed' kettle to him. The 'bad energy' can also be delivered by talking negatively about the person, or wishing them bad luck. According to Orochens, spoken words can become 'placings' conveying 'good' and 'bad' energies, and can be employed to influence different situations (for the power of words among the Orochen *see* Varlamova 2004: 57-63, and for Siberia *see* Zelenin 1929).

Chapter Seven: *Spirits, Taiga Medicine, and the Practical Engagement of the Landscape among Orochen-Evenkis*

There are ways to protect against negative influences or to reduce the harm done, such as smudging (cleansing one's body) with the smoke of Labrador Tea (*Ledum palustre*) [Oro. *senkire* Rus. *chiushachii bagulnik*]. This was often done by herders and hunters before leaving and after they left the village, as well as before visiting the dead or during rituals. Another old way to protect one's well-being involved 'placing his or her soul' into a certain object, called an *omiruk* [Oro. *omi-soul*]. This could be a doll made from bone, wood, or iron, and it is said that 'if one's soul is placed in another item, then one can be wounded but can recover quickly' (Vasilevich 1969:225). A few Orochen tales and stories I recorded tell of strong people who could not be killed, partly because their strength was located in one of these items (Voskobonikov 1965:335). However, it is also said to be very dangerous for an individual if their *omiruk* is destroyed. One family told me that a river flood in Rossoshino Village destroyed their son's *omiruk*, shortly before his tragic death. In addition to this personal protection, amulets and permanent idols exist in various mountain passages, which protect one's subsistence practices in these areas from evil activities.

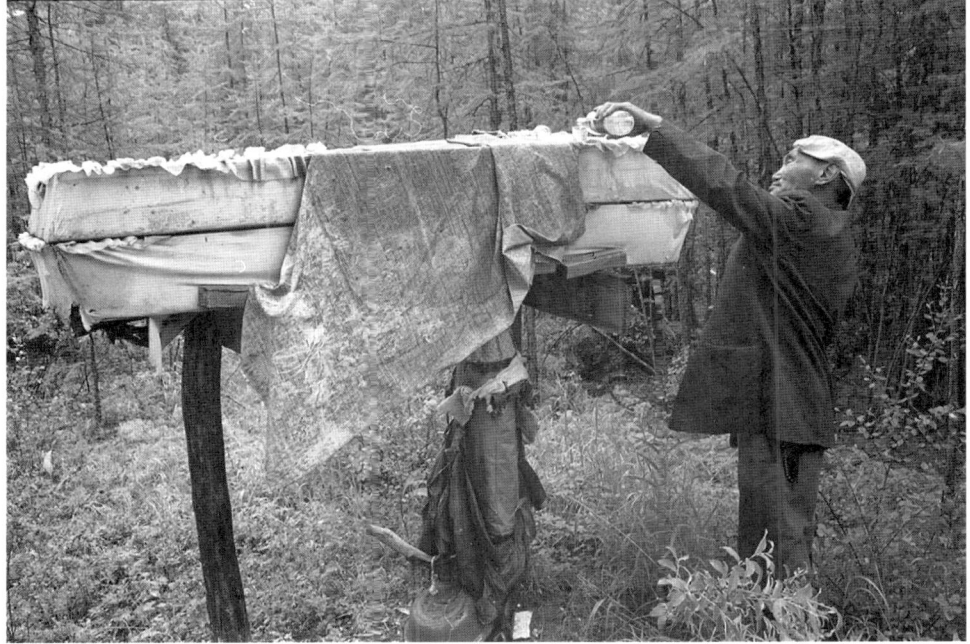

Figure 7.3. *Nikolai Dimitrov from Bugunda village leaving vodka offerings near the mortuary scaffold of his deceased relative.*

Hunters also mistrust others and prefer to keep their plans secret from villagers in order to avoid violence and the chance that their luck would be spoiled by magic. They avoid 'evil people' and '*porcha*' when entering and leaving the village, and also seek to mislead evil spirits. Indeed, whenever I was about to leave the village with Orochen, we never spoke about our route; occasionally, we even waited for darkness before leaving the village. Once, when we were packing our stuff on a river bank, other people were constantly looking at our work from far away, with great interest. This kind of curiosity [Rus. *liubopytsvo*] is also seen as a kind of harm, and I was told to make various signs or *kukish* using all five fingers, or to say very 'bad words' in order to send the people away [Rus. *poshli ikh podalshe*]. We did not manage to kill anything that week and I was told that this was because of the curiosity shown by the other people. Ethnographies reveal that

Orochens also change or conceal their names using nicknames in order to maintain their luck or protect their well-being, to mislead evil spirits or following negative events (Shirokogoroff 1929:266,284; Tugolukov 1962:37; Kureiskaia 2000).[9] There are other, much more elaborate, rituals and discourses employed to protect hunting or herding grounds.

Various methods, such as the interpretation of dreams, are also used to predict illness (Voskoboinikov 1965). If one sees blood in the dream, an illness is imminent. Also, Tungokochen Orochens perform a divination during mortuary rituals. Typically, a fire is kept burning all night near a mortuary scaffold; in the morning, animal tracks found in the ashes are used to foretell the future (Fig. 7.3). For instance, bear tracks may mean an oncoming illness or the death of a relative. Illness can also be foreseen in divination.

Autonomy and the Knowledge of Medicine

In winter, most hunters leave their villages to hunt animals for fur, staying in tents or log houses in remote taiga areas for up to five months. The success of subsistence depends on one's ability to dwell in the taiga alone; therefore, Orochen pedagogy teaches that one should be skilled in all kinds of craftwork and in curing disease. Further, one should avoid becoming an obstacle to the realization of someone else's goals, based on their own autonomy and not through the aid of others. Hence, one's autonomy among Orochens also calls for respect of the autonomy of others (for autonomy among Dene Ta *see* Goulet 1998:37-39).

The elders say that, although the shamans were killed in the Soviet period and therefore much knowledge died with them, this knowledge can be rediscovered by observing animals and learning from them. This observation can reveal which sources of water can be used for healing and which plants have efficacy for fighting disease. In this way, different medicinal items such as animal parts, oil, fat, rocks and plants are rediscovered and used in treating illness in the taiga and villages.

The most valued medicines are the so-called 'stone-oil,' velvet antler products [*pantakrin*], and parts of bears, such as the gall bladder and inner fat. They are used widely in the region and referred to as 'most powerful ones.' These are well-known for strengthening health and fighting a huge range of diseases.

'Stone-oil' [Oro. *delaniusa;* Rus. k*amenoe maslo*, also known in Russia as *mumio*], is a very rare, dark, oil-like mineral harvested from cracked rocks.[10] Sites of 'stone-oil' are shown only to very close relatives and friends, and it is often kept secret. The rocks only exude the oil in winter, but it is harvested all year round—a dangerous business as it involves climbing high through steep rocks, or using ladders. It is said that one should always leave offerings in exchange for the 'stone-oil,' and using a knife or rifle to scrape it from the cracks is not recommended. Orochen hunters believe that 'stone-oil' can hide from humans if they do not show the proper respect or talk too loudly of harvesting it.[11]

---

[9] The Orochen female hunter Iulia Semirekonova was named Aiulchik (a male name) by a shaman aiming to mislead an evil spirit that caused her sickness.

[10] [Editor's note] In Himalayan traditional medicine, *mumeo* is known by the Sanskrit word *shilajit*. The terms *asphalatum* and mineral pitch are also used in English to describe medicinal deposits gathered in high mountains.

[11] Hunters and herders do not talk about non-human beings and animals or their plans, so that they are not heard and therefore will have a successful hunt. Also, most of the events that are spoken of are discussed far away from the places where they occurred. Similarly, the ethnographer Suslov (*see* Batashev 2007:99) describes his 'difficulties of communicating' with Evenki of Tunguska in his expedition

Chapter Seven: *Spirits, Taiga Medicine, and the Practical Engagement of the Landscape among Orochen-Evenkis*

Small pieces of this medicine are shared only between very good friends and close relatives; it cannot be sold. 'Stone-oil' is mostly used for strengthening one's health and, more specifically, as a remedy for stomach aches and diarrhoea.

Bear gall bladder [Oro. *dzhɔ*] is used to heal liver problems including cirrhosis, and is a popular medicine among the Southern Buriat and Chinese people. The inner fat of a bear, meanwhile, is used in various ways. It is said to increase strength; hunters often say that eating it is good for combating physical exhaustion. It is also used to fight coughs, a common complaint among the hunters as they tend to smoke many strong cigarettes without filters, and as a cream for healing skin problems such as burns. Other bear products—e.g., paws and hides—can also be used in medicine; however, these are often sold to traders [*komersanty*], for export to China (Fig. 7.4).

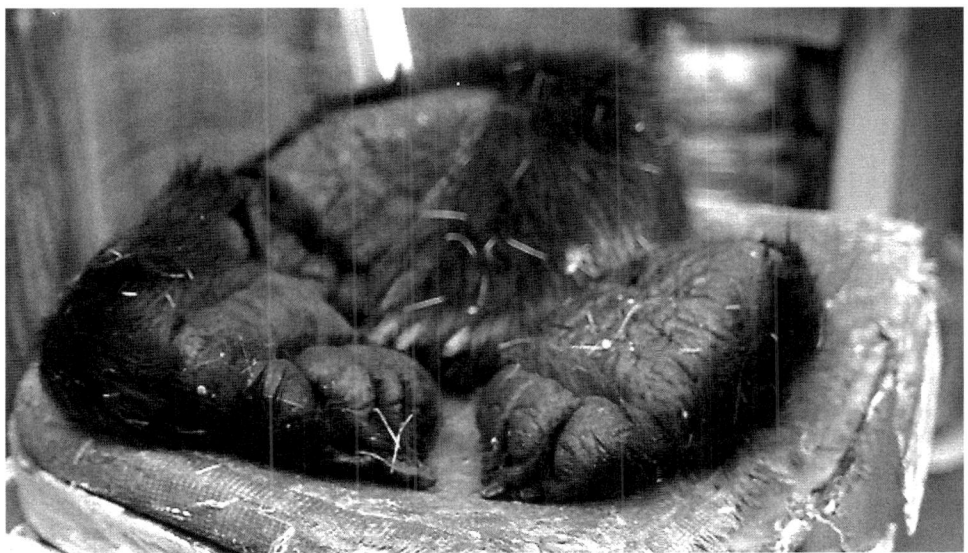

Figure 7.4. *Bear paws cut to be traded to* komersanty *and exported to China.*

Velvet antlers, called *panty*, are processed and made into *pantakrin* in pharmaceutical factories in Irkutsk, Kirov, the Moscow Okhotovodsk Scientific Institute, and China.[12] Hence, the *panty* of wild reindeer, moose, and elk are always cut and cooked, then dried to preserve them for export.[13] *Pantakrin* is widely used in Russia; it is popular as a strong medicine that helps 'strengthen the metabolism' and is used as a medical supplement for sportsmen. In the taiga and villages, medicines are produced from the *panty* of wild animals and vodka (Fig 7.5). Reindeer herders, however, do not cut the *panty* of domesticated reindeer since 'it makes reindeer sick.' Elk penises and tails are also exported to China, or

---

diaries (1926-1927), saying that Evenki usually talk about events indirectly [Rus. *inoskozatel'no*] and only if there is some kind of spatial distance from the object they are talking about. Suslov (1926-1927) points out that Evenki believe that spirits can hear them, recognize their personality and become angry at them [Rus. *gnevo ego (dukha) ne budet predela*].

[12] A few elk farms were established in Zabaikal'e in the Imperial era for *pantakrin* production.

[13] *Panty* is a Russian term that has spread around Siberia, referring to the buds of a growing antler.

used to produce similar medicine for strengthening one's metabolism and balancing blood pressure. Prostate problems have been treated with a soup made from the hoofs of large animals [Oro. *chimchen*].

A variety of medicines exist that can be used on a daily basis for preventing serious diseases, or treating simple ones. A birch fungus (*Inonotus obliquus*) called *chaga* is consumed for fighting cancer, while a tea made from the Siberian dwarf pine (*Pius pumila*) is used constantly as a blood enhancer. I used to walk with hunters for 20 to 30 km per day and often developed sores on my feet, which were treated using larch gum. Puffballs are used for treating saddle sores on reindeer and horses. The common cold was treated with the blood of the white ptarmigan [Oro. *elaki*], while a soup made from partridge [Oro. *oribko*] was consumed for coughing, to clean one's lungs and even avoid tuberculosis. When I had toothache, I was given a sable's gall bladder to put on the aching tooth to reduce the pain. A hunter named Aleksei Aruneev used a variety of plants and different shrubs as a compress to help aching joints. He had recently learned from the elders how the clay of certain hills had been used in healing for ages among Orochens, hence he was planning to try it too.

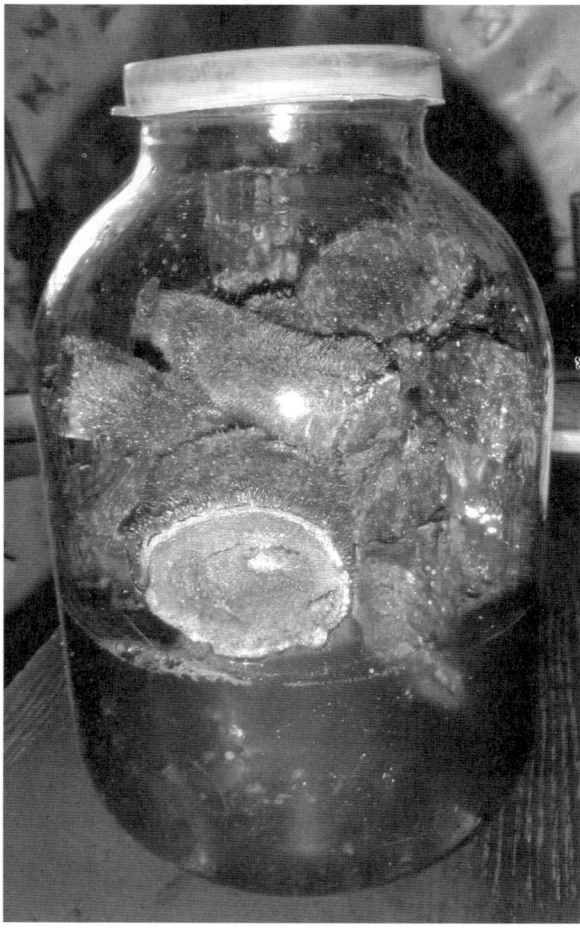

Figure 7.5. *Conserved fresh velvet antler* (panty), *valued as powerful medicine.*

Hunters also mistrust others and prefer to keep their plans secret from villagers in order to avoid violence and the chance that their luck would be spoiled by magic. They avoid 'evil people' and '*porcha*' when entering and leaving the village, and also seek to mislead evil spirits. Indeed, whenever I was about to leave the village with Orochen, we never spoke about our route; occasionally, we even waited for darkness before leaving the village. Once, when we were packing our stuff on a river bank, other people were constantly looking at our work from far away, with great interest. This kind of curiosity [Rus. *liubopytsvo*] is also seen as a kind of harm, and I was told to make various signs or *kukish* using all five fingers, or to say very 'bad words' in order to send the people away [Rus. *poshli ikh podalshe*]. We did not manage to kill anything that week and I was told that this was because of the curiosity shown by the other people. Ethnographies reveal that Orochens also change or conceal their names using nicknames in order to maintain their luck or protect their well-being, to mislead evil spirits or following negative events (Shirokogoroff 1929:266,284; Tugolukov 1962:37; Kureiskaia 2000). There are other, much more elaborate, rituals and discourses employed to protect hunting or herding grounds.

A Landscape of Spirits

Orochens see the landscape as being full of places marked by recent social conflicts, drunken rivalry and tragic deaths that include homicide and accidents caused by water or lightning. The herder of the largest reindeer herd, Nikolai Aruneev, often referred to the damage done to the landscape by Soviet industrial activities, as well as widespread poaching, as violence against local spirits. People say that the spirits have become angry because of mining and military activities, and deliberately set forest fires in the taiga, making the landscape even more dangerous. Places of misfortune and mishap are perceived to require new victims constantly. Hence, people can experience constant misfortune when using these areas. Illness is also believed to result from encounters with evil spirits or bears sent by masterspirits. People often tell how several hunters lost their way [*kruzhilsia*] and behaved and spoke erratically [*zunduglit*] after encountering non-human beings in the taiga.

There is a common idea that master-spirits will visit the camp or winter log house where one is camping if one does not establish a positive relationship with them. Hunters, herders, and villagers say that the contemporary taiga is full of spirits or ghosts, called *arenkil*, who can influence people dwelling in different places (*see also* Shirokogoroff 1935:137-138). Orochens define *arenkil* as the souls of hunters or herders who did not reach the world of the dead because of sudden or accidental death, or because their souls were not escorted there by rituals (Ermolova 2010). These souls are forced to stay in this world and can be either benevolent or malevolent (Tsintsius 1975:51). According to herders, during the time the Soviet state prohibited public ritual practices, very few shamans were available to perform the necessary rituals to transport the souls to the world of the dead [Oro. *buny*].[14] Several shamans were killed with the help of their own kinsmen during early Soviet political rule, while others died under repressive Soviet policies. The legacy of these tragic deaths permeated the landscape with angry souls. These 'bad places,' where the

---

[14] According to the Orochen hunter and herder Nikolai Aruneev, the souls of the dead go to the underworld, which he used to call 'the world of dead people.' He used to tell how one could meet souls coming back from a cave from the underworld. Vasilevich (1969:212) describes the Evenki worldview as divided into *ugu buga* [Upper World] and *hergu buga* [Underworld]. Varlamova (2002:180) reports the Orochen world as divided into *ugu buga* [Upper World], *dulin buga* [Middle World] and *hergu buga* [Underworld].

The Healing Landscapes of Central and Southeastern Siberia

deaths happened, are thought to demand new victims. Some elders told me that they always fear camping in new and unfamiliar places for this reason.

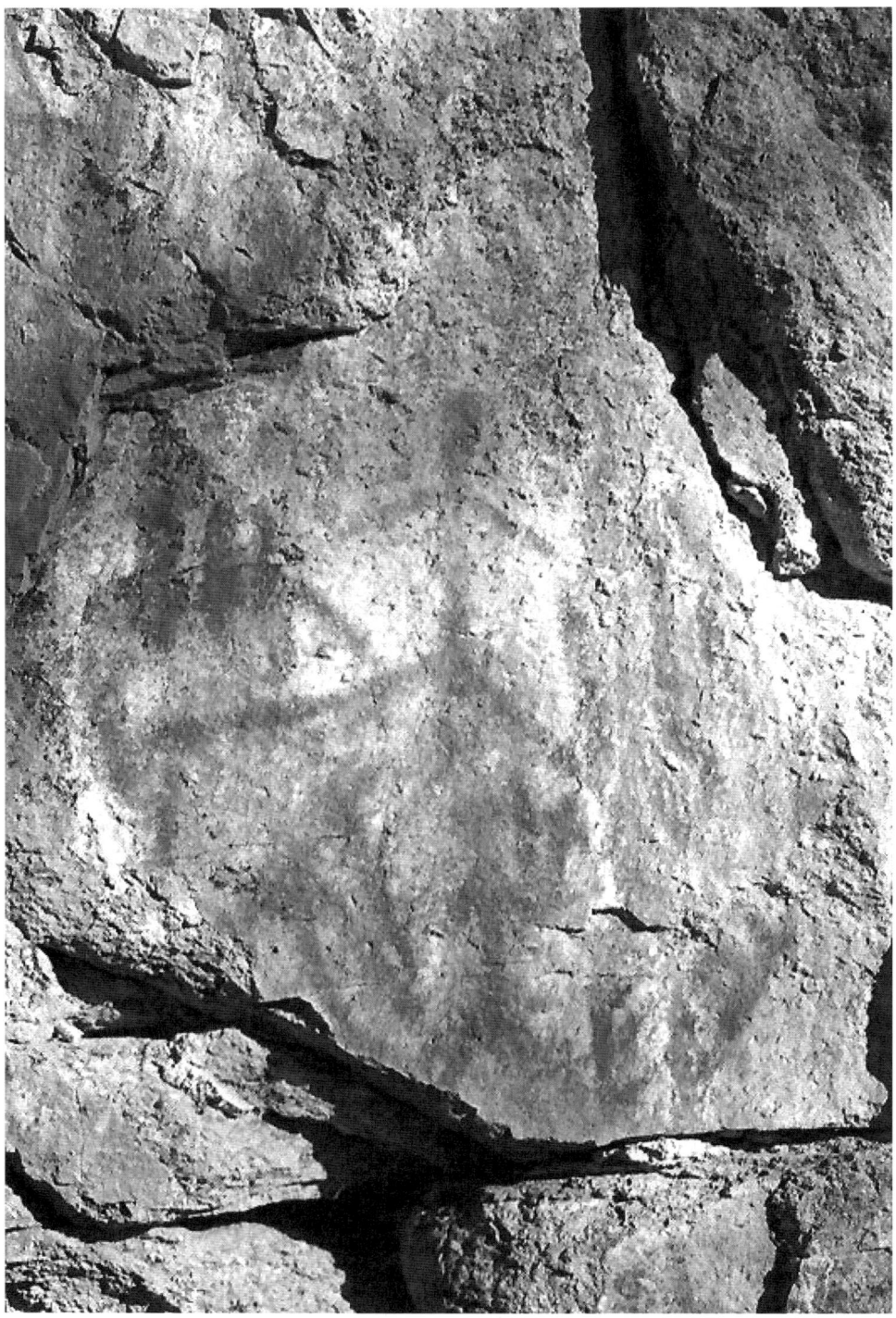

Figure 7.6. *Rock drawings: an important place for Orochen rituals.*

Chapter Seven: *Spirits, Taiga Medicine, and the Practical Engagement of the Landscape among Orochen-Evenkis*

The danger of dwelling on the land has increased even more as the knowledge and memories of mortuary sites or 'sacred places' has faded, and the elders say this is the reason people constantly encounter *arenkil*. An *arenki* can weaken an individual;[15] the hunter will fall ill and may even die, so the appearance of an *arenki* can herald an imminent journey to the world of the dead. Orochens also say that one can easily lose strength [Oro. *chinen*] and become ill by encountering a bear sent by spirits.[16] People tell elaborate stories about how *arenkil* or bears come for revenge when one stays overnight in old camping sites without giving gifts to the master-spirit, or if one destroys a cache or mistreats a mortuary site. When I asked herders why they rarely camp near the Buktokon River, Nikolai Aruneev explained to me that reindeer refuse to graze on the Buktokon and "if you push them hard they will start to get ill." He added that reindeer herders who migrated to the area in the early 1950s observed that reindeer avoided the site. Nikolai remarked that it is a 'bad place' [Rus. *plokhoe mesto*] and the reason may be revealed only in the future. Shirokogoroff (1935:88) noted that Tunguses used to explain their choice of camping site by saying: 'this is a good place; no bad spirits are around.'

Orochen hunters and herders also associate different landscape features, known as 'places of strength' [Rus. *mesta sily*], with health issues. These may include lakes, rocks, caves, rivers, valleys or water sources that are seen as inhabited by master-spirits. Today, these sites are widely known in villages and are specially attended with rituals performed by hunters and herders. People tell of many extraordinary events experienced during visits to such places. A few rock art sites, called *dukuvuchi* [Oro. 'one who drew'], are located in Buriatiia (near the Sali River) and Zabaikal Province (near the Muishin River) and have been visited by local hunters and reindeer herders for ritual observances for hundreds of years (Fig. 7.6). The performance of rituals near the rock art sites are documented among many groups of Evenki all over Eastern Siberia.[17]

The *dukuvuchi* near Muishin River is referred to as a place where a master-spirit communicates to humans, and has had a huge impact on many generations of hunters and herders (*see* Arbatskii 1978). People from the villages of Tungokochen, Krasnyi Iar, Lumurchen and Bugunda visit rock-art sites; sometimes the hunters of Tungokochen visit rock arches before going to the rock art sites, believing that a ritual of going through the arches will cleanse them of 'sins' (*see* Kagarov 1929 for such Evenki rituals in Kagarov). At the rock art site, they spend a few hours near a fire, boiling tea and sprinkling it on the ground, and offering food for the master. Hunters and herders also leave other offerings such as coins, cigarettes and bullets near the rock drawings. They typically expect that new drawings will appear on the rocks after the gifts have been given, providing them with answers to many questions that relate to their personal life.

Orochen hunters stress that the master-spirit, not humans, makes these drawings and that the pictures change all the time. Therefore, after boiling tea and sprinkling it near the

---

[15] *Chinen* can indicate notions such as 'spiritual strength' [Rus. *dukhovnaia sila*], 'energy' [Rus. *energiia*], 'capability' [Rus. *umenie*], 'physical strength' [Rus. *fizicheskaia sila*] and 'strength of movement' [Rus. *sila dvizhenie*].

[16] Orochen say that bears bring messages or come to take away a person's strength [Oro. *chinen*]. Therefore, bear-visits often foretell the illness or the death of a certain person. As hunters say, 'a bear comes to the camp looking for *buni* [a dead person].'

[17] Georgi (1779:38), Kochmar (2002:52-55), Lopatin (1895:249-50), Mainov (1898), Okladnikov and Mazin (1976:112), Tugolukov (1977:41-44), Vasilevich (1957:62). From archaeological excavations, we know that rock art sites have been used as important ritual sites since the Neolithic (*see* Okladnikov and Mazin 1979:99).

site, one must approach the rock and observe the different signs on the rock surface. These signs can bring messages and even visions that can foretell future hunting luck, illness or births. The rock is said to be so powerful that children are told not to walk there, since 'it can drive them crazy.' People say that the strength of the place can be felt with one's whole body as soon as one enters it, and many hunters describe a strong 'inflow of energy' [Rus. *pritok energii*] when visiting rock art sites. However, if one is disrespectful, for instance by speaking loudly, polluting ritual places, cutting down trees, shooting, quarrelling with dogs, horses, or reindeer, hunting, etc., they can easily fall ill.

Several hunters in the village told me how their mistreatment of different sites resulted in long-term negative consequences, such as pain in the legs or a temporary inability to walk. People also refer to the remains of an all-terrain vehicle that was accidentally burned there and to a plane that crashed there. These remains and the stories that accompany them serve as a sign of the strength of these sites, teaching people to fulfil their moral responsibilities toward the local spirit-masters.

Morality and Illness

Illness is often described as a result of inappropriate behaviour and unethical interactions with other humans, master-spirits and animals in the taiga. Orochen elders often teach that certain activities are 'sins' [Oro. *ngelomel*, Rus. *grekh*]. Anyone who behaves inappropriately, for instance by failing to leave gifts for the master-spirits, poaching, or destroying old graveyards or storage platforms, can experience disease or misfortune sent by the master-spirit. Hunting, wastage, or mistreating animals are also often seen as very dangerous activities; it is believed that the master-spirits can start hunting the hunter in return, or cause the hunter to become ill. Local hunters believe that even a skilful hunter has limits for hunting success. Orochen hunter Aleksei Aruneev explains this as 'when a hunter can only kill what he is given by the master-spirit or he can't kill anything after a very lucky hunting period.' His brother, Nikolai Aruneev, says, 'you will not be able to gain luxury or earn much cash from such hunting.' If one has no relationship with the master-spirit, they have no such limits and can kill an enormous number of animals, but this is also seen as dangerous and can often cause a hunter's illness or even death. Aleksei Aruneev related various stories to me in this vein, saying 'when you start to push the taiga hard, then the spirits will also push you back hard' [Rus. *kogda kruto s taigoi nachinaesh, togda i taiga s toboi kruto mozhet postupit'*].

Hence, according to Oleg Taskerov, 'one who does not care about the masters can hunt as much as he is able to take.' However, people tell stories of how 'spirits push hunters off the place when they kill many animals drastically' [Rus. *ugrobit*]. Therefore, Nikolai says that hunting has no benefit for villagers, as most of them lose their health and even their lives. A hunter named Baran used to complain to me, when telling about his life, that he had had no hunting luck at all for the last several years. He interpreted this as having reached his limit, set by master-spirits, for killing a great number of animals in the past when he was a collective farm hunter, trading meat for money. Today, Baran tries to follow his moral responsibilities, treating master-spirits well, and is only able to kill a few animals.

The hunter Aleksei Aruneev explained: 'we can take as much as *buga* gives us, but no more. If *buga* is not giving to us, then we will have no chance to hunt successfully.'[18]

---

[18] Georgi (1779:38), Kochmar (2002:52-55), Lopatin (1895:249-50), Mainov (1898), Okladnikov & Mazin (1976:112), Tugolukov (1977:41-44), Vasilevich (1957:62). From archaeological excavations, we know that rock art sites have been used as important ritual sites since the Neolithic (*see* Okladnikov & Mazin 1979:99).

He told me of how they had once spent more than a week traveling to different places and hunting moose and elk unsuccessfully, but finally managed to kill a large male roe deer. When riding back to the village, they saw a few roe deer grazing in the remote open field. There were four hours left before sunset, just long enough to get home. However, since they usually brought many more animals to the village, Aleksei kept suggesting they slaughter the roe deer seen grazing in the field. They tried hard to surround the animals, without success. After half an hour, they saw another group of roe deer and again he insisted they hunt them, saying, 'Let's try, we can do it.' However, their last attempt ended with shooting and misfiring. When they returned to the track leading to the village, all of the dogs were away searching for a 'killed animal,' having heard the rifle fire. They waited for half an hour and then started to move, aiming to get home before midnight. A few dogs did not appear even after half an hour. Soon, they saw wolves running in a remote field and decided to stop and camp for the night. Their mood was getting worse with every minute, since the most experienced and valued dogs were lost, which was a rare event. Aleksei did not talk much and went directly to sleep without cooking food or eating. He also told me, 'You see yourself what happens if one pushes hard to take, we should have been happy with what had been shared. We found this dog lying ill in the morning near our tent. I was told that next time one of us could get ill instead of the dog.'

Caches belonging to dead people can also have an impact on the health and well-being of the living; they can be seen as retaining the deceased's soul [Oro. *omi*] and many people tell of how violations of caches have brought punishments such as lack of hunting success, incapacity, dangerous bear attacks, the appearance of spirits and death. Some people kept their idols in caches during the Soviet times, feeding and smudging them. Nadia Taskerova, who was a shaman's daughter, also considered these caches a safer place to store these items than having idols in the herders' camp. Turov (1975:198) also states that Evenkis built special caches that were designed to display sacred items and serve as protection for the hunting territory. Hence, Nikolai was among many storytellers who told of how personal items stolen from the deceased, or from living Orochens, can bring great harm to people. All these stories are retold in part for strategic purposes. Hunters and herders discuss how violence and disrespect toward the master-spirits of different places call for revenge. The landscape is invested with meaning through narration and mnemonic representations that shape present-day human activities.

Conclusions

Although Orochen shamans were repressed during the 1930s when most indigenous people were moved by state authorities to live in sedentary villages, Orochen practices of subsistence such as reindeer herding and hunting persist. Their beliefs and rituals, linked to the master-spirits of the taiga, and traditional ways of curing diseases or escaping misfortune also remain. These beliefs and practices are linked to ideas that evil spirits or 'bad energies' can dwell in different locations and can be emplaced into material objects as well as into words, which are then transferred to the human body causing illness or misfortune. Most people of the northern villages have lost their trust in the collapsing medical care system and have become more dependent on taiga resources, contesting among themselves for land and hunting. In today's unpredictable socio-political environment, it has become important to protect health and hunting territories through moral teachings, storytelling, and rituals of reciprocity with spirits as well as with the guidance of a variety of healers, be they Orochens or other nationalities (*see* Brummond, this volume). Today, it is important for people to find their own ways of avoiding evil spirits and misfortune and to use defensive strategies. Furthermore, knowledge of taiga medicine and individual choices and strategies of healing have become important for Orochen autonomy and self-reliance. Although an early account from officials of the Tsar and Soviet regimes maintained that the nomadic way of life caused illness and that the land was unsuitable for humans, I have shown in this chapter how Orochen knowledge of landscape and awareness of non-human beings can restore their sense of well-being. Hence, one's illness and well-being cannot be perceived as independent of successful social interactions within human communities and also with non-human persons (*see* Anderson, this volume). Instead of addressing healing as the province only of healers or shamans, I have argued that we cannot analyze Orochen ideas of healing and illness without their knowledge and experience of practical engagement with the landscape and interactions with non-human beings, guided by reciprocal relationships and the morality of respect.

Acknowledgements
This field research that formed this chapter was part of my PhD project, which focused largely on the variety of skills and knowledge, including the ritual practices necessary for success or luck in hunting and reindeer herding (Brandišauskas 2009). It was supported by grants from the Social Sciences and Humanities Research Council of Canada (SSHRCC MCRI 2000-1000), the Wenner Gren Foundation (Dissertation fieldwork grant 7260), and The Committee for Central and Inner Asia (University of Cambridge), and a Postdoctoral Fellowship (Research Council of Lithuania).

Chapter Eight

Public Health and Folk Medicine Among North Baikal Evenkis

Vladimir Davydov

This chapter discusses the creation of public health institutions in the North Baikal region, and the boundary between them and folk healing practices. The field material for the chapter was collected in the Evenki village of Kholodnaia in the Severobaikal'skii district [*raion*] of the Republic of Buriatiia. The archival and field research took place over fifteen months from 2007 to 2009. During my fieldwork, I observed that the local population relied on both public health institutions and folk medicine. Moreover, local nurse-practitioners [*fel'dshery*], who are employed in public health institutions, used both scientific and local knowledge in their healing practices. Neither patients nor nurse-practitioners perceived these two domains of medical knowledge as contradictory. They used both in healing practices and daily life. This chapter will explain the use of public and folk medicine in healing, examine the use of local medical knowledge in the post-Soviet period and describe how rare medicinal herbs have become objects of accumulation within the market economy.

In the late Tsarist period (late 19th and early 20th centuries), public medicine was incorporated into the routine of hunters and reindeer herders in the North Baikal region. There was no professional medical help in indigenous administrative districts [*inorodcheskie upravy*] for the majority of the 19th century and people relied mostly on their own skills and knowledge. The first medically trained specialist appeared in the region in 1864 (Anonymous 1939), and he was only an inoculation assistant [*ospennyi uchenik*] who vaccinated North Baikal Evenkis against smallpox. He left the area after only a short time. The first permanent nurse practitioner [*fel'dsher*] came to the region in 1903 (Anon. 1939). These early nurse practitioners also worked as school teachers. A common Evenki surname in Kholodnaia is Lekarevs, derived from the word *lekar'* [doctor]. Hence, people with this surname believe that they are descended from physicians who married Evenki women.

One of the first steps toward the creation of public medicine in the region was made in 1925, when special mobile medical groups from the Russian Society of the Red Cross and the National Commissariat of Public Health [*Narodnyi Komissariat Zdravookhraneniia*] started to work in the region (Shubin 2001:104). During the early Soviet period, regional authorities organized several surveys to collect data on Evenki health: the physicians Perevodchikov (1925), Agrovskii (1926-27) and Ogint (1927) worked with Baunt Evenkis (NARB 247-1-5:49). In 1927, Dr. Agrovskii, a graduate of Saratov's medical institute, was the first physician to work in a newly opened small hospital in Dushkachan serving Evenkis from the Kindigir clan (Shubin 2001:104,105: AMAE RAN 12-1-51).

In the early 1920s, Shamagir Evenkis were registered at clinic №7, located 133 kilometres from Tompa (NARB 247-1-73:26). Initially, their registration was a formality. Not many people visited the clinic because of its remote location. The local population needed permanent medical stations in the settlements. A small medical station with five beds was opened in the Evenki village of Tompa in 1926. However, a nurse-practitioner only visited the village for one month, in August 1927, and a midwife visited it for only one week in an eight month period (NARB 247-1-73: 26).

An expedition was organized by the Anthropological Institute and the Moscow State Museum of Ethnological Studies [*muzei narodovedeniia*] to study Tunguses [Evenkis] in 1927. The members of the North Baikal module of this expedition were Soviet ethnographers B.A. Kuftin, Ia.Ia. Roginskii and M.G. Levin. They teamed up with Dr. Agrovskii in Nizhneangarsk who helped them find boat transportation to Dushkachan. The initial goal of the expedition was to collect ethnographic artefacts while Dr. Agrovskii vaccinated Evenkis against smallpox. However, he also helped the researchers identify people to interview and arranged for the sale of ethnographic material to the museum. After completing his work in Dushkachan, Dr. Agrovskii moved to Tompa and invited Kuftin to visit this settlement with him. Kuftin's diary describes the boat trip to Tompa, which took several days (AMAE RAN 12-1-51).

A researcher named Neupokoev worked with Kindigir Evenkis in Dushkachan in the early part of the 20th century during an epidemic of scabies. Women and children, in particular, were so susceptible to the disease that some of their bodies and faces 'were completely covered with scabs' (Neupokoev 1928:10). Evenki patients acknowledged that medical treatment was necessary and took all the medication, prepared by a medical assistant [*lekpom*] from Nizhneangarsk and delivered by Neupokoev. However, Neupokoev's instruction to wash with warm water surprised them (Neupokoev 1928), as the idea of washing their faces and hands with ordinary water was unfamiliar to them (Tugolukov 1969:98-99). He demonstrated to Evenkis what it meant to 'wash' [*umyvat'sia*] and gathered them near a brook. It is interesting to note that while the local Evenkis showed scepticism as Neupokoev washed himself with water and green soap, that they were well aware of the healing properties of a hot spring near the eastern shore of Lake Baikal. As a confirmation of this, another early Soviet researcher A. Comaritsyn wrote: 'it would be beneficial for them to spend one or half month on these hot springs because they do not have an opportunity of visiting a hospital' (NARB 247-1-73:26).

According to Neupokoev, the most typical and common illnesses among North Baikal Evenkis were trachoma, rheumatism, malaria, and stomach diseases. Epidemics of typhus, smallpox and dysentery, however, appeared to be the most serious, responsible for an increasing death rate (NARB 247-1-73). Sixty seven Shamagir Evenkis died in 1914 from smallpox, one hundred and twenty people from typhus in 1920 and many children from dysentery in 1923 and 1925 (NARB 247-1-73:15). In 1928, Comaritsyn documented that dysentery, common among Evenkis, mostly occurred during spring and autumn and usually broke out in combination with the common cold. Evenkis from Tompa were also very susceptible to gastrointestinal complaints and rheumatism.

Venereal diseases were absent among North Baikal Evenkis (Neupokoev 1928:10). According to Neupokoev, there was not one case of venereal disease reported by medical assistants in Nizhne- and Verkhne-Angarsk (Kumora), and Evenkis told researchers that they did not have 'the bad' disease [*durnaia bolezn'*] (Neupokoev 1928). Nazagaev also documented this in his report (NARB 247-1-18:102-103), where he wrote that venereal diseases were not typical for the population of the *aimak* [district]. Neupokoev (1928:10) also mentioned that tuberculosis was not common among Evenkis in the 1920s. However, this contradicted Nazagaev's report, which stated that there had been many tuberculosis patients, especially among Evenkis (NARB 247-1-18:102-103).

Early Soviet administrators introduced a plan to develop a public health system in the North Baikal area. Plans were made to build special stationary medical stations in all large settlements, despite the lack of medical specialists. Frequently, the first medical assistants

Chapter Eight: *Public Health and Folk Medicine Among North Baikal Evenkis*

had no special education and did not know how to treat patients well. According to Nazagaev (NARB 247-1-18:102-103), the director of Nizhneangarsk's medical station, Nikulin, 'was not competent in medicine' and 'local people were afraid of visiting him as he regularly gave wrong medicines by mistake.' Two other medical stations opened in Kumora and Goremyka in the mid-1920s but the local residents also did not trust the medical assistants who worked there (NARB 247-1-18) and often preferred to seek alternative medical help from *znakhari* [sorcerers] and *kolduny* [magicians] (NARB 247-1-18). They would invite a shaman, or self-treat illnesses using medicinal herbs (Neupokoev 1928:10). Early in the 20th century, it was said that every Evenki knew how to use medicines prepared from medicinal herbs, minerals or animal parts. Therefore, this type of knowledge was shared by all members of a local community. Consequently, people at that time relied mostly on these alternatives rather than on public medicine.

Until the early 1930s, North Baikal Evenkis frequently invited a shaman to heal diseased people. For example, in 1927, B.A. Kuftin, Ia.Ia. Roginskii and M.G. Levin observed two shamanistic rituals performed by Aleksei Aeul'ev and Annushka, known as *Briukhataia Starukha* ['Potbellied Old Woman'] (AMAE RAN 12-1-38, 39, 40, 51, 52). Kuftin also documented that people invited Aleksei Aeul'ev to heal a woman with a nervous disorder (AMAE RAN 12-1-51:46). Generally, shamanism is associated with the knowledge of how to use 'traditional medicines' and it is often taken for granted that they possess a wide knowledge of medicinal herbs. However, in Kholodnaia, local people respected them for their ability to heal through the use of power [*sila*] without the use of medicines. Pana Lekareva stressed that shamans did not usually work with herbs or other medicines; rather they used their own power and healed through communication with spirits. This was unique to shamans and, according to Fana Lekareva, the scale of the healing effect depended on a shaman's sila. Arkadii Lekarev told me that Aleksei Aeul'ev, who did some rituals and was sometimes invited to Dushkachan in order to heal people, was a 'weak' [*slabyi*] shaman. In contrast, according to Kholodnaia villagers as well as the records of Neupokoev (1926, 1928) and Kuftin (AMAE RAN 12-1-38, 39), Annushka was considered to be a 'Big Shaman' [*Bol'shoi Shaman*]. Neupokoev wrote that North Baikal Evenkis considered this old woman to be their main shaman (Neupokoev 1926:29). Neupokoev visited Annushka in 1925 and saw her shamanic clothes in her *iurta* [conical mobile lodge]. He describes a leather mask, a leather dress decorated with ribbons, beads, bells and pieces made from iron and tin. He also saw a drum [*buben*], bunches of reindeer and bear teeth and bones hanging nearby. Finally, there was a wooden stick with an iron trident on the end (Neupokoev 1926:29). Shamans employed these objects as mediators of their power in healing. Some shamanic objects have now become exhibits in school museums, however people still respect them as the 'embodiment of shamanic power' and perceive them as dangerous objects.

The Soviet authorities argued against 'old religious traditions and shamanistic beliefs.' Consequently, early Soviet public propaganda was extremely anti-religious, and shamanistic rituals were perceived by the Soviet authorities as a resistance to the political regime. The 1930s was a period of persecution and oppression of shamans in the North Baikal region, with many Siberian shamans being denounced as 'enemies of the people' [*vragi naroda*], 'exploitative conjurers' and 'psychologically deranged individuals' (Vitebsky 2005:231). Shamans were 'deprived of the vote, kicked out of meetings, stripped of their regalia and exiled' (Slezkine 1994:227). The elders from Kholodnaia remember that the last shaman was imprisoned in the early 1930s.

What I have observed in the region is that people believe not only in shamanic power but also in the ability of *znakhari* [sorcerers] to heal people. *Znakhari* existed among the

The Healing Landscapes of Central and Southeastern Siberia

Russian population in the region before the Revolution of 1917 and even though Soviet authorities imprisoned 'anti-Soviet elements' such as shamans in the 1930s, *znakhari* continued to heal people afterward. For instance, in the 1950s a *znakharka* named Tkacheva treated people in the village of Kumora, trying to heal villagers from tuberculosis, nervous twitches, toothaches and gastric diseases (Koroleva 1950). The local authorities were aware of the existence and activity of *znakhari* but did not punish them. In fact, *znakhari* also heal people in contemporary Kumora and have been known to use their help in treating styes.

Although public medicine had become widely available for villagers during the Soviet period, there was no permanent medical help available to semi-nomadic reindeer herders, who continued to use local knowledge and folk medicine. According to Pana Lekareva, North Baikal Evenkis were taught medicinal herbs and special methods of healing from their childhood. For instance, Evenkis treated headaches using rounded birch sticks (Neupokoev 1928:10). However, folk medicine was not always successful, so Evenkis willingly accepted treatment from medical assistants and physicians who worked in the region. The elders in Kholodnaia still remember one of the first medical professionals, a Russian named Anna Fedorovna Komaritsyna. She worked as a nurse practitioner [*fel'dsher*] in Kholodnaia for more than 40 years and people called her 'The Evenki Doctor.'

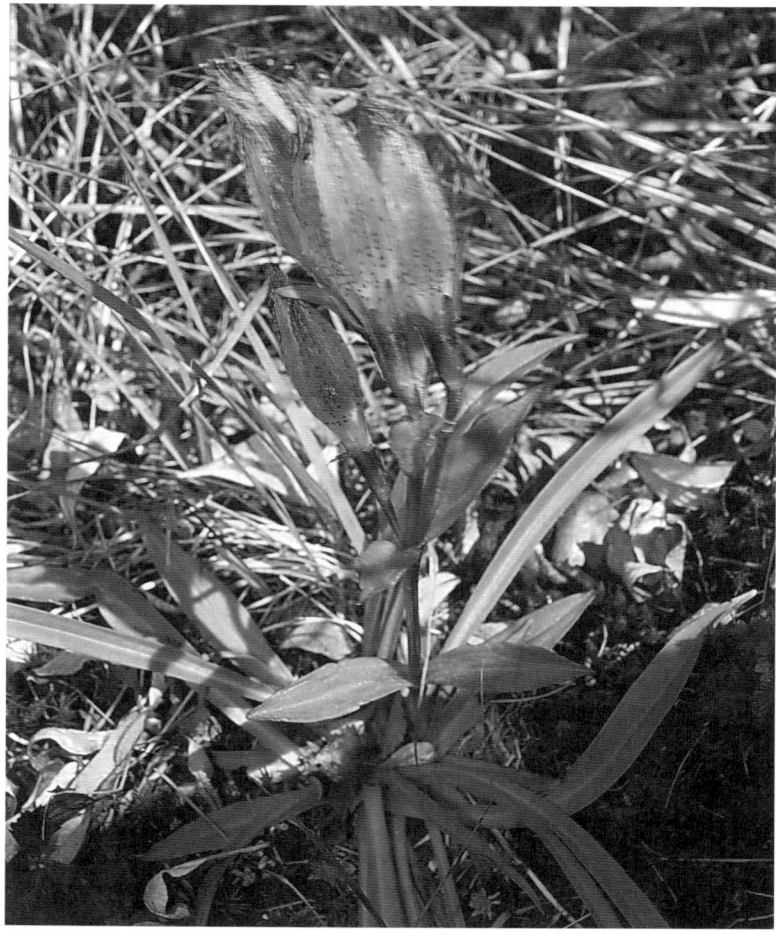

Figure 8.1. Ianda. *Nomama Lake, August 2009.*

Thus, historically, local people combined three main ways of treatment: folk medicine using local knowledge of medicinal plants, minerals and animal parts, healing by the 'power' of shamans and *znakhari*, and visiting medical assistants and physicians. The elders in Kholodnaia stressed that the system of public medicine introduced by the authorities benefitted the people, as medical treatment was free. However, the price of medicine soared after the collapse of the Soviet Union, forcing people back to relying mainly on folk medicine.

Contemporary medical assistants are especially respected in the villages. Today, two Evenki women work in Kholodnaia in a first-aid post, which has two medicine cabinets located in a separate building. However, the doctors prescribe traditional 'Evenki medicines' to their patients along with 'official' medication, and healing using medicinal herbs continues to be relied upon widely in Kholodnaia. Tugolukov (1969:97) wrote that Evenkis knew how to heal fever, heart and skin diseases using folk medicine, and they prepared most of their remedies from plants. Local medical assistants frequently recommend a flowering plant known as *ianda* (*Gentiana algida*) as a medicine for many diseases and infections. It is a rather rare herb and only several villagers know where it grows. The medical assistants usually keep it on hand (Fig. 8.1).

During my fieldwork, I was surprised by the popularity of this herb in the village. Most people considered *ianda* to be the most effective and valuable medicine for all diseases. Today, it is the most frequently used and most valuable medicinal herb in Kholodnaia. For example, Pana Lekareva said the elders told her that *ianda* 'could heal any disease; except torn entrails' [*vse vylechit, tol'ko ciorvannye kishki ne mozhet soedinit'*]. Reindeer herders in a central base near the Nomama River told me that a hunter used it to cure appendicitis; he was two days' walk from the village and unable to get first aid when he felt a strong pain in the right part of his belly. Luckily, he had *ianda* in his winter log house [*zimov'e*] so he prepared a tea from it, which he drank until he felt much better and was able to move to the village. *Ianda* is brewed and drunk for fever, sore throats, chronic tuberculosis or prophylaxis, and consumed to normalize blood pressure. However, it does not suit everybody. Some people with high blood pressure prefer not to drink it because it can increase blood pressure. Nevertheless, it is considered to be especially useful for children and the elderly. For instance, a reindeer herder named Leonid Tulbukonov remembers that as a child his grandmother prepared a tincture [*rastoika*] of this herb and gave him a spoonful almost every day; he still remembers the bitter taste. His parents would also drink this tincture.

Arkadii Lekarev stated that *ianda* is 'the main Evenki medicine' [*osnovnoe lekarstvo Evenkov*], adding that *ianda* in the Evenki language means 'the best medicinal herb' [*samaia khoroshaia trava, lekarstvennaia*]; however, Pana Lekareva translated *ianda* generically as a 'mountainous herb.'

According to Tugolukov (1969:98), Evenkis know how to treat not only themselves, but also their reindeer. People who previously worked in the *kolkhoz* [collective farm] as reindeer herders said they used to give *ianda* to young reindeer to drink, and reindeer herders from Kholodnaia treated weak reindeer using ground *ianda*.

People often learn about medicinal herbs by watching which plants the animals eat and where. For example, people saw that moose like to eat *ianda*, and Pana Lakareva said that diseased dogs also treat themselves with this plant. Another example is *Cladonia rangiferina* [Rus. *iagel'*] collected from the trees and used to ease pain in the stomach; local people say that moose and Manchurian deer treat themselves the same way in winter. Thus, local residents conclude that if a plant helps treat animals, logically the same medicine could be useful for humans.

Leonid's father and uncle worked at a reindeer farm that was a separate *kolkhoz* unit; it was called 'a nomadic reindeer farm' because its location changed from year to year. They used the valleys of the Gasan-Diakit, Niurundukan, Chaia, Tyia and Andoka Rivers—all locations where *ianda* could be found. Thus, Leonid Tulbukonov's relatives knew the location of the plant, and supplied their relatives in the village with medicinal plants, minerals and animal parts. People who work at 'Oron' and 'Uluki' reindeer farms today still usually supply their relatives with various medicines. For instance, Leonid Tulbukonov usually visits the village twice a year, and brings *ianda* in the autumn to his relatives who live there. People may share medicinal herbs and other medicines with their neighbours as well as relatives, and form part of a culture of reciprocity in the village. When people receive *ianda* from their neighbours, they may give them other medicinal herbs or animal fats in exchange and as a sign of respect. Pana Lekareva remembers that hunters and reindeer herders shared *ianda* with the elders. She added that if anyone asked *Iandikan bishin?* [Ev.: 'Do you have a little *ianda* on hand?'], Evenkis always shared it with them. Some people may have surpluses of herbs which they sell to other villagers or to customers in the district [*raion*] centre, Nizhneangarsk.

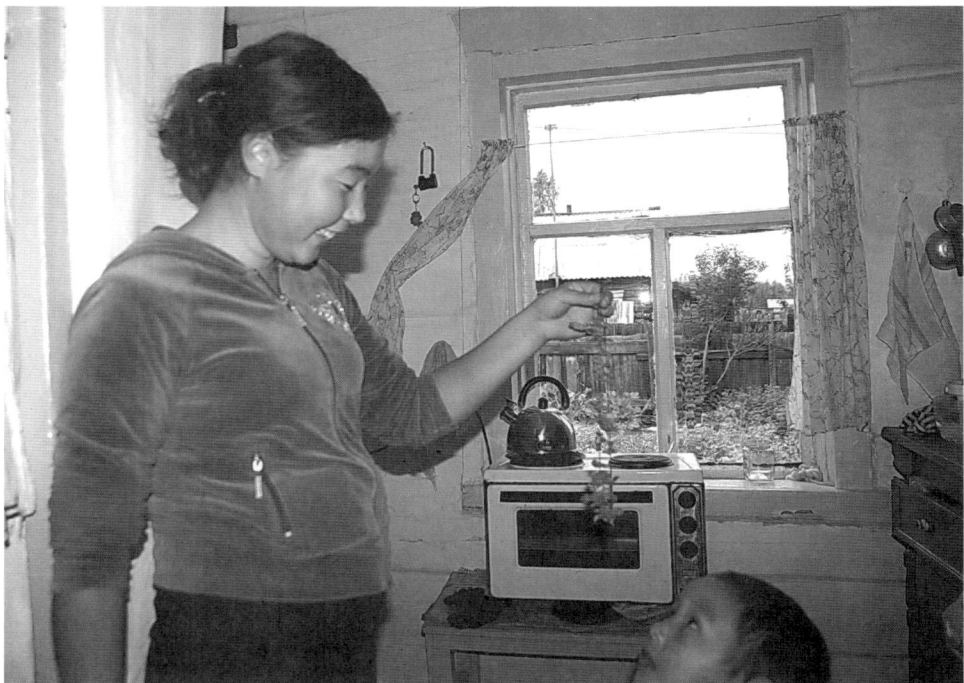

Figure 8.2. *A granddaughter of Pana Platonova holds a bundle of* zolotoi koren'.

Medical assistants in Kholodnaia frequently recommend another 'Evenki medicine' to their patients called by its Russian name *zolotoi koren'* (*Rhodiola rosea*) (Fig. 8.2). Pana Platonova said Evenkis called it *uildyn*, meaning 'emergent' or 'raised,' while Pana Lekareva said that people previously called this plant *uildyun* and thinks that the name came from an Evenki word *u* that means 'liver' or 'pluck.' She interprets *uildyun* as 'the liver healer.' The dictionary prepared by Vasilevich (1958:433) defines *uildyn* as 'bound,' 'connection,' 'bundle,' and 'bunch.' These definitions make sense when the practice of drying *zolotoi koren'* is considered, as people usually cut it into small pieces and connected them like beads.

Chapter Eight: *Public Health and Folk Medicine Among North Baikal Evenkis*

Pana Lekareva remembers that her grandparents used *zolotoi koren'* for treating flatulence; however, today people drink tea made from the roots of this plant as a medicine for many types of disease [*ot vsego p'iut*]. Local people consider both *ianda* and *zolotoi koren'* to be 'universal' medicines and try to keep a store of them.

Both *ianda* and *zolotoi koren'* grow in mountain valleys located some distance from Kholodnaia, and can be found on the shores of mountain lakes and springs. I have observed people gathering them near the foot of the mountains close to Nomama Lake (Figs. 8.3 and 8.4). Hunters and reindeer herders gather *ianda* here from early August to early September, when it is green; in September both plants become red and the *ianda* loses its sap. According to Arkadii Petrovich Lekarev (the eldest man in Kholodnaia), Evenkis gathered *ianda* while hunting marmots (*Marmota sibirica*).

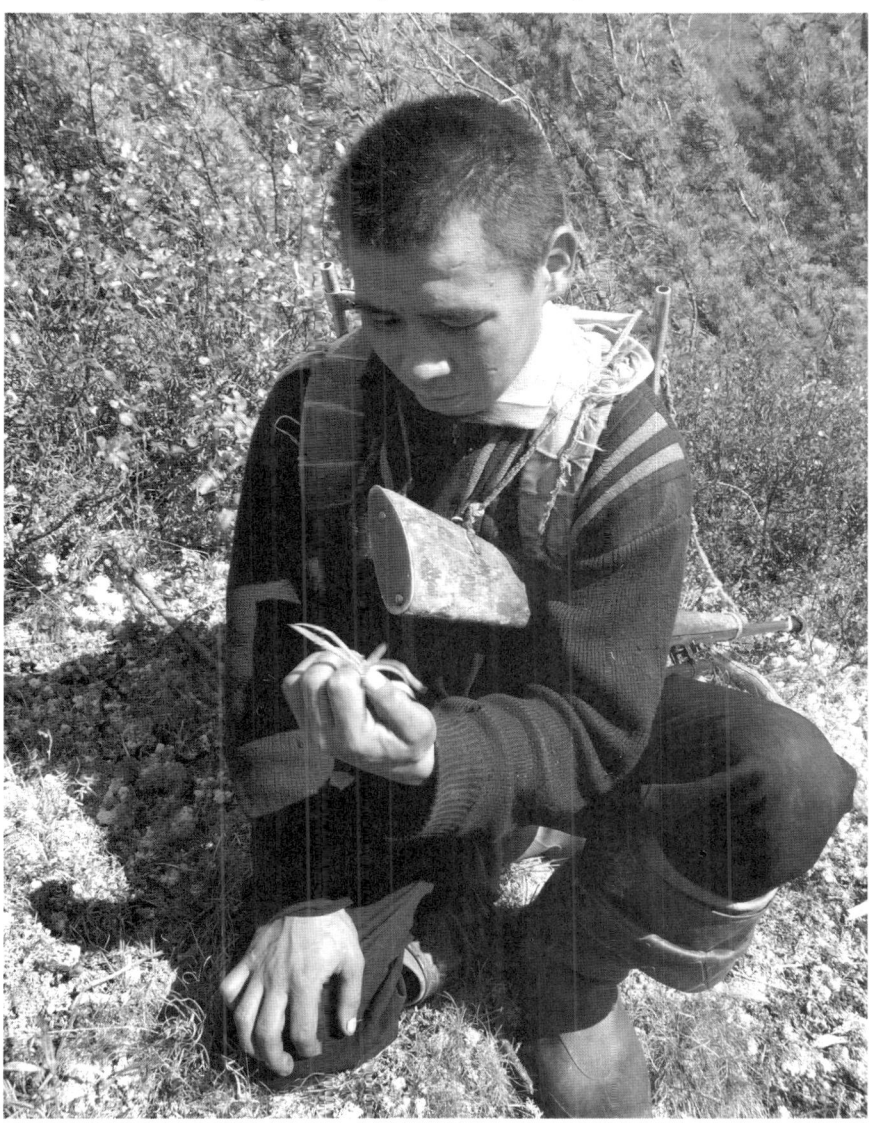

Figure 8.3. *Valerii Falimonov with 'the Evenki medicine'* (ianda).
Nomama Lake, August 2009.

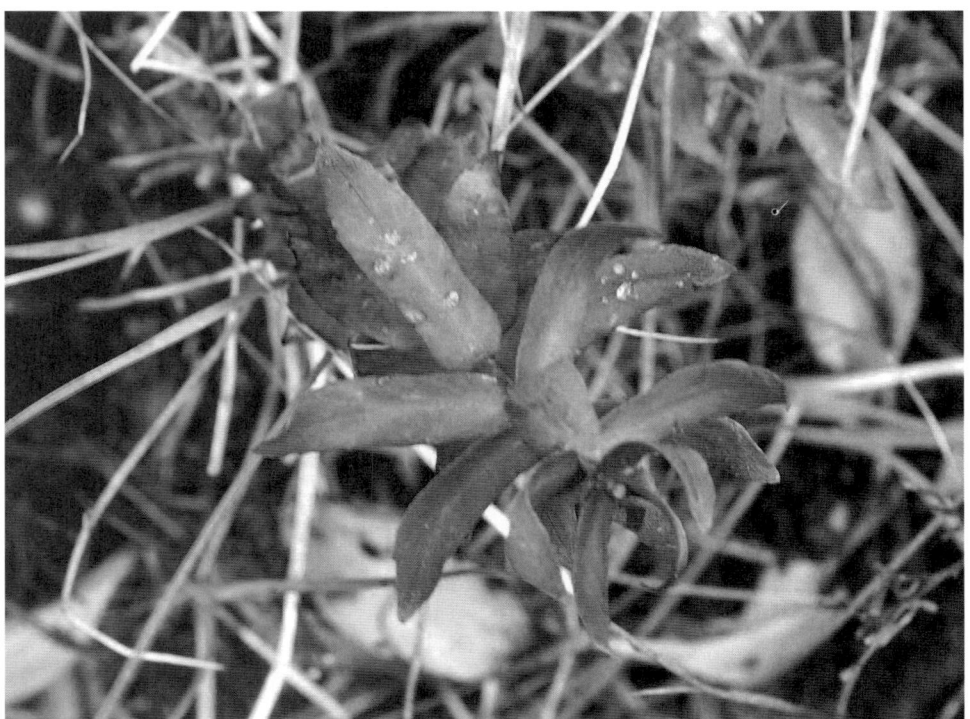

Figure 8.4. Zolotoi koren' (Rhodiola rosea). *Nomama Lake, September 2009.*

The gathering of medicinal plants at Nomama usually involves the preparation of food, a knife [Ev. *kato*], matches and a special Evenki frame backpack [Ev. *poniaga*]. They usually take tea [Ev. *chaimi*], bread [Ev. *kolobo*] and sugar, which are carefully packed in a bag together with the knife and matches, and attached to a *poniaga*. Valerii Filimonov said that his *poniaga* brings him luck [*fartovaia*] in gathering herbs, believing that it helps him to find *ianda*. People also usually take a rifle and cartridges with them to ward off bears [Ev. *amikan*] and to be able to shoot a moose or a Manchurian deer (Fig. 8.5).

Reindeer herders and hunters gather medicinal herbs either collectively or individually. They usually leave early in the morning and it takes about forty minutes to get from the central base of the *obshchina* 'Uluki' to Nomama Lake. This lake is four kilometers long and *ianda* can be found near the water on the opposite shore, as well as along the edges of mountain springs. The shores of the lake are swampy, and so the preference is to travel to the other side by boat. It usually takes an hour and a half to get to the places where *ianda* can be found, but if it's very windy it may take up to three hours to get to the opposite shore. *Ianda* grows only in particular places, which people keep secret, and it is extremely difficult for people traveling to the lake for the first time to find it. It is interesting that I did not observe anyone leaving specific items in return for the plants, however at each site a campfire was made and the plant-hunters fed a piece of bread or bread with paté to the fire. They said that if they had had vodka they would have fed it that instead. *Ianda* is a perennial plant and the older plants have distinctive blooms. Other plants in the area look very similar to it and newcomers often mistake these for the *ianda*. However, *ianda* has a specific bitter taste that the other plants do not. In August 2009, I took part in several trips for gathering medicinal plants. The first time I saw *ianda*, I wasn't sure whether it was the correct plant; Valerii Filimonov tasted it and confirmed that it was *ianda* because of the

Chapter Eight: *Public Health and Folk Medicine Among North Baikal Evenkis*

bitter taste. He added: 'There are some plants that look like *ianda*; however, they are not bitter at all.' Therefore, people usually taste the plants in order to determine whether they are the correct ones.

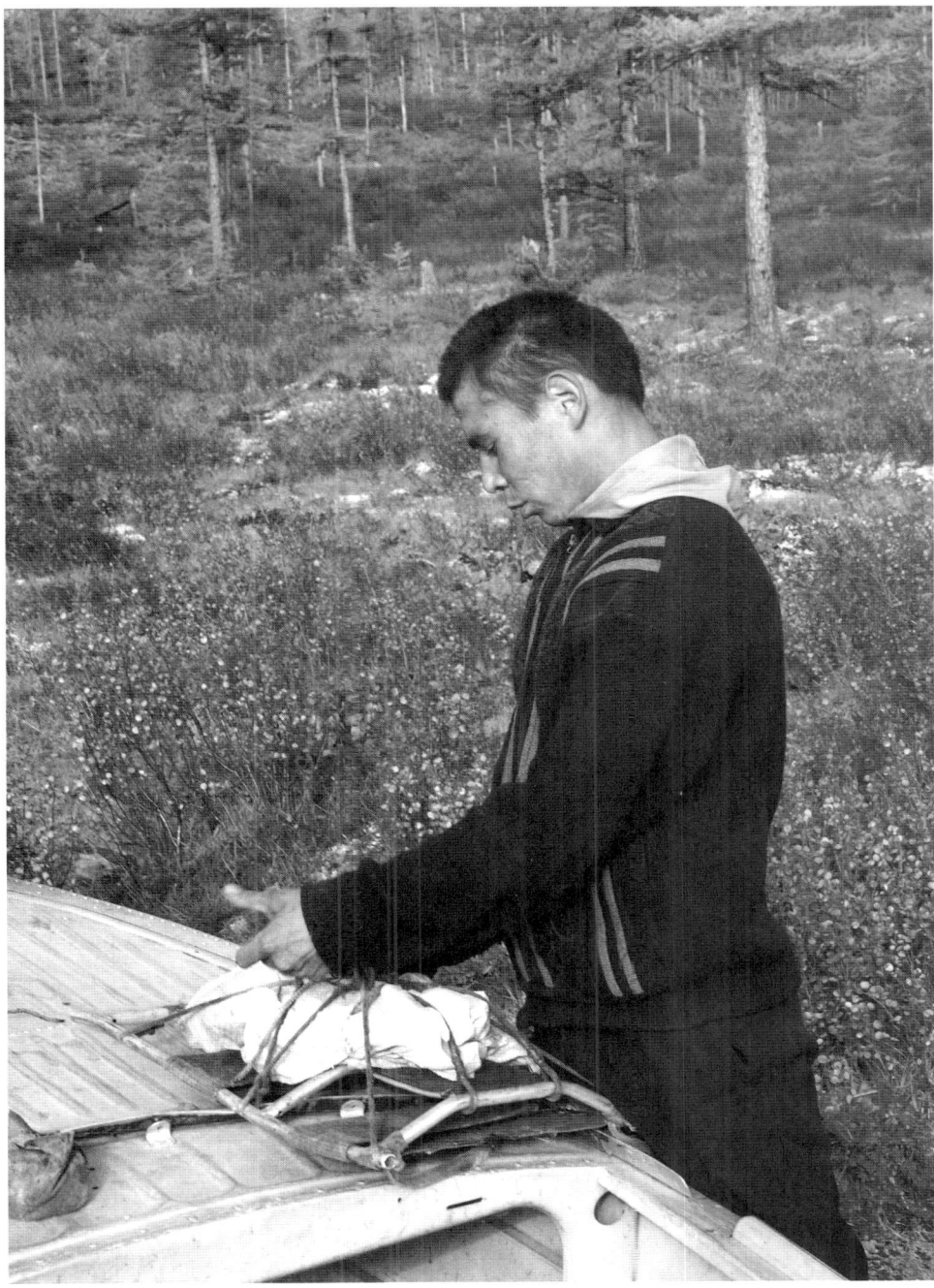

Figure 8.5. *Valerii Filimonov binding a pack with* ianda *to his 'lucky'* poniaga. *Nomama Lake, September 2009.*

The hunters and reindeer herders from the *obshchina* 'Uluki' usually gather these medicinal herbs at the head of the Nomama River as well as on the shores of the lake. The whole plant can be used as a medicine, but Kholodnaia villagers gather only the roots, digging them out using a knife or their fingers, and leave stems with leaves. It is much easier to dig out roots growing on moss-covered hummocks than those growing in the ground.

Gathering *ianda* and *zolotoi koren'* may take several hours; usually both plants are collected on the same trip, but sometimes people will collect only one or the other. People are careful never to take too much of these herbs; they obey the rule of the local environmental ethics and leave some plants for the future. Similar 'voluntary limits' exist in hunting (Sirina 2008:130). Hunters follow certain 'limits on the harvesting of animals, even if they are not codified in such an explicit manner as the wildlife management agencies prefer' (Anderson 2000b:126). Similarly, those who gather medicinal plants never take more than they actually need. Telling funny stories about greedy gatherers serves as a mechanism of social control (Ventsel 2005:269-299).

People do not usually rest until they have gathered enough plants; in fact, to have a rest before completing a task is considered to be bad luck. I was told a comical story about one hunter from Kholodnaia who had started drinking tea just after crossing a tributary of the Nomama River one hundred meters from the main base. People perceive such breaks as undesirable if a hunter wants to return with meat. I argue that the perception of luck in gathering medicinal herbs has many similarities with the perception of luck in hunting. In this sense, local people 'hunt' *ianda*, rather than merely gathering it. When people have gathered enough herbs and are tired, then they usually stop to drink hot tea and have a snack. After drinking tea, people bind a pack with ianda to a *poniaga* and move back to the main base. During my fieldwork I often observed how people bound different things to a *poniaga* carefully and in a masterly fashion (Fig. 8.6).

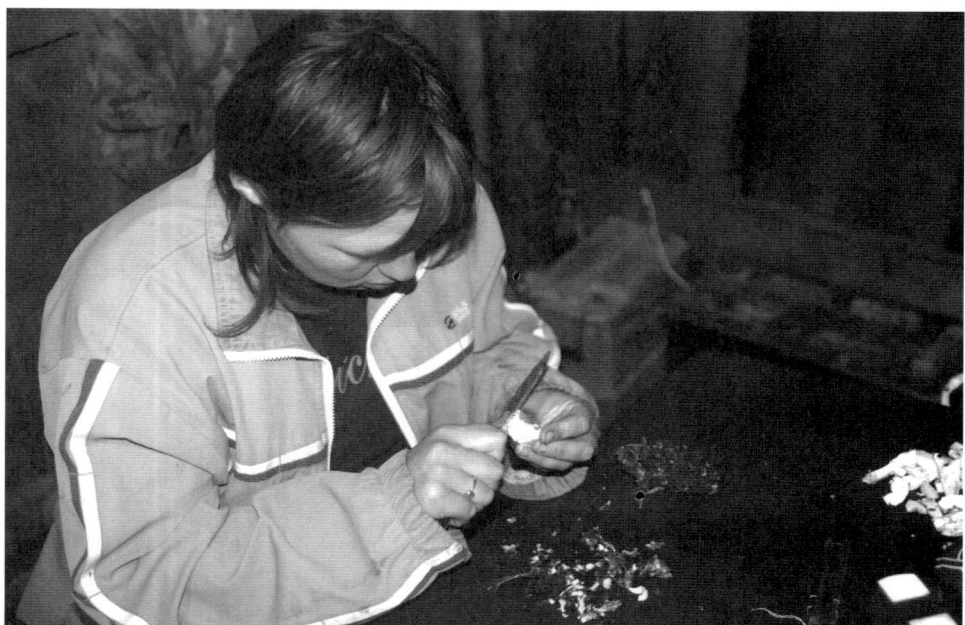

Figure 8.6. *Anastasiia Shangina cleaning* zolotoi koren'. *Nomama, September 2009.*

Chapter Eight: *Public Health and Folk Medicine Among North Baikal Evenkis*

On the return trip, people cross the lake by boat once more, and after beaching it they usually leave a kettle and cups in the boat. The road back to the main base goes downhill, so it usually takes less time than the outward journey. Hence, local people say: "The way back is always shorter!" [*Doroga nazad vsegda koroche!*]. I observed that people usually returned home in the evening when it was getting dark. After their return, they start cleaning the mud from the plants they have gathered using knives, and then sew them together in bunches.

Today, most people dry *ianda* and *zolotoi koren'* for their own consumption. However, the herbs are highly valued and can therefore be sold in times of financial hardship, serving as a reserve resource for many people. Many sell their surplus to other villagers in Nizhneangarsk and Severobaikal'sk, and some even have a circle of regular clients who purchase medicinal herbs from them (Sirina and Fondahl 2006:20) (Fig. 8.7).

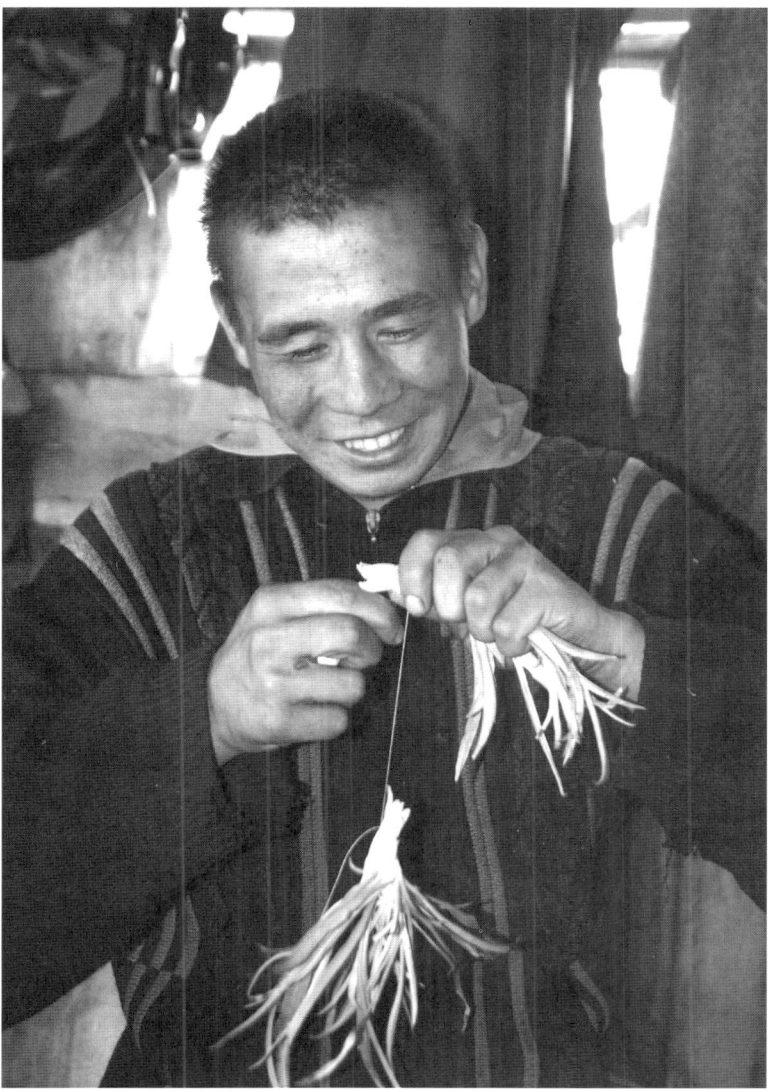

Figure 8.7. *Valerii Filimonov makes bunches from* ianda. *Nomama, August 2009.*

The elders in Kholodnaia say that people previously gathered medicinal herbs mostly for their own consumption, but now they can be easily converted to money or can be exchanged for food or pure grain spirit. I heard from locals that a physician from Nizhneangarsk recommended this 'old Evenki medicine' to his patients and that he regularly buys some medicinal plants from Kholodnaia villagers for his own use and to sell to his clients. In 2008-2007, one small tuft of *ianda* cost from fifty to one hundred roubles in Kholodnaia. Anastasiia Shangina said that in 2007 she sold small bunches of *ianda* in Nizhneangarsk for one hundred and fifty roubles. This is about the price of one litre of vodka in the local stores, and *ianda* can be easily exchanged for vodka. Thus, Valerii joked when he tied *ianda* up in order to make bunches: "This is one bottle of vodka! This is another one! [*Puzyr', eshche puzyr'!*]" (Fig. 8.8).

The growing number of immigrants in the region during the late Soviet period created a situation of competitiveness between the local population and the newcomers. Now, they use the same places and compete for resources such as meat, fish, pine nuts, berries and medicinal herbs. In the first part of the 20th century, a similar competition over resources existed for the gathering of berries and nuts. For example, B.E. Petri wrote that the Russians and Evenkis from the Tutur district in the Irkutsk province vied with each other when visiting berry fields, each trying to get there first in order to start gathering early. In addition, Evenkis were often not able to find berries in the usual places because Russians and Buriats had already cleaned them out (Petri 1930:68).

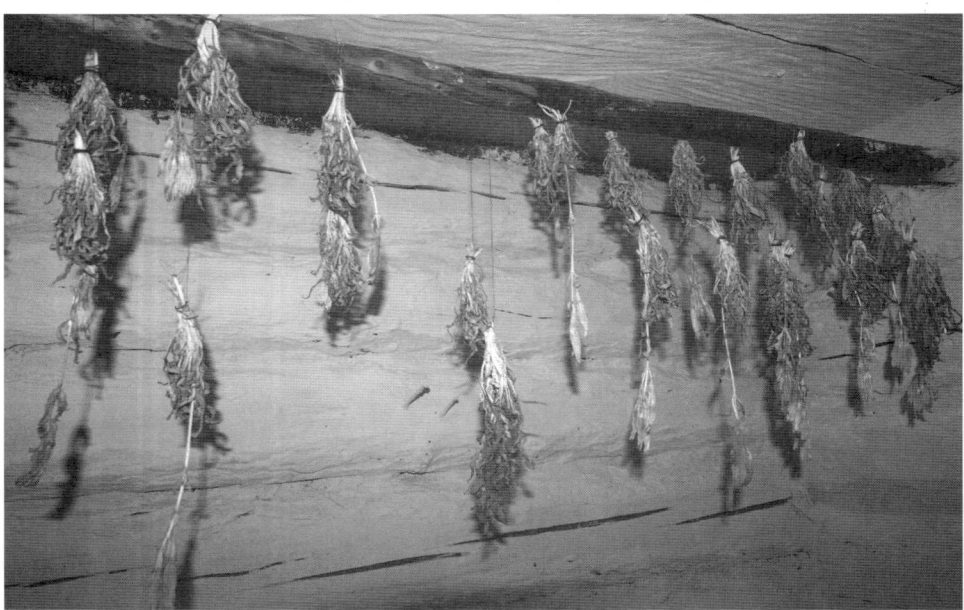

Figure 8.8. Ianda *drying under the ceiling in the* zimov'ie. *Nomama, August 2009.*

The same sort of competition exists today between villagers and newcomers in medicinal herb gathering. The former Baikal–Amur Railway (BAM) builder Sergei Petrovich, who stayed in Kholodnaia and works now as a cook at the reindeer farm, said that *zolotoi koren'* was one of the most popular medicinal herbs among his colleagues who worked as Magirus truck drivers.' Sergei said that BAM builders [*bamovtsy*] 'took everything out near the mountain Dovyren and, as a result, this plant almost disappeared from there.' Now Sergei has to gather *zolotoi koren'* on the territory of the *obshchina* 'Uluki,' located more than fifty kilometers from Kholodnaia. As a result of these kinds of events, people try to keep the knowledge of places rich in medicinal herbs a secret and avoid telling outsiders of the locations. Thus, after visiting the places where *ianda* and *zolotoi koren'* were abundant, I was asked by hunters and reindeer herders not to share the information about the exact locations with other people [*Ty im-to khot' tam ne rasskazyvai!*].

Kholodnaia villagers believe that sunlight reduces the effectiveness of these herbs and therefore recommend drying them in the dark. They also prefer to dry them in small bunches; as mentioned above, *zolotoi koren'* is cut into small pieces and threaded onto a string, like beads. Some people, however, put the pieces on a sheet of paper laid on a flat surface. Hunters dry *ianda* in the space under the ceiling in winter log houses (*zimov'ia*), and it takes about one week to dry (Fig. 8.9).

Pana Lelareva stated that this method of drying *ianda* has been used by Evenkis for many years, since the time when reindeer herders lived mostly in *iurty* [conical mobile lodges], the only difference being that the tendons [*zhily*] of animals were used instead of thread. Keeping the herbs in small bunches was practical, given their constant mobility. In Kholodnaia, people often dry different kinds of herbs in the same place.

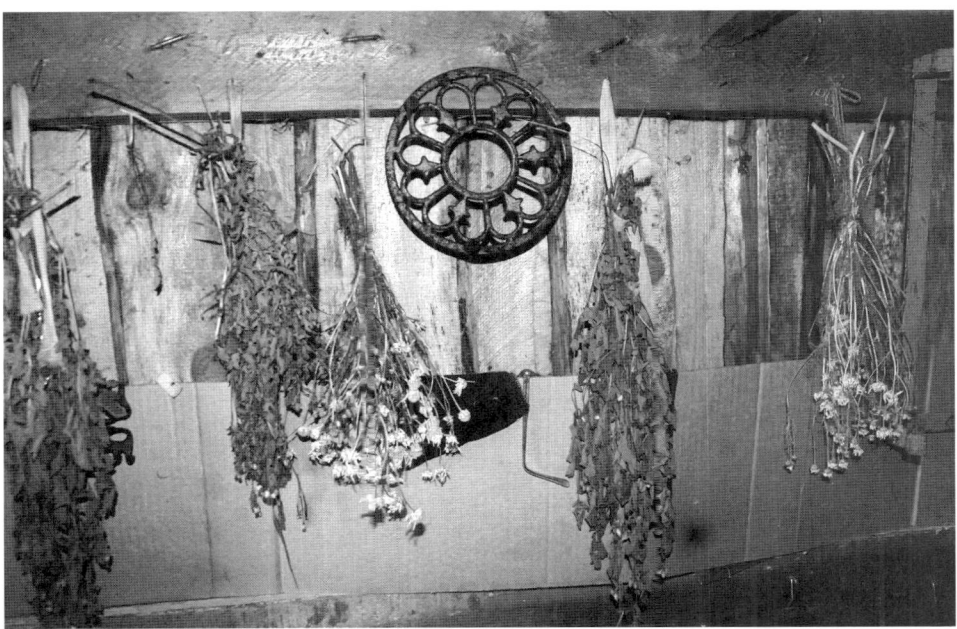

Figure 8.9. *Medicinal herbs drying in a veranda of a house. Kholodnaia, September 2009.*

Every herb has its own spectrum of use. While people use *ianda* and *zolotoi koren'* for healing a wide range of diseases, others are used only for one illness. A type of wild thyme known in the region as *bogorodskaia trava* [Rus.] or *chabrets* [Rus.] (*Thymus serpyllum*) is used for several complaints: short breath, coughs, treating nervous disorders and liver disease. This plant has a strong and pungent smell, so it is also used to 'smudge' [*okurivanie*] a cow after calving in order to avoid a 'bad smell.' Finally, it is used in burial rituals for 'smudging' the dead. The people of Kholodnaia also use another herb as an expectorant, known as Labrador Tea, *sviniachii bagul'nik* [Rus.] or *senkire* [Ev.] (*Ledum* sp.). Pana Lekareva recommends putting both Labrador Tea and wild thyme into a cup and filling it with boiling water. Rita Arpeul'eva said that children used to eat Labrador Tea for fun, despite its bitter taste.

The Healing Landscapes of Central and Southeastern Siberia

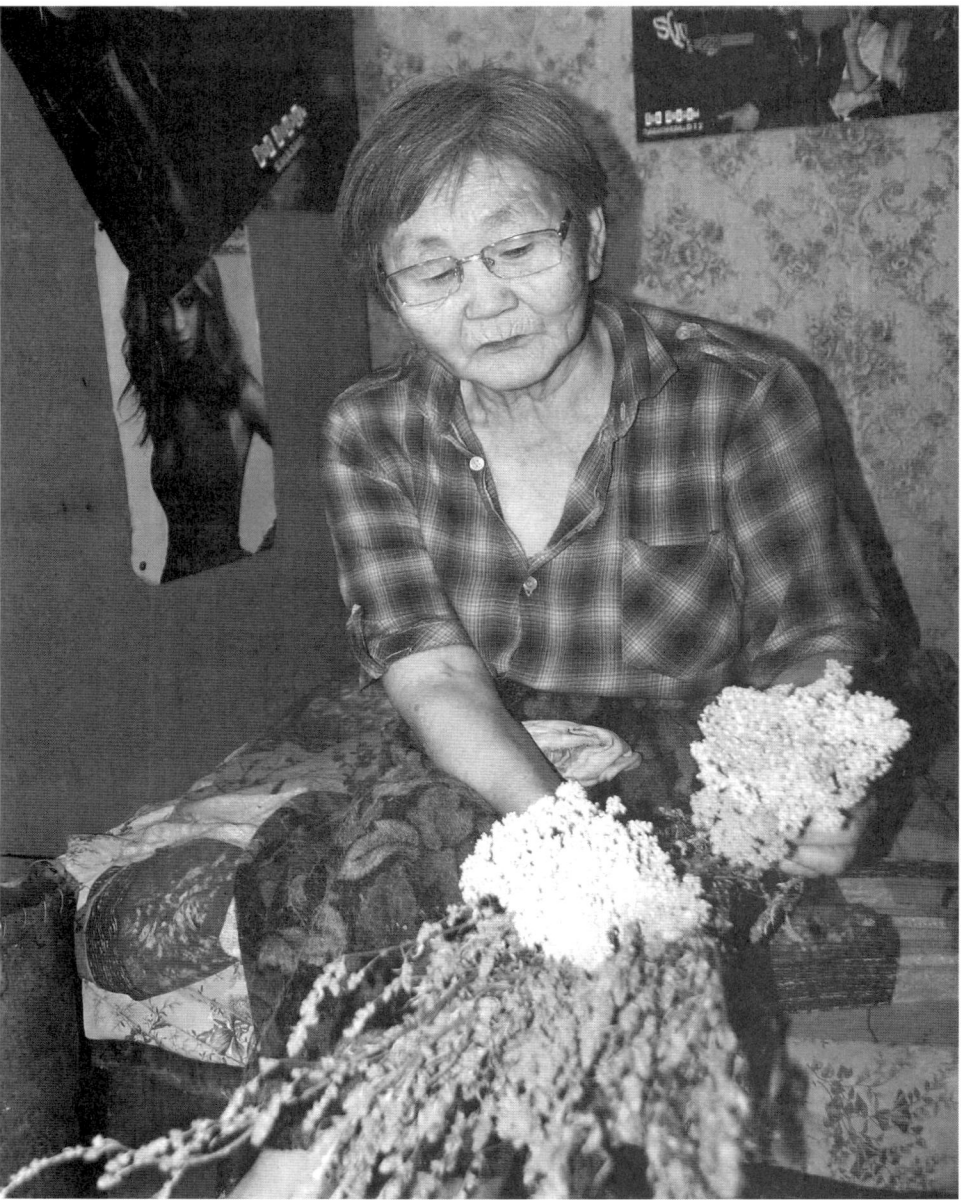

Figure 8.10. *Oktiabrina Uronchina with* polyn' *(Artemisia) and* tysiachelistnik *(Achillea) she had gathered two days before. Kholodnaia, August 2009.*

Other medicinal plants gathered by local people are a wild rhododendron *sakhan-dalia* [Buriat] (*Rhododendron adamsii*) and a cliff fern known as *kamennyi zveroboi* [Rus.] [Ev. *erekte*, *Dryopteris fragrans*]. The wild rhododendron is rather rare in the North Baikal area; it can be found in the mountains near the Chaia River as well as near the former geologists' village of Pereval and looks similar to Labrador Tea. It is drunk as a tonic to normalize low blood pressure and help insomnia. According to the elders, Evenkis have only recently begun to gather *sakhan-dalia*; they learned of it from Buriats and its name came from the Buriat language. The cliff fern is much easier to find, as it grows on scree.

Chapter Eight: *Public Health and Folk Medicine Among North Baikal Evenkis*

Pana Platonova remembers that reindeer herders used to mix *zveroboi* with salt and give it to reindeer, but people also used it to treat themselves (Shubin 2007:169). The plant can be gathered from spring to autumn, and it is considered to be less valuable than *ianda* and *sakhan dalia*. According to local people, *kamennyi zveroboi* helps coughs and it is especially useful for lung diseases and tuberculosis. A plant called *gol'tsevaia polyn'* (*Artemisia* sp.) has a similar medicinal quality. This plant has a strong bitter taste and the mix of *polyn'* and *bogorodskaia trava* is considered to be an effective medicine for habitual drunkenness as it is thought to create an aversion to alcohol. However, people emphasized that the person should want to stop drinking, otherwise the treatment will not help. The elders stress that any type of treatment is effective only when the person wants to be healed.

I observed the gathering of other herbs, *kamennyi zveroboi* and roots of *badan* [Rus.] (*Bergenia* sp.), at the beginning of May. As described above, most people consume a brew of the medicinal herbs and plants when they are ill; however, some of the elderly Evenkis, for example, Viktor Tsyvilev who was born in Tompa Village, used to gnaw the roots of *badan* instead of brewing it. This particular herb is said to help an upset stomach. It is also used to turn leather, used for clothing, black. Other medicinal herbs are not used to cure disease, but for strengthening health. Thus, every summer Oktiabrina Uronchina gathers *tysiachelistnik* (*Achillea* sp.), which increases immunity and helps gastritis (Fig. 8.10).

Some medicinal plants can be extracted at any time of the year, but hunters gather them only when they are needed. For instance, the medicinal herb *chilitkan* [Ev.] grows in the birch forest near the village; it prevents the appearance of pus and also helps drain any pus already present from a wound. When a person is wounded, *chilitkan* can even be gathered from the snow in winter. Oleg Ganiugin from Kholodnaia said he used *chilitkan* on a hand wound sustained during muskrat hunting one autumn and that it helped even better than the special ointment from the local medical centre.

Several other herbs are gathered for different diseases, for instance in order to heal women's diseases, people gather *borovaia matka* [Rus.] (*Orthilia secunda*). Some gather a plant known as *siniukha golubaia* [Rus.] or *ortiliia odnobokaia* [Rus.] (*Polemonium caeruleum*), considered to be useful for people with heart diseases, but it is rather rare in the forests near Kholodnaia. Pana Lekareva told me that stomach diseases, bowel complaints and diarrhoea could be treated with *troelistka* [Rus.] or *vakhta trekhlistnaia* [Rus.] (*Menyanthes trifoliata*), which grows in swampy areas and around lakes. As with *ianda* and other herbs, people observed that moose eat this plant frequently.

Another rare plant, known as *baiunchuka* [Ev.], may be found in the remote, stony, treeless mountains and foothills and is used the same way as *ianda*. It is known mostly to elderly people but they do not know the Russian name of this herb. *Sopchokty* [Ev.] is another herb that the elders of Kholodnaia used to gather; according to Pana Lekareva, the Russian name of this herb is *gornaia valeriana* (*Valerian* sp.) and translates as 'shaggy' [*lokhmataia*]. Both *ianda* and *sopchokty* are high-altitude herbs found in particular locations. These two plants often grow in the same places, but taste quite different. The pedicle of *sopchokty* is similar to those of carrot; however, the leaves are longer and a different colour. It is used instead of iodine as an antiseptic. Wounds can be disinfected using a special powder prepared from this herb; it can also be consumed as a tea. People say that *sopchokty* is even more effective than the disinfectants available in the pharmacy. Arkadii Lekarev emphasized that iodine was not previously available for most Evenkis. Even though there was a small medical centre [*meditsynskii punkt*] in the village when he was young, people who worked at the *kolkhoz* reindeer farm far from the village relied mostly on folk medicine and local knowledge.

Pana Platonova gathers *chistotel* [Rus.] (*Chelidonium* sp.), used to help purify the blood [*ochishchaet krov'*] and treat liver disease. Pana Lekareva said that Evenkis did not previously gather this herb; they only started after learning about it from newcomers. The herb is dried and used to make special tinctures: Pana Lekareva puts dry *chistotel* into a bottle with one glass of sugar, adds vodka and leaves it for ten days. She learned of this tincture when she worked as a cook in a kindergarten and was given this remedy from the local medical centre. Having tried it and felt better the same day, she started making it herself. While medicines were given for free in the Soviet period, tinctures today are rather expensive in the pharmacy so she makes several herself.

Minerals are also used for healing. For broken bones, villagers rely on 'stone-oil' [*kamennoe maslo*], a specific mineral collected from rocks in the mountains (Fig. 8.11). It is extremely rare, and intensive gathering over the last few years has depleted the resources even further, but experienced hunters know where it can be found. It is gathered by shooting a rifle at a rocky outcrop and collecting the mineral from the ground afterward. A local hunter said it appeared on shale [*slantsy*]. People recommend stirring it into water and drinking it; it tastes sour and chewing it is likely to result in damage to the teeth. It is said that parents should be careful when giving this mineral to their children because it can spoil their tooth enamel. Those who have consumed 'stone-oil' say that 'the bones knitted rather rapidly; yet, it was harmful for the teeth.' I met many people who complained about this negative effect of 'stone-oil;' however, they still recommended it to people with fractures believing that 'bones will knit within a week.' Another possible side-effect of consuming 'stone-oil' is constipation. A hunter named Anatolii Shishmarev said that it can also be used externally, for example, it can be made into a compress or a lotion for applying to bruises. Like *ianda*, 'stone-oil' is highly valued by local people and can be sold in Kholodnaia or in the *raion* [district] centre Nizhneangarsk.

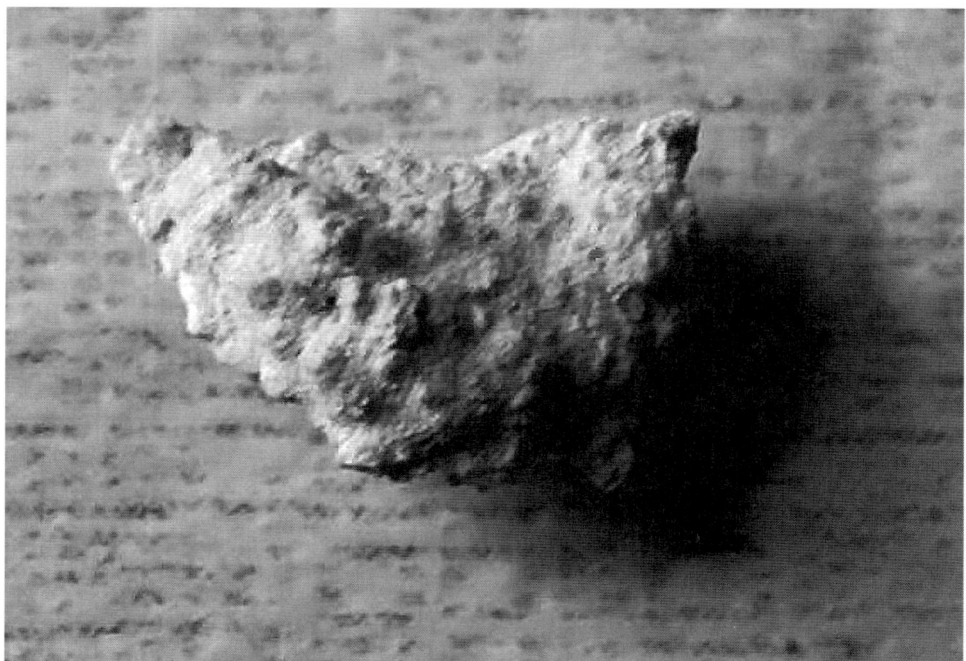

Figure 8.11. *A piece of 'stone-oil' gathered by Leonid Tulbukonov. Kholodnaia, September 2009.*

Chapter Eight: *Public Health and Folk Medicine Among North Baikal Evenkis*

Local people also use animal parts as medicines, and people prepare remedies both for their own consumption and for sale in Nizhneangarsk and Severobaikal'sk. Hunters know the medicinal qualities of bear's gall bladder [*zhelch'*], which is used as a medicine for liver pain, as well as velvet antlers [*panty*] and bears' paws (*see also* Brandišaukas, this volume). The fat of bears, marmots and dogs is used to treat lung diseases. Tuberculosis remains a common and dangerous disease for Evenkis in Buriatiia (Sirina and Fohndal 2006:9). In 2007-2008, there were four chronic tubercular patients [*khroniki*] in Kholodnaia Village. A technician with a mobile X-ray station in the *raion* visits the village regularly and many people have X-ray tests taken every year. However, some people avoid being tested. Generally, eating together with guests from one plate or a frying pan and drinking from one cup is common for many villagers, and this is believed by some to help ward off the disease. Moreover, if one refuses to join, it can be classified as 'disrespect' [*brezglivost'*]. This tradition is common for hunters and reindeer herders, who boil the meat in one pot. In the village, I heard the opinion that a person will never be infected by tuberculosis when he or she eats from one plate with a diseased person and regularly consumes dog meat or fat (Davydov and Simonova 2008: 221).

Consumption of marmot and bear fat is also recommend to those with tuberculosis, and Tugolukov wrote that Evenkis who had tuberculosis consumed not just bear fat, but they also drank bear blood (Tugolukov 1969:97). Mixing the fat with pine nuts is said to increase successful healing.

Many people in the village, however, emphasized that even though folk medicine is extremely useful for healing many diseases, it is 'better not to joke around with tuberculosis' and the best decision for a diseased person is a combination of folk and Western medicine. An Evenki woman from Kholodnaia said: "Of course dog's and bear's fat could help. However, people need also special medicines in order to kill the bacillus. Tuberculosis is of great vitality [*zhivuchii*]." For instance, one person from Kholodnaia who regularly ate dog's meat 'as preventive medicine' [*dlia profilaktiki*], contracted the serious form of tuberculosis intoxication in the summer of 2008 and the medical assistants sent him to a hospital in Ulan-Ude. Many people in the village do not have passports or, consequently or medical insurance certificates [*polisy*]; however, the local medical assistants help them even without these documents.

Finally, people in Kholodnaia believe that fresh air and water can serve as medicines as well. Thus, the reindeer herders say that skin wounds heal much more rapidly in the mountains near the river Nomama compared with in the Southern part of the Republic of Buriatiia during their military service. As a young hunter—Valerii—said, "the lack of bacteria in the mountainous taiga means that 'all skin wounds disappear like on a dog (*zazhivaet kak na sobake*)." He added people never become ill in this place because "the mountainous air is clean and people do not need any other medicines." A phrase I heard repeated many times when people had no opportunity for washing their hands or tableware was: 'There is no dirt in the taiga [*V taige griazi ne byvaet*].' People meant that the environment itself in the mountainous taiga does not support the existence of microbes.

In summary, this chapter outlined the main remedies of Evenki folk medicine used by the people of Kholodnaia. The villagers use a combination of both public and folk medicine. In the case of illness, people consult many different specialists, such as *znakhari*, *shamany* and *fel'dshery*, as well as find remedies in the forest on their own. In other words, both nurse-practitioners and specialists in folk medicine are actively engaged into healing practices, demonstrating the existence of medical pluralism in northern Buriatiia as identified by K. Metzo. It follows that local medicinal knowledge is not set in opposition to state medicine. There is no strict border between these domains of knowledge for local people; rather folk medicine has become an integral part of the public health system. However, this integration was not initiated from above, because local nurse practitioners [*fel'dshery*] did not acquire special training in folk medicine as part of their formal training and studies in college. Rather, they possess this knowledge as members of the local community. Consequently, the use of this knowledge in combination with remedies from the drugstore is a result of their own experience. Even though it is possible to buy medicines at Kholodnaia's first-aid post, many people continue to rely on 'Evenki medicines' too. Furthermore, as D. Brandišauskas has shown in his chapter, medicinal knowledge is not a property of a narrow circle of specialists, but it is shared by all representatives of the local community and can be considered part of their daily knowledge of subsistence. At the same time, local people try to keep secret the knowledge of the location of various forest medicines, which became the objects of accumulation, from the BAM newcomers who became their main competitors in the taiga. Gathering 'medicines in the forest' helps local people save money and acquire extra economic reserves, and they continue to be reliable medicines in remote locations such as reindeer herders' and hunters' base camps, where permanent and professional medical first aid is not available.

Acknowledgements

I would like to thank the School of Social Sciences, University of Aberdeen and the Social Sciences and Humanities Research Council of Canada (SSHRCC MCRI 412-2005-1004) for funds supporting my ten months of fieldwork and five months of archival and library research in 2007-2008.This chapter was prepared in 2010 during a research fellowship at the University of Tromsø sponsored by The Research Council of Norway (Yggdrasil, project no. 195702).

Chapter Nine

The Categories of Ket Spiritual Healing

Edward Vajda

Ket Healing Practices in a North Asian Context

The Ket family groups who traveled near the Enisei River and its tributaries in Russia's Turukhansk District were some of the last hunter-gatherers of Inner Eurasia (*see* Figs. 9.1 and 9.2).

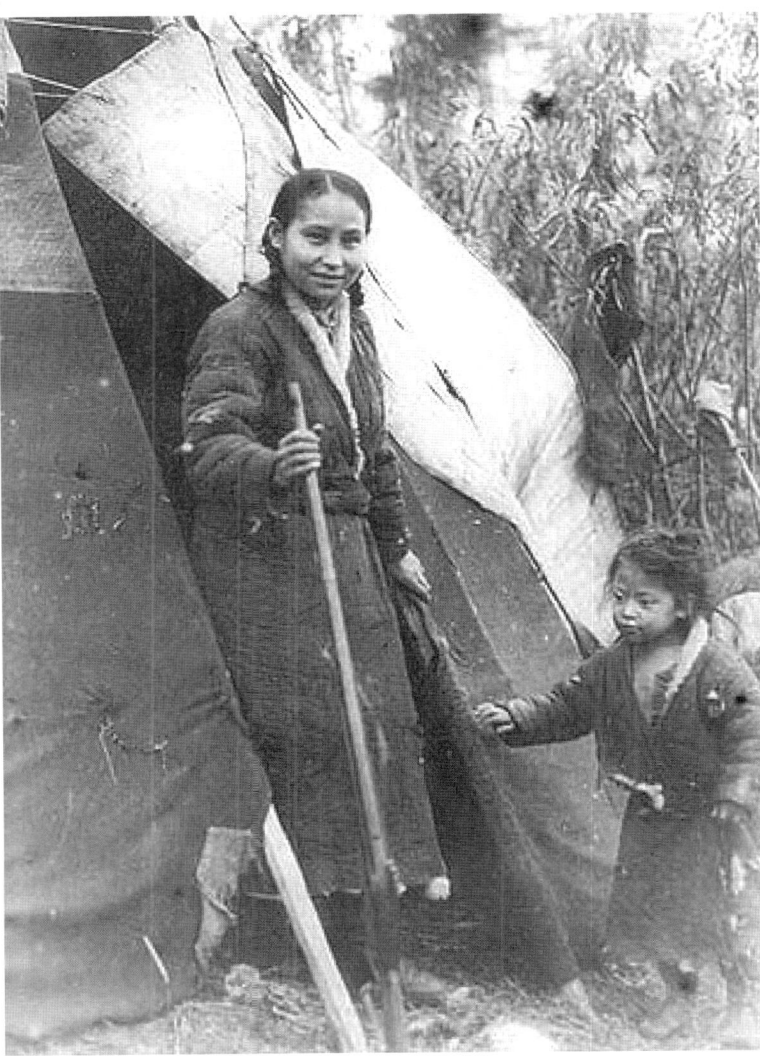

Figure 9.1. *Ket woman beside birchbark tent.* Photo by V.I. Anuchin, 1906.

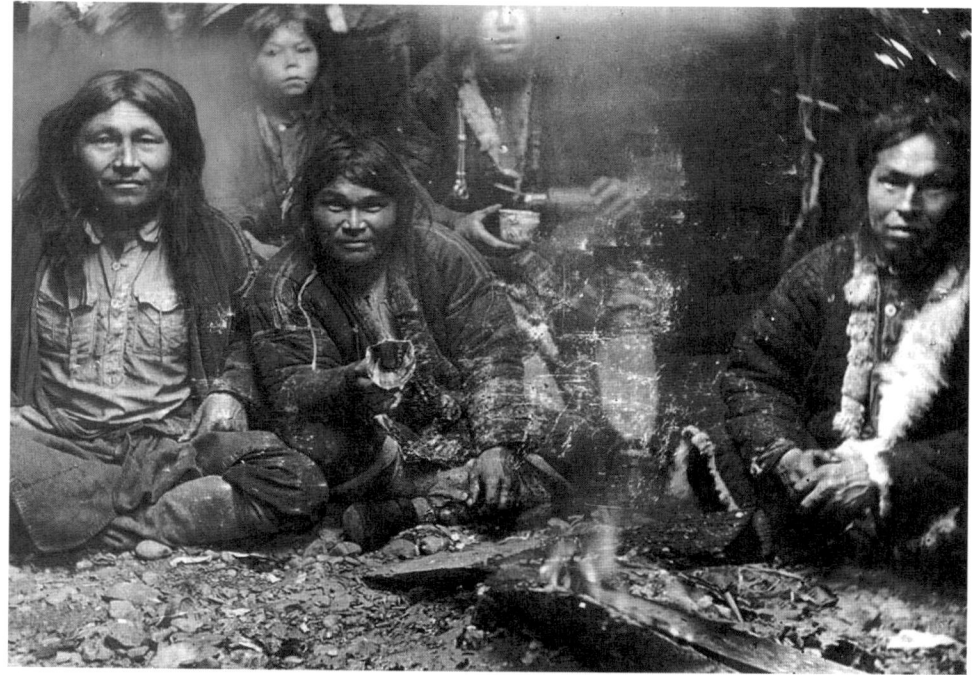

Figure 9.2. *Ket men inside a tent. Photo by Hans Findeisen, 1927.*
Photo by Janina Findeisen.

Ket traditions of spiritual healing are particularly interesting, as they can shed light on the ancient cultures of the North before the advent of reindeer domestication. Beliefs about the spiritual nature of human illness were closely tied to the methods employed to heal various maladies. Spiritual healing was practiced primarily by the *sening*—the Ket shaman. There were five categories of shamans, each with its own spirit and animal helpers as well as distinct paraphernalia. Kets also had a category of folk healers called the *bangos* whose healing practices were not connected with shamanistic rituals and who specialized in curing different types of illnesses. The sections that follow discuss what is known in Ket traditional lore about illness and healing, describing the various specialties and practices of the *sening* and *bangos*.

A Word About Kets and Those Who Have Studied Them

Kets today are the last remaining Eniseian people. Their southern relatives—the Iugh, Kott, Assan, Arin and Pumpokol—all died out during the last three centuries, and little is known of the distinct shamanistic practices of these tribes. Kets have survived because they chose to live in one of the most isolated parts of modern Siberia. The Turukhansk District has yet to see modern development based on the exploitation of underground reserves of oil, natural gas or minerals, although exploration is underway. There are no cities or even roads or railroad links in this vast area, which is much larger than the territory of modern Germany. Nearly all of the 1,200 or so people recorded in the 1989 census as ethnic Kets live in small villages near the Enisei or its tributaries, where they were settled during the Soviet collectivization of the 1930s. Detailed and relatively current available demographic information can be found in Krivonogov (1998, 2003).

Chapter Nine: *The Categories of Ket Spiritual Healing*

Traditional ethnographic accounts such as Shrenk (1883:256-7) place Kets among the 'Paleosiberians' or 'Paleoasiatics' together with Iukagirs, Iupiks, Itelmens, Nivkhs, and Ainu sea-mammal hunters and fishers of the North Pacific Rim, though Ket origins and language are in fact separate from these peoples. Though Ket shamanism reveals a number of unique aspects, particularly in its distinction between categories of shamans, the features shared with other West Siberian forest peoples such as Sel'kups and Khantys, as well as with South Siberian Turks (Khakases, Altaians, Shors), place it squarely within the cultural heritage of spiritual traditions from aboriginal central Siberia.[1]

Originally referred to as the Enisei Ostiak, they were studied first-hand ethnographically only in 1905-1908, when V. Anuchin of the Imperial Academy of Sciences recorded detailed information about their material and spiritual culture. The objects Anuchin brought back to St. Petersburg are the basis of the Peter the Great Museum of Anthropology and Ethnography's collection of Ket artifacts. Anuchin's (1914) monograph on Ket shamanism contains a wealth of information on both the *sening* and *bargos*, much of it not recorded again by subsequent fieldworkers. The Finnish linguist Kai Donner visited Kets in 1912 during the second of the three years he spent in central Siberia. Donner (1933) contains valuable remarks on shamanism, some of it collected from Ilia F. Dibikov, a young Ket man who visited the author in Finland for three months in 1926. Writings left by 18th or 19th century explorers deal primarily with the Ket language, though some include brief anthropological observations pertinent to the study of shamans (cf. Vajda 2001:1-17, 92-94).

The next researcher of Ket ethnography was from Germany. After the establishment of the USSR, the new Soviet Government invited Berlin Museum worker Hans Findeisen to spend 13 months in 1927-28 among Kets in the area of the Podkamennaia Tunguska River. Findeisen's chief interest was shamanism, and he collected a vast amount of data, including songs, photographs (*see* Figs. 9.2 and 9.3), artifacts, and folkloric texts. Much of Findeisen's material remains unpublished and some of it seems to have been destroyed by Allied bombing raids in the Second World War (Janina Findeisen, personal communication). Findeisen's pioneering and invaluable work on Ket shamanism remains largely unknown, aside from what he included in his general monograph on shamanism (Findeisen 1953).

The next major advance in the study of Ket shamanism began in the 1960s in connection with three decades of ethnographic fieldwork conducted by Evgeniia A. Alekseenko on behalf of the same Peter the Great Museum of Anthropology and Ethnography that houses the earlier collections by Anuchin and Karger (*see* Fig. 3). Some of her most important findings derived from fieldwork conducted during expeditions in the summers of 1970 to 1972, undertaken primarily to gather new data on Ket shamanism. The essential readings on Ket shamanism are Alekseenko (1967, 1978, 1979, 1981a, 1981b, 1984a, 1984b, 1992, 1997), though this list far from exhausts that author's published works. Vajda (2001:20-41) contains an annotated bibliography of Alekseenko's numerous publications on Ket ethnography between 1959 and 1998.

Invaluable information on the five categories of Ket shamans appears in English for the first time in Alekseenko (1978). Each category was distinguished by specific differences in their dress and paraphernalia. Dr. Alekseenko was able to show that the detailed description of the shaman's costume found in Anuchin (1914) actually described only one particular category of shaman, the *qaduks* or reindeer shaman. Each of the five categories also had distinctive spirit helpers. They also differ as to their ability to travel up to the sky or to other realms during their shamanic trances (*see below*). Because shamanism throughout the North was actively suppressed by Soviet authorities beginning in early 1930s, only

---

[1] For more on Ket ethnic origins and historical interactions *see* Vajda (2010a).

Anuchin, Donner and Findeisen were able to observe traditional Ket spiritual life in open practice, and even this picture was likely no more than a remnant of what had once existed before the social dislocations brought on by the importation of European diseases and the imposition of *iasak* (the fur tax) beginning in the 17th century. Nevertheless, the salvage ethnographic studies conducted by Alekseenko beginning in the late 1950s have uncovered many previously unknown facts about Ket shamanism. It is to Evgeniia Alekseenko that the present author wishes to dedicate this overview of traditional Ket healing practices.

Other studies conducted during the second half of the 20th century also mention previously undocumented aspects of Ket shamanism, notably Kreinovich's (1969) description of the traditional economic life-cycle of Kets living as nomads in the vicinity of the Podkamennaia Tunguska River. Nikolaev (1985) traces the ethnic origins of different aspects of Ket culture, some apparently connected with the forest, others with steppe pastoral peoples farther to the south. Ivanov and Toporov (1969) compare Ket mythological elements with other Native Siberian traditions. Werner (2006:51-63) analyzes shamanism along with other aspects of traditional Ket culture by comparing Ket vocabulary with that recorded from the extinct southern Eniseian languages. Werner's work is also valuable for its compilation of shamanic lexicon—special words used by shamans during their songs and séances. The annotated bibliography in Vajda (2001) provides descriptive commentary on all publications dealing with Ket shamanism through 1998 (*cf.* especially the indexed listing on pp. 384-5).

Life Essence and its Spiritual Link to the Nature of Illness

Anuchin (1914:11) reported that Kets possessed "amazingly few healing resources" as well as an unexpectedly sparse knowledge of plant lore, given the fact that they were forest hunter-gatherers. Plant lore is also weakly represented in the Ket language, and even the best speakers of Ket today have but a limited repertoire of names for individual herbaceous plants. Because healing practices among Kets were documented only in the 20th century, however, it is plausible that some earlier traditions disappeared unrecorded. One reason for the lack of medical practice is that Kets attributed all illnesses not to physical problems with the human body itself but rather to the condition of its *ulvei*—the immortal life essence thought to animate each human being. Kets believed every person possessed an *ulvei*. This word literally means 'water-wind' and is often translated as 'soul' [Rus. *dusha*] in descriptions of Ket spiritual culture. Kets believed that every person was inhabited by seven spirits, the number seven figuring prominently throughout Ket folklore and belief. Among these seven, only the *ulvei* was absolutely essential to the person's well-being. The rest were acquired from eating various plants and animals and little is known about their individual characteristics. Unlike the other spirits, which could inhabit plants and animals as well as humans, the *ulvei* could only inhabit a human being or a bear, the latter being regarded as a lost human relative. According to Pavel Sutlin (personal communication), the *ulvei* possessed the form of a small person. A similarly anthropomorphic image of the *ulvei* appears in Anuchin (1914:10), who relates how the evil witch Hosedam imprisoned the *ulvei* of the great shaman Doh by nailing its hands and feet to a tree, after which Doh lost his shadow and was unable to remain on the earth, thereafter dwelling in the second layer of the sky. Illness typically occurred when an *ulvei* wandered too far from its owner. Chills were diagnosed as a sign that the *ulvei* had gotten lost in a cold place, while fever resulted if the *ulvei* became overheated. Serious illness such as paralysis or coma indicated that the *ulvei* had lost its way completely or had been captured by Hosedam, the evil witch of the north who devoured lost human souls. Long-term absence of the *ulvei*, unless remedied by shamanic rituals, eventually caused the death of its human host.

When a person died, his *ulvei* could pass into the sky or descend to the underworld, later returning to inhabit another individual. The *ulvei* itself was considered to be immortal. One of the shaman's duties at funerals was to divine whether the *ulvei* had departed to the sky or to the underworld. An *ulvei* outside a human body experienced neither torment nor ecstasy, but simply waited in a sort of limbo for the next incarnation. Typically, the *ulvei* was reincarnated when it entered the body of an unborn baby near the time of birth by passing through the sex organs (Anuchin 1914:10). A chief task of the shaman-healer was to locate a missing *ulvei* and return it to its owner, thus curing severe illness. This quest was one of the main aims of the shaman's singing and dancing. The shaman was also able to discover why an *ulvei* was ill or out of sorts, in which case the person it animated would show the same symptoms. Hosedam, evil goddess of the North, hunted down and consumed *ulvei* that wandered too far, causing the illness and death of their owners. Hosedam and her many servants were principal adversaries of the shaman.

As mentioned above, two categories of people in Ket society were traditionally involved in healing the sick. These were the shaman (known as *sening*) and the sorcerer [*bangos*, or *bangoket*, a term meaning 'earth person']. The *sening* operated exclusively through magical intervention involving contact with the spirit world and did not resort to the use of natural medicines, while the *bangos* treated the sick with the help of talismans containing various plants and minerals. Certain categories of shamans were connected with the upper, heavenly world and were helped by myriad spirits [*esdeng*] who dwelled in the seven layers of the sky. The *bangos* by contrast, was confined to the earthly realm and also had knowledge of the underworld. Such people were said to be able to see no higher than the flight of a bat, yet they could peer far down into the earth (Anuchin 1914:19). The bat, mole, and snake were animals associated with the *bangos* and his earthly power. The *sening*, by contrast, was able to ascend up to the sky or fly far across the earth in order to commune with the spirit world, and each *sening* had his unique path, secret from that of other shamans. According to Anuchin, (1914:25) there were no 'black' or evil shamans among Kets, whereas a *bangos* could cast both good and bad spells on people. For example, the *bangos* was thought to be able either to cure or induce rheumatism in people. Both *sening* and *bangos* claimed to be able to foretell the future and predict good fortune for hunters. This suggests that *sening* and *bangos* were social roles, rather than invariably distinct personages or entirely unrelated traditions. Anuchin (1914:32) reports that of fourteen shamans operating among Kets during his 1906-08 expedition, several functioned as *bangos*, as well. The latter role was most effective on moonless nights, whereas *sening* typically began their séances in the evening, preferably when both sun and moon were visible in the sky. In general, the practice of *sening* as opposed to *bangos* magic was kept in separate spheres, and even *bangos* talismans were disallowed during shamanic séances (Anuchin 1914:19). Unfortunately, no detailed study of the *bangos* was ever made and it is possible that this social role represents the survival of a more ancient healing tradition.

To recapture lost or stolen *ulvei* and return them to their owners, the shaman resorted to a trance-like state that assisted his flight into other realms. During my stay on the Elogui River in August, 2009, one elderly woman told me that shamans used to ingest the fly agaric mushroom, *Amanita muscaria*, which is called *hango* in Ket, in order to achieve the trance-like state needed to conduct spiritual healing. It was the shaman's task, assisted by his spirit helpers, to fight Hosedam or any other malevolent entities that stood in the way of accomplishing this feat. Ket lore held that the great shamans of the past could induce Hosedam to regurgitate the souls she had swallowed, after which they could be reunited with their owner. If the owner had already died, the *ulvei* would become free to be born into a new human baby. The Ket culture hero Alba, a figure with folkloric parallels among the South Siberian Turks (Ivanov and Toporov 1969; Nikolaev 1985), was said to have liberated many souls by inducing vomiting and diarrhea in Hosedam. Generally only shamans had the capacity to traverse the dangerous northwest trail into the realm of the northern witch to battle her for control of the *ulvei*. The shaman's ability to undergo the shamanic trance and travel to the spirit world was thus considered crucial to the health of all members of society.

According to Kets, there were also material causes behind certain diseases. Chronic maladies afflicting people were thought to be caused by a rock getting into the sick person. The shaman was able to remove the rock with the help of the spirit of the gray crane [*tau*], which extracted the object with its long beak. The loon [*bit*] was also seen as a shamanic bird in light of its keen ability to dive from the air into the water to get food. Shamans would employ their loon spirits to find wayward ulvei who had become lost in the underworld realm.

The Shaman's Gift

Among Kets, both men and women could become shamans. Anuchin (1914:23) claims that the shamanic gift was passed on to a member of the opposite sex in the next generation so that it alternated between males and females in the same family line. Alekseenko, however, noted that while the shaman's gift was inherited within the confines of a single family group, the preponderance of shamans were men, as were all great shamans, so that a strict gender-based intergenerational skewing does not appear to have been a universal norm, at least not by the 20th century. Women shamans were unable to travel up to the sky and were limited to the earthly realm in their shamanic quests (Alekseenko 1978, 1981b).

Shamans differed from ordinary people through family inheritance of the shaman's gift, or *qut*. The *qut* is conceptualized as an anthropomorphic spirit that is passed from one generation to the next. The *qut* also brought special 'sky people' [*esdeng*], shamanic helper spirits whose power likewise passed from one shaman to a relative in the next generation (Alekseenko 1981b:99). The *qut* was immortal, with each bearer merely representing a single link in the chain of its earthly manifestation. It could not be shared by two shamans in the same family simultaneously, but passed on only after the death of the older shaman. The shaman's song is also known as *qut*, and the same root appears in verb forms expressing shamanic dancing and singing: *duqut* 'he shamanizes,' *dilqut* 'he shamanized.' Finally, this root also forms the basis of the word *quttyn* (or *qutn*), used as a synonym for *sening*—'shaman.' The latter word appears to be more ancient in that it is found in some of the extinct southern Eniseian languages as well as in Ket.

The shaman's gift sometimes became evident at a young age, when a child proved to be high-strung and unsociable. More often it manifested itself in young adulthood, when the individual would fall into a sort of mental illness called *dariy*. This word is translated as 'shaman's illness,' though it is also used in modern Ket to refer to any sort of mental illness. According to Anuchin (1914:24), the *qut* might appear to a twenty-year old and summon him to begin shamanizing. Other spirits would follow, causing the inchoate shaman to become unsociable, to laugh or cry without obvious cause, and to feel the urge to sing or dance. According to Anuchin's informants, a person beset with *dariy* who resisted the shamanic call might become permanently insane or even die, but one who heeded it spent the next few months or years learning to master the spirits that had come to him. It was considered that every shaman had a choice of seven spiritual trails, one of which was fatal to him. Finding one's proper trail, the secret path to be taken during shamanic trances, was essential for the beginning shaman, as was composing the proper song [*qut*]. Generally, a person called by the spirits to become a shaman would succeed in finding his proper trail and in composing his unique song. He would master the spirits that had induced *dariy* and would regain his mental health. As a sign to the community that this had occurred, the beginning shaman would request that a beater stick [*hatbul*] be made for him. A man or woman who received this first *hatbul*, which was typically fashioned from semi-rotten wood to symbolize its temporary character, was called a 'minor shaman' [*hyna sening*]. There was no other custom of shamanic initiation among Kets, no public ceremony. Minor shamans had no drum and simply sat beside the fire singing their spirit song, keeping tempo by hitting the beater stick against the left shin to summon the spirits (Anuchin 1914:26).

According to Anuchin (1914), the shaman grew increasingly powerful with practice. Shamans destined to possess the greatest power would go through seven stages of three-year cycles to finally become a 'great shaman' [*qa sering*], capable of traveling to the upper levels of the sky. With each successive stage, the shaman acquired more spirit helpers. Great shamans were uncommon, and always were old men (Anuchin 1914:25). Such a powerful spirit gift was greatly prized by the families that possessed it. Alekseenko (1981b) explains how the majority of shamans did not follow this complex path of maturation but remained what she called 'family shamans,' that is, minor shamans [*hena sening*] who shamanized only occasionally and, as a rule, only within the confines of their own family group. A minor shaman who later refused to acquire a drum progressed no further in the development of his shamanic powers. Such shamans appear much closer in function to the *bangos*, since they likewise healed minor ailments. Both minor shamans and *bangos* were able to foretell the future or divine answers to questions by tossing a bear paw up into the air, the palm landing skyward denoting an affirmative answer to whatever yes-or-no question had been posed to the spirits. Minor shamans often lacked both drum and special clothing. Great shamans equipped with the full accoutrement of shamanic regalia were much less common. When a shaman died, his basic regalia were placed by his grave to decay—a sign that the spirits were ready to pass to the shaman's descendant. But a great shaman's iron pendants and perhaps his crown and the top of his staff were handed down directly rather than left to the elements. As important family heirlooms they were kept in a special box called a *qossul*. The contents and form of one *qossul*, translated as 'shaman's sled,' is described in detail in Alekseenko (1981a), an article containing illustrations of the various iron spirit images that once belonged to a great shaman.

Anuchin (1914:33) described the clothing and paraphernalia associated with the stages of becoming a full-fledged 'big' shaman. The individual elements were received in a specific order, as the shaman became increasingly more powerful through the acquisition of more and more spirit helpers. The first item was the temporary beater stick [*hatbul*], followed by a headband [*tuneng*]. This was followed by the acquisition of a breast pendant [*qutn*], then boots and gloves [*senda tesing* and *senda boon*]. A crucial stage in becoming a stronger shaman was receiving a drum [*has*] and a new beater stick. This was followed by a shaman's staff [*tagoks*], then by a coat and crown [*senda qat* and *senda dy'*], the latter two objects being acquired simultaneously. As shamans gained more spirit helpers, they also received an increasing number of iron pendants symbolizing these spirits. Pendants were placed on the shaman's coat during shamanic séances. Shamans destined to become great shamans would eventually receive a second drum. The round drum shape is shared between Kets and most other peoples of south-central Siberia, notably the Altai Turks and the Samoedic Sel'kup. According to Findeisen (1953), the drum of the Ket shaman is larger than that of other Siberian tribes (*see* Fig. 9. 3).

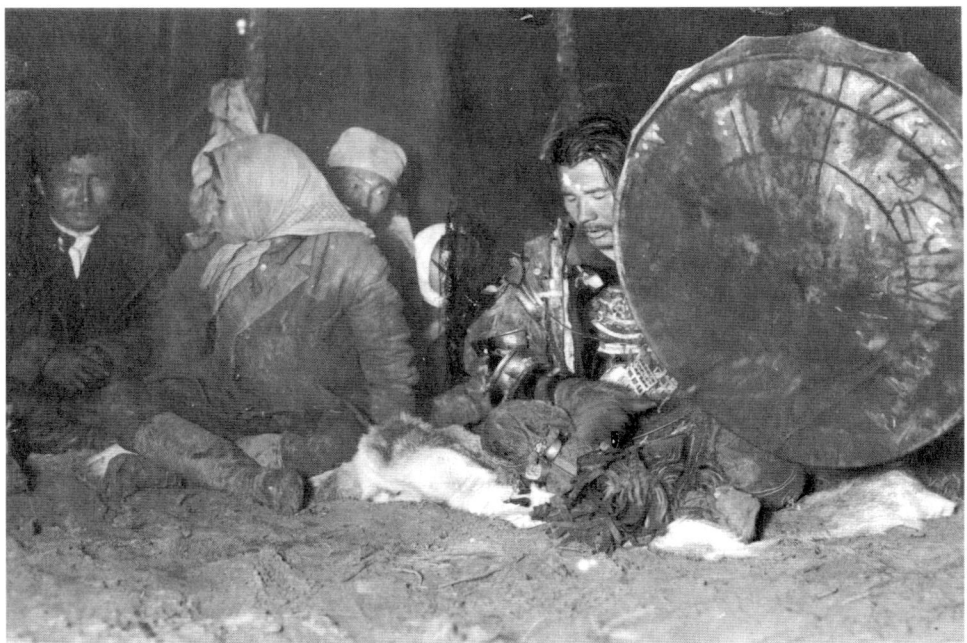

Figure 9.3. *Ket shaman with drum.*
Photo by Hans Findeisen, courtesy of Janina Findeisen.

The fieldwork performed by Alekseenko in the early 1970s added an important new dimension to our understanding of the Ket shaman by elucidating the presence of five distinct categories of shamans, distinguished by different primary animal helpers and consequently by different types of clothing and other regalia (Alekseenko 1978). The shaman costume described so elaborately in Anuchin (1914) is, in fact, typical for only one particular category. This happened to be the most widespread type, called the *qaduks* shaman, whose main spirit helper is a flying female reindeer, known as *qaduks*, a word not found outside of shamanic parlance. This category of shaman ascended to the sky world by transforming his drum into a female reindeer as his mount. The membrane of *qaduks* shaman's drum was made of reindeer skin. A *qaduks* great shaman typically had reindeer horns made of iron as part of his headgear (*see* Fig. 9.4).

In contrast to the *qaduks* shaman, the bear shaman generally did not ascend into the sky but rather took horizontal paths across the earth, especially in a direction leading to the forbidding northwest, where Hosedam was thought to keep the stolen souls of unfortunate people. The bear shaman possessed no drum and used a bear paw instead of a drumstick. When shamanizing he sometimes fastened the dried nose and mouth portions of a bear over his face, keeping them in place with a rawhide strap. His clothing was made of bearskin and contained iron images of the bones of bears. There was also a category of shaman whose patron spirit was an anthropomorphic being called *kandelok*, an enigmatic figure that sported bear paws instead of hands. The *kandelok* shaman also had an iron headdress described by Alekseenko (1978:261) as resembling a sort of helmet. Bear shamans and *kandelok* shamans possessed bear spirit helpers. They were also assisted by the *allel* family guardian spirits and by the *dangols*, or spirits of dead ancestors.

Chapter Nine: *The Categories of Ket Spiritual Healing*

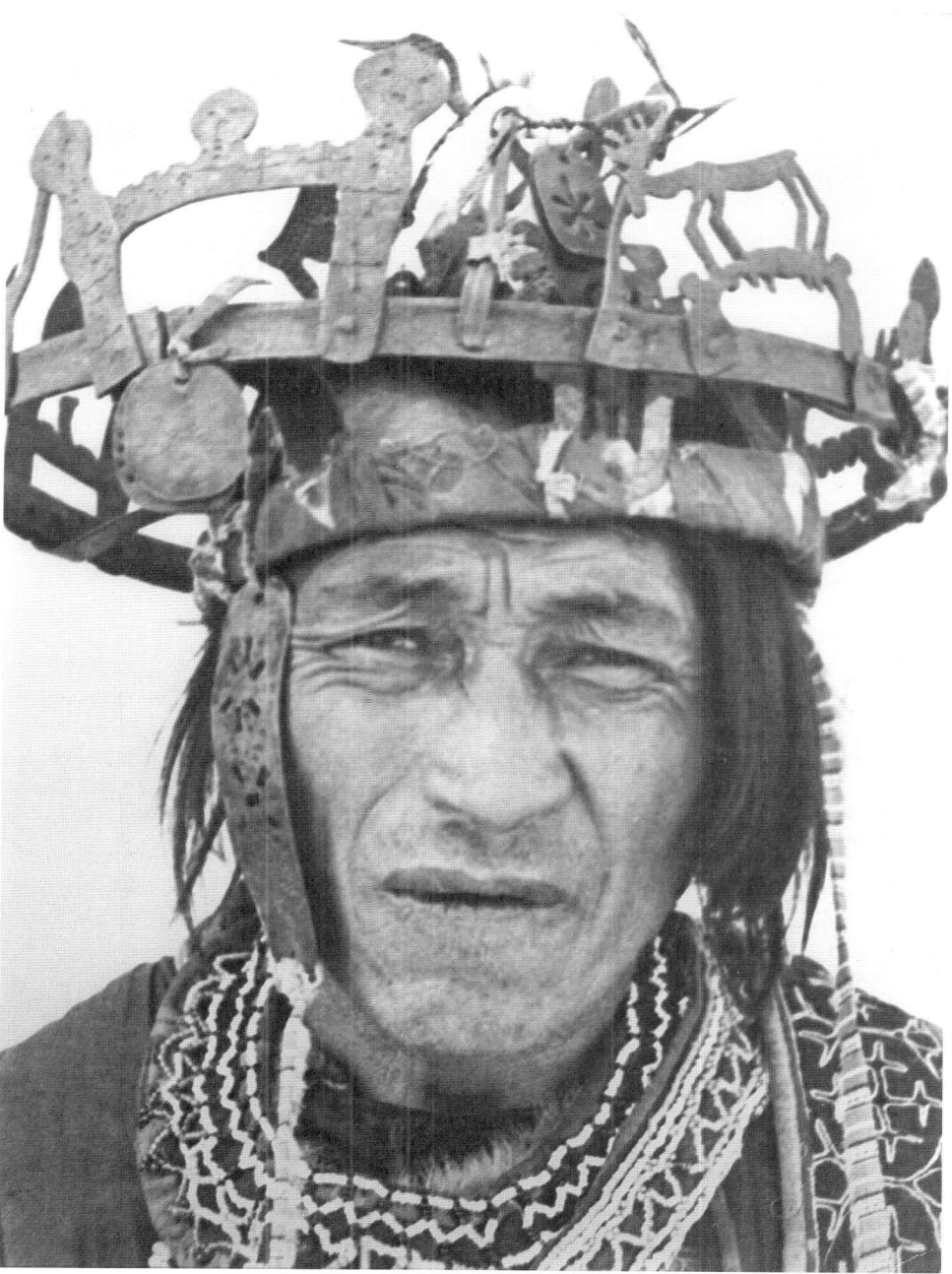

Figure 9.4 .*Reindeer shaman's headgear, Kellog Village 1976.*
Photo courtesy of Heinrich Werner.

Another category of shaman was associated with a mythical giant eagle known as *dagh*, said to be large enough to cover the sun. Iron images of eagle claws often adorned the eagle shaman's coat. Eagle feathers were especially prized by this type of shaman, who, like the *qaduks* shaman, could ascend to the sky and receive assistance from spirits there. Interestingly, the eagle was said to have first taught humans how to shamanize. In one version, the first shaman had originally been an eagle; in another version a two-headed eagle taught humans to shamanize and was punished by losing one of his heads, in a sort of Siberian analog to the Prometheus myth. Two-headed eagle images are often found among the shaman's iron pendants. The first great shaman Doh seems to have been an eagle shaman, as an eagle often perched on his shoulder. Among Kets it was taboo to kill eagles, and eagle feathers that happened to be found on the ground were displayed in special places of honor in the tent.

The final category of shaman was the dragonfly [*dynd*] shaman, whose coat tapered to a point in the back, symbolizing the insect's shape. A photograph in Alekseenko (1967:191) illustrates the dragonfly shaman's headdress, which sported iron plates formed in the shape of thunderclouds. This type of shaman was thought to be the most powerful, and could ascend to the highest levels of the sky accessible to humans. His patrons were the dragonfly, the swan, and also Tomam, benevolent goddess of the south revered for sending the migrating birds northward every summer. The swan [*tigh*], a sacred bird that could not be hunted, served as special spirit helper to the dragonfly shaman. Dragonfly shamans could only operate in warm months, however, during the brief summer when the dragonfly, swan, and other migratory birds sent by Tomam were present. Dragonfly shamans seem to have been the least common type of shaman, whereas minor shamans most often belonged to the *qaduks* category. These did not acquire a drum or headdress and practiced with a drumstick, wearing regular clothing and the special headband known as *tuneng* (Aleskeenko 1981b:104).

The seven trails accessible to shamans for use in their spiritual healing quests were apportioned differently according to the category to which the shaman belonged (Alekseenko 1978:261). The *qaduks*, bear, *dagh* and *kandelok* shamans all were capable of traveling from southwest to northwest, into the frozen realm of Hosedam. The dragonfly shaman could travel only to the southwest, along two different trails. All shamans except the bear shaman could travel east toward the sunrise. Bear shamans were confined to the earth, while the other categories could also fly up to the sky during their quests, though the *kandelok* shamans, like the bear shaman, normally operated in the earthly realm.

The Evolution of Ket Shamanism—In Place of a Conclusion

Kets are broadly similar to other early hunter-gatherers across the globe, where certain members of the tribe are regarded as being endowed with special powers to heal the sick through spiritual intervention, normally accomplished through magical singing. The root of the word sening 'shaman,' appears related to words meaning 'sing shamanically' in the languages of the North American Athabaskans, Eyak, and Tlingit (Vajda 2010b). If correct, this linguistic comparison reveals the deep antiquity of shamanic practice in the Northern Hemisphere. At the same time, many features of Ket shamanism reveal close parallels with the peoples of the Altai-Sayan Mountains of south-central Siberia notably the Altai, Khakas and Shor Turks. The round shape of the Ket shaman's tamborine is very similar to that of Altai-Sayan peoples, and the name of this instrument [*has*] is possibly shared with languages of steppe pastoralists. The Buryat Mongol word for 'shaman's drum' [*xese*] and the Teleut and Tubalar Turkic word for 'hoop' [*kash*] may represent the same word as Ket has, 'shaman's drum.' Alekseenko (1984b:81) suggests these words originated from the expansion of steppe nomads in the Hunnic Era, before the rise of the First Turk Kaghanate in 552AD. Alongside the word *sening*, the Ket shaman is also known as *quttyng*, a term apparently derived from *qut,* a loanword into Ket meaning 'shaman's gift' or 'shaman's song' that in Turkic seems to have originally meant 'spirit.' The whole complex of belief in the sacred sky world and the ascent of the shaman skyward to find spirit helpers there appears borrowed from interaction with Turkic steppe peoples. The word *qaduks* 'flying female reindeer,' a figure associated most obviously to the ability of shamans to ascend to the sky, likewise appears to lack any Native Ket etymology. The vertical axis of sacred sky and profane underworld duplicates the probably more ancient Ket horizontal dichotomy, whereby the upriver south appears as sacred in contrast to the downriver north, the location of Hosedam and the area where souls are lost or devoured (Vajda 2010c). A later Turkic origin for more elaborate social forms of shamanism also coincides with the arrival of iron from the steppe peoples and its association with details of the shaman's costume. The original Ket shaman, the *sening*, was probably more like the *bangos* sorcerer, with lore of the earth being central to the most ancient traditions of spiritual healing

The mixed forest and steppe shamanic heritage of the Ket tribes encountered by the Russian state in the early 17th century was left mostly unchanged, despite interference from the Russian Orthodox Church. Only in the 19th century did Christian proselytizers begin to make inroads into the traditional world of Ket spiritual belief (Alekseenko 1979). Even here, however, reported baptisms resulted at most in a conversion in name only, as Kets generally maintained their beliefs in shamanism and other pre-Russian traditions. edical knowledge from the Russians was slow to penetrate the rth, due to the extreme isolation of the forests through which most Ket lived as nomads, so that before the mid 20th century it did not significantly compete with shamanic, spiritual-based cures. Until the latter half of the 20th century, family shamans and *bangos* appear to have undertaken the largest share of healing in the community.

Only when Soviet power became firmly established in the North did this scenario rapidly begin to change. Bolshevik rule first suppressed the Russian Orthodox Church, a change that actually granted the local shamans a respite from competition by a state-sponsored ideology. Then shamanism was attacked during the 1930s, and Kets forced to settle in Russian-style villages. One of the most elderly informants recalls seeing a pile of broken drums and other profaned shamanic attributes left lying in the mud by the post office in Kellog Village during the first wholesale anti-shaman campaign. Everyone saw this destruction as the loss of power by the shamans, since a broken drum symbolized the death of the shaman who owned it. The establishment of modern medical personnel in the North undermined reliance on traditional forms of spiritual healing, though Kets continued regularly to make recourse to shamanic magic within the confines of their own family, especially when living as nomads through the forests during the fall and winter hunts. The small-scale family practice of shamanism went underground, where it barely survived. The age of 'great shamans' known far and wide was over forever.

The last shaman in Kellog Village died in the 1970s, and his costume, modeled by his son, appears in Fig. 9.4. According to my informants, there are no longer any true shamans among Kets. The survivals of active Ket shamanism into the last quarter of the 20th century reported by Alekseenko (1997) appear to have largely disappeared by now. One hunter told me there would be no more shamans, because "*Es* [the sky deity] will never again send shamans to the people after how they were treated." Even basic knowledge of shamanic lore survives among no more than a select few of the oldest generation of Ket. This makes the ethnographic descriptions by Anuchin, Donner, Findeisen, and Alekseenko all the more invaluable as the sole surviving record of a tradition of folk healing that is partly unique among indigenous peoples.

Acknowledgements
Dedicated to Evgeniia A. Alekseenko (Peter the Great Museum of Anthropology and Ethnography, St. Petersburg, Russia), whose decades of fieldwork have provided a far richer portrait of traditional Ket healing practices than would otherwise have survived.

References

Aiusheeva, L.V. (2007). *Tibetskaia meditsina v Rossii*. Ulan-Ude: Izd-vo BTS 'Rinpoche-bagsha.'

Alekhin, K.A. (1999). *K voprosu o traditsionnoi meditsine taezhnykh evenkov*. Gumanitarnye nauki v Sibiri. Seriia: Arkheologiia i etnografiia, Vol. 3: 93-96.

Alekseenko, E.A. (1967). *Kety: etnograficheskie ocherki*. Moscow: Nauka.

Alekseenko, E.A. (1978). 'Categories of the Ket shamans,' pp. 255-264 in V. Diószegi and M. Hoppál, eds., *Shamanism in Siberia*. Budapest: Akademiai Kiadó.

Alekseenko, E.A. (1979). 'Khristianizatsiia na Turukhanskom severe i ee vliianie na mirovozzrenie i religioznye kul'ty ketov,' pp. 50-85 in I.S. Vdovin, ed., *Khristianstvo i lamaizm u korennogo naseleniia Sibiri*. Leningrad: Nauka.

Alekseenko, E.A. (1981a). 'Shamanskaia narta (qossul) u ketov,' pp. 169-178 in I.S. Vdovin, ed., *Material'naia kul'tura i mifologiia*. In series: Sbornik Muzeia Antropologii i Etnografii tom XXXVII. Leningrad: Nauka.

Alekseenko, E.A. (1981b). 'Shamanstvo u ketov,' pp. 90-128 in I.S. Vdovin, ed., *Problemy istorii obshchestvennogo soznaniia aborigenov*. Leningrad: Nauka.

Alekseenko, E.A. (1984a). 'Etnokul'turnye aspekty izucheniia shamanstva u ketov,' pp. 50-73 in C.M. Taksami, ed., *Etnokul'turnye kontakty narodov Sibiri*. Leningrad: Nauka.

Alekseenko, E.A. (1984b). 'Iuzhnosibirskie paralleli v shamanstve ketov,' pp. 77-82 in I.N. Gemuev and Iu.S. Khudiakov, eds., *Etnografiia narodov Sibiri*. Novosibirsk: Nauka.

Alekseenko, E.A. (1992). 'Zhenskoe shamanstvo i mirovozrenie ketov,' pp. 5-11 in I.S. Gurvich and R.F. Its, eds., *Rannie formy religii narodov Sibiri*. St. Petersburg: Muzei antropologii i etnologii.

Alekseenko, E.A. (1997). 'K izucheniiu shamanstva u ketov,' pp. 195-202 in C.M. Taksami, ed., *Kul'tura narodov Sibiri. Materialy III sibirskikh chtenii*. St. Petersburg: Muzei antropologii i etnologii.

Alekseev, N.A. (1992). *Traditsionnye religioznye verovaniia tiurkoiazychnykh narodov*. Novosibirsk: Nauka.

Anuchin, V.I. (1914). *Ocherk shamanstva u eniseiskikh ostiakov*. St. Petersburg: Imperial Academy of Sciences.

Altman, N. (2000). *Healing Springs*. Rochester, VT: Healing Arts Press.

Alves, R. and I.L. Rosa (2005). Why study the use of animal products in traditional medicines? *Journal of Ethnobiology and Ethnomedicine* 1:5 doi:10.1186/1746-4269-1-5

Alves, R.R.N., M.D.G. Oliveira, *et al*. (2010). An ethnozoological survey of medicinal animals commercialized in the markets of Campina Grande, NE Brazil. *Human Ecology Review* 17(1): 11-17.

Anderson, D.Dz. (2001). *Narodnaia Meditsina*. Novosibirsk: Sibprint.

Anderson, D.Dz. and Iu.V. Popkov, eds. (2001). *Bezopastnaia pit'evaia voda v usloviakh Severnogo poselka: Kanadskii i mezhdunarodnii opyt'*. Novosibirsk: Sibprint.

Anderson, D.G. (2000a). 'Surrogate currencies and the wild market in central Siberia,' pp. 318-344 in P. Seabright, ed., *The Vanishing Rouble: Barter Networks and Non-Monetary Transactions in Post-Soviet Societies*. Cambridge: Cambridge University Press.

Anderson, D.G. (2000b). *Identity and Ecology in Arctic Siberia: The Number One Reindeer Brigade*. Oxford: Oxford University Press.

Anderson, D.G. (2010). 'Shamanic revival in a post-socialist landscape: Knowledge, luck and ritual among Zabaikal'e Orochen-Evenkis,' pp. 71-97 in P. Jordan, ed. *Landscape and Culture in Northern Eurasia.* Walnut Creek, CA: Left Coast Press.

Anisimov, A.F. (1963). 'The shaman's tent of the Evenki and the origins of shamanistic rite,' pp. 84-123 in H.N. Michael, ed., *Studies in Siberian Shamanism.* Toronto: University of Toronto Press.

Anonymous (1939). *Nash Aimak.* Krasnyi Baikalets, №110, 7 November, p. 2.

Anthropac (2010). *Anthropac* version 4.98 (searched 4 Sept 2010) http://www.analytictech.com/anthropac/apacdesc.htm.

Arakchaa, K.K. (1995). *Slovo ob arzhaany Tuvy.* Moskva: Polikom.

Arbatskii, A.I. (1978). 'Nekotorye dannye o religioznyh perezhitkakh Vitimskikh evenkov,' pp. 177-180 in G.I. Medvedev, ed. *Drevniaia istoriia narodov iuga vostochnoi Sibiri.* Irkutsk: Irkustkii gosudartstvennyi universitet.

Arnold, D. (1988). *Imperial Medicine and Indigenous Societies.* Manchester, UK: Manchester University Press.

Asad, T. (2003). *Formations of the Secular: Christianity, Islam and Modernity.* Stanford, CA: Stanford University Press.

Aseeva, T.A., D.B. Dashiev, A.D. Dashiev, S.M. Nikolaev, N.A. Surkova, G.V. Chekhirova, and T.A. Iurina (2008). O.D. Tsyren-zhapova, ed., *Tibetskaia meditsina u buriat. Novosibirsk:* Institut obshchei i eksperimental' noi biologii SO RAN.

Badmaev, P. (1991 [1903]). *Osnovy vrachebnoi nauki Tibeta.* Zhud-Shi. Sankt-Peterburg–Moskva: Reprintnoe vosproizvedenie izdaniia 'Glavnoe rukovodstvo po vrachebnoi nauke Tibeta. Zhud-Shi.'

Baer, H.A. (2001). *Biomedicine and Alternative Healing Systems in America: Issues of Class Race Ethnicity, and Gender.* Madison, WI: University of Wisconsin Press.

Balick, M.J. and P.A. Cox (1996). *Plants, People and Culture: The Science of Ethnobotany.* New York: W.H. Freeman & Company.

Bazaron, E.G. (1987). *Ocherki Tibetskoi meditsina, Buriatskoe kn.* Ulan Ude: Izdvo.

Banzarov, D. (1955 [1846]). 'Chernaia Vera, ili shamanstvo u mongolov' in D. Banzarov *Sobranie sochinenii.* Moscow: Izdatel'stvo Akademii Nauk SSSR.

Banzarov, D. (1997). *Sobranie sochinenii.* Ulan-Ude: BNTs CO RAN.

Basharov, I.P. (2003). 'Predstavlenie o dukhakh-khoziaevakh mestnosti u russkogo promyslovogo naseleniia Vostochnogo Pribaikal'ia,' pp. 4-14 in A.G. Generalov, ed., *Narody i kultury Sibiri. vzaimodeistvie kak factor formirovaniia i modernizatsi.* Irkutsk: Mezhregional'nyi Institut Obschestvennykh nauk.

Batashev, M.S. (2007). Materialy Krasnoiarskogo muzeia po kul'tovym sooruzheniiam Evenkov. *Eniseiskaia provintsiia* 2: 77-106.

Bawden, C.R. (1968). *The Modern History of Mongolia.* London, UK: Kegan Paul International.

Boddy, J. (1989). *Wombs and Alien Spirits: Women, Men and the Zar Cult in Northern Sudan.* Madison, WI: University of Wisconsin Press.

Bogdanova, K.M. and M.P. Bichikhanov (1991). *Lekarstvennye rasteniia Buriatii i ikh okhrana.* Ulan-Ude: Buriatskoe knizhnoe izdatel'stvo

Bold, S. and M. Ambaga (2002). *History and Fundamentals of Mongolian Traditional Medicine.* Ulaanbaatar, Mongolia: Sodpress, Inc.

Borre, K. (1991). Seal blood, Inuit blood, and diet—a biocultural model of physiology and cultural-identity. *Medical Anthropology Quarterly* 5(1): 48-62.

Botoroev, K.S. (1991). *Kurort Arshan.* Ulan-Ude: Buriatskoe Knizhnoe Izdatelsvo.

Bourguignon, E. (2004) Suffering and healing, subordination and power: Women and possession trance. *Ethnos* 32(4): 557-574.

Brainerd, E. and D.M. Cutler (2005). Autopsy on an empire: Understanding mortality in Russia and the former Soviet Union. *The Journal of Economic Perspectives* 19(1): 107-130.

Brandišauskas, D. (2009). Leaving Footprints in the Taiga: Enacted and Emplaced Power and Luck among Orochen-Evenki of the Zabaikal Region in East Siberia. PhD Thesis. Department of Anthropology, University of Aberdeen.

Caldwell, M.L. (2002). The taste of nationalism: Food politics in postsocialist Moscow. *Ethnos* 67(3): 295-319.

Crapanzano, V. (1973). *The Hamadsha: A Study in Moroccan Ethnopsychiatry*. Berkeley, CA: University of California Press.

Csordas, T.J. (1994). *The Sacred Self: A Cultural Phenomenology of Charismatic Healing*. Berkeley, CA: University of California Press.

Danzanova, A.A., K.P. Dulganov, and V.K. Dulganov (2001) 'K istorii Tibetskoi meditsiny v Zabaikal'e,' pp 32-34 in I.D. Buraev, ed., *Tibetskaia meditsina: teoriia i praktika*. Ulan-Ude: Izd. Buriatskogo nauchnogo tsentra SO RAN.

Daribazarova, S.O. (2001). 'Pitanie v traditsionnoi kul'ture buriat,' pp. 34-40 in I.D. Buraev, ed., *Tibetskaia meditsina: teoriia i praktika*. Ulan-Ude: Izd. Buriatskogo nauchnogo tsentra SO RAN.

Dashiev, D.B. (2004). 'Tibetskaia meditsina v Buriatii,' pp. 451-459 in L.L. Abaeva and N.L. Zhukovskaia, eds., *Buriaty*. Moscow: Nauka.

Dashizhapova, S. (2007). Tibetskii lekar'. *Gazeta «Ekstra»*, Ulan-Ude, 17 oktiabria.

Davydov, V.N. and V.V. Simonova (2008). Sobach'e serdtse: Antropologiia sobakoedeniia v post-sovetskoi evenkiiskoi derevne. *Izvestiia Laboratorii drevnikh tekhnologii* 6: 213-230.

Donner, K. (1933). *Ethnological Notes About the Yenisey-Ostyak*. Helsinki: Finno-Ugric Society.

Dorzhiev, Ts.Z. and Ts.B. Namzalov (2001). *Baikal: The Wonderland of Live Nature*. Ulan-Ude, Buriatiia: Buriat Research Centre.

Dugarov, D. (2002). 'Foreword,' pp. vii-ix in V. Tkacz with S. Zhambalov and W. Phipps, *Shanar: Dedication Ritual of a Buriat Shaman in Siberia as conducted by Bair Rinchinov*. New York: Parabola Books.

Eliade, M. (1964). *Shamanism: Archaic Techniques of Ecstasy*. Princeton: Princeton University Press.

Ermolova, N.V. (2010). 'Predstavleniia o dushe, smerti i zagrobnoi zhizni v traditsionom mirovozrenii evenkov,' pp. 93-158 in Y.E. and L.R. Pavlinaskaia, eds., *Ot bytiia k inobytiiu: Fol'klor i pogrebalnyi ritual v traditsionnykh kul'turakh Sibiri i Ameriki*. St. Peterburg: MAE RAN.

Fernandez-Gimenez, M.E. (2000). The Role of Mongolian Nomadic Pastoralists' Ecological Knowledge in Rangeland Management. *Ecological Applications* 10(5): 1318-1326.

Field, M.G. (1957). *Doctor and Patient in Soviet Russia*. Cambridge: Harvard University Press.

Finch, C. (1999). *Mongolia's Wild Heritage*. Boulder, CO: Avery Press.

Findeisen, H. (1953). *Sibirische Schamanentum und Magie*. Augsburg: Institut für Menschen und Magie.

Fisher, I.E. (1774). *Sibirskaia istoriia s samogo otkrytiia do zavoevaniia sei zemli Rossiiskim oruzhiem*. St Peterburg: Imperatorskoi Akademii Nauk.

Foucault, M. (2004). *Cours au Collège de France 1978-1979: La Naissance de la biopolitique.* Paris: Seuil.
Fridman, E. and J. Neumann (2003). Coming together: Buryat and Mongolian healers meet in post-soviet reality. *Cultural Survival* 27(2): 40-44.
Galdanova, G.R. (1987). *Dolamaistckie verovaniia buriat.* Novosibirsk: Nauka–sibirskoe otdelenie.
Garmaeva, Ch.Ts. (2001). 'Traditsionnaia Tibetskaia meditsina na sovremennom etape,' pp. 9-19 in I.D. Buraev, ed., *Tibetskaia meditsina: teoriia i praktika.* Ulan-Ude: Izd. Buriatskogo nauchnogo tsentra SO RAN.
Georgi, I.G. (1779). *Opisanie vsekh v Rossiiskom gosudarsve obitaiuchikh narodov.* St. Petersburg: Imperatorskoi Akademii Nauk.
Gerasimova, K.M., G.R. Galdanova, and G.N. Ochirova (2000). *Traditsionnaia kul'tura buriat.* Ulan-Ude: BELIG.
Gordon, D.R. (1988) 'Tenacious assumptions in western medicine,' pp. 10-56 in M.M. Lock and D.R. Gordon, eds., *Biomedicine Examined.* Dordrecht, Boston: Kluwer Academic Publishers.
Goulet, J.G. (1998). *Ways of Knowing: Experience, Knowledge, and Power among the Dene Tha.* Lincoln: University of Nebraska Press.
Gurvich, I.S. (1977). *Kul'tura severnykh iakutov-olenevodov.* Moskva: Nauka.
Gusev, B. (2000). *Petr Badmaev: Krestnik Imperatora, Tselitel, Diplomat.* Moskva: Olma.
Hamayon, R.N. (1990). *La chasse à l'âme.* Nanterre: Société d'ethnologie.
Hamayon, R. (1994). 'Shamanism in Siberia: From partnership in supernature to counter-power in society,' pp. 76-89 in: N. Thomas and C. Humphrey, eds., *Shamanism, History and the State.* Ann Arbor: University of Michigan Press.
Han, G.S. (2002). The myth of medical pluralism: A critical realist perspective. *Sociological Research Online* 6(4): U92–U112.
Heath, D.B. (1987). Anthropology and alcohol studies: Current issues. *Annual Review of Anthropology* 16(1): 99-120.
Heissig, W. (1980 [1945]). *The Religions of Mongolia.* Berkeley, CA: University of California Press.
High, M. (2008). Dangerous Fortunes: Wealth and Patriarchy in the Mongolian Informal Gold Mining Economy. PhD Thesis, Department of Social Anthropology, University of Cambridge.
Hope, R.C. (1968 [1893]). *The Legendary Lore of the Holy Wells of England Including Rivers, Lakes, Fountains and Springs.* Detroit, MI: Singing Tree Press.
Hruschka, D.J. (1998). Baria healers among the Buriats in eastern Mongolia. *Mongolian Studies* XXI: 21-41.
Hsu, E. (2008). Medical pluralism. *International Encyclopedia of Public Health* 4: 316-321.
Humphrey, C. (1998). *Marx Went Away—But Karl Stayed Behind: Updated Edition of Karl Marx Collective: Economy, Society and Religion in a Siberian Collective Farm,* 2nd Ed. Ann Arbor, MI: University of Michigan Press.
Humphrey, C. (2002). 'Shamans in the City,' pp. 202-221 in *The Unmaking of Soviet Life: Everyday Economies after Socialism.* Ithaca: Cornell University Press.
Humphrey, C. and U. Onon (1996). *Shamans and Elders: Experience, Knowledge and Power among the Daur Mongols.* Oxford, UK: Clarendon Press, Oxford University Press.

Hutton, R. (2001). *Shamans: Siberian Spirituality and the Western Imagination*. London: Hambledon and London.
Illich, I. (1977). *Limits to Medicine, Medical Nemesis: The Expropriation of Health*. Harmondsworth: Penguin Books Ltd.
Il'ina, I.V. (2008). *Traditsionaia meditsinskaia kul'tura narodov evropeiskogo severo-vostoka* (konets XIX-XX vv.). Sykhtyvkar: Komi Nauchnyi Tsentr.
Ingold, T. (1992). 'Culture and the perception of the environment,' pp. 39-56 in Croll and D. Parkin, eds., *Bush Base: Forest, Farm, Culture, Environment and Development*. London, UK: Routledge.
Ivanov, V.N. and V.N. Toporov (1969). 'Komentarii k opisaniiu ketskoi mifologii,' pp. 148-166 in Viachslav Ivanov et al., eds., *Ketskii sbornik. Mifologiia, etnografiia, teksty*. Moscow: Nauka.
Jakobsen, M.D. (1999). *Shamanism: Traditional and Contemporary Approaches to the Mastery of Spirits and Healing*. Oxford: Berghahn Books.
Janes, C.R. (2002). *Buddhism, science, and market: The globalisation of Tibetan medicine*. Anthropology and Medicine 9(3): 267-289.
Jokic, Z. (2008). The wrath of the forgotten Ongons: Shamanic sickness, spirit embodiment, and fragmentary trancescape in contemporary Buriat shamanism. *Sibirica* 7(1): 23-51.
Kagarov, E.G. (1929). *Shamanskii obriad prokhozhdeniia skvoz' otverstie*. Doklady Akademii Nauk SSSR, pp. 189-192.
Kalland, A. (2000). 'Indigenous knowledge: Prospects and limitations,' pp. 319-335 in R. Ellen, P. Parkes and A.Bicker, eds., *Indigenous Environmental Knowledge and its Transformations: Critical Anthropological Perspectives*. Canterbury, UK: Harwood Academic Publishers.
Khakarainen, M.V. (2007). Lokal nye predstavleniia o bol'nykh i lechenii (Poselok Markovo, Chukotka). Kandidatskaia dissertatsiia. Kafedra istorii. European University at Saint Petersburg.
Khangalov, M.N. (2004 [1958]). *Sobranie Sochinenii*. Ulan-Ude: Buriatskoe knizhnoe izd-vo.
Kochmar, N.N. (2002). 'Issledovanie zhertvenikov pisanits srednei Leny,' pp. 42- 55 in T.N. Kononova, ed., *Narody i kul'tury Sibiri: Vzaimodeistviia kak faktor formirovaniia i modernizatsii vyp. 1*. Irkutsk: Ottisk.
Koester, D. (2003). Drink, drank, drunk: A social-political grammar of Russian drinking practices in a colonial context. *The Anthropology of East Europe Review* 21(2): 41-48.
Koledneva, N.V. (2009). *Planeta Evenkiia: nauchno-populiarnaia literatura*. Chita: Ekspress- izdatel'stvo.
Koroleva, K. (1950). Universal'naia znakharka. *Krasnyi Baikalets* 28, 25 May, p. 2.
Kravchenko, S.A. (2007). *Sotsiologiia moderna i postmoderna v dinamicheski meniaiushchemsia mire*. Moskva: Izd-vo «MGIMO-Universitet».
Kreinovich, E.A. (1969). 'Obriad kormleniia 'dorozhnoi starukhi' u ketov,' pp. 236-242 in V. Ivanov et al., eds., *Ketskii sbornik. Mifologiia, etnografiia, teksty*. Moscow: Nauka.
Krivonogov, V.P. (1998). *Kety na poroge III tysiacheletiia*. Krasnoiarsk: Izd-vo KGPU.
Krivonogov, V.P. (2003). *Kety: desiat'let spustia (1991–2001 gg.)*. Krasnoiarsk: Izd-vo KGPU.
Kureiskaia, E.A. (2000). *Kak zovut tebia bee? Slovar' evenkiiskikh imen*. Krasnoiarsk: LAA.

Kwon, H. (1998). The saddle and the sledge: Hunting as comparative narrative in Siberia and beyond. *Journal of the Royal Anthropological Institute* 4: 112-147.

Lambek, M. (1980). Spirits and spouses: Possession as a system of communication among the Malagasy speakers of Mayotte. *American Ethnologist* 7(2): 318-331.

Lamoreaux, P.E. and J.T. Tanner, eds. (2001). *Springs and Bottled Waters of the World: Ancient History, Source, Occurrence, Quality and Use.* Berlin, Germany: Springer-Verlag.

Law, J. (2004). *After Method: Mess in Social Science Research.* London: Routeledge.

Leete, A. (2004). 'Invasion of materialism into the Soviet North: Sedentarisation, development of professional medicine and hygiene in the 1920-40s,' pp. 69-86 in E. Kõresaar and A. Leete, eds., *Everyday Life and Cultural Patterns. International Festschrift for Elle Vunder.* In Series Studies in Folk Culture, Vol 3. Tartu: Tartu University Press.

Lenkhoboev, G.L. and N.Ts. Zhambaldagbaev (1983). 'K izucheniiu buriatskoi narodnoi meditsiny,' pp. 72-80 in K.D. Basaeva, ed. *Sovremennost' i traditsionnaia kul'tura narodov* Buriatii. Ulan-Ude: BF SO AN SSSR.

Lenkhoboev, G.L. and NTs. Zhambaldagbaev (2003). *Praktika tibetskoi meditsiny v Buriatii: iz opyta i vozzrenii emchi-lam.* Novosibirsk: Izd-vo OOO «RTF».

Leslie, C. (1976). *Asian Medical Systems.* Berkeley, CA: University of California Press.

Leslie, C. (1980). Medical pluralism in world perspective. *Social Science and Medicine* 14B(4): 191-195.

Lewis, I.M. (2003). *Ecstatic Religion: A Study of Shamanism and Spirit Possession,* 3rd Ed. New York: Routledge.

Ligaa, U. and D. Tsembel (2003). 'Medicinal plants of Mongolia and their use in traditional medicine,' pp. 114-140 in D. Badarch, R. Zilinskas, and P.J. Balint, eds., *Mongolia Today: Science, Culture, Environment and Development.* London, UK: Routledge Curzon Press.

Lindenau Ia.I. (1983 [1742]). *Opisanie tungusov, kotorye zhivut u Udskogo ostroga 1744-1745. Opisanie narodov Sibiri (pervaia polovina XVIII veka). Istoriko-etnograficheskie materially o narodaks Sibiri i Severo-Vostoka.* Magadan: Kniga.

Lindquist, G. (2002). Healing efficacy and the construction of charisma: A family's journey through the multiple medical field in Russia. *Anthropology and Medicine* 9(3): 337-358.

Lindquist, G. (2006). *Conjuring Hope: Healing and Magic in Contemporary Russia.* New York: Berghahn Books.

Lock, M.M. and D.R. Gordon (1988). *Biomedicine Examined.* Dordrecht, Boston: Kluwer Academic Publishers.

Long, J. (2010). Negotiating Belonging: Ritual, Performance and Buriat National Culture in Pribaikal'e, Southern Siberia. PhD Thesis, Department of Anthropology, University of Aberdeen.

Lopatin, I.A. (1895). *Dnevniki Vitimskoi Ekspeditsii 1865.* In series: Vestnik Imperatskogo Russkogo geograficheskogo obshchestva 28 (1). St. Peterburg: IRGO

Lukina, T.A. (1982). G.V. Steller o narodnoi meditsine Sibiri (neopublikoannyi traktat 40-kh godov XVIII). *Strany i narody Vostoka.* vyp. 24: 127-148.

Lux, M.K. (2001). *Medicine that Walks: Disease, Medicine and Canadian Plains Native People, 1880-1940.* Toronto, Buffalo: University of Toronto Press.

Mainov, I.I. (1898). *Nekotorye dannye o tungusakh Iakutskogo kraia.* In series: *Trudy Vostochnogo Sibirskogo Otdeleniia Russkogo geograficheskogo obshchestva,* Vol. 2. Irkutsk: VSORGO.

Manzanov, G.E. (2005). *Religioznye traditsii v kul'ture buriatskogo naroda.* Ulan-Ude: Izd-vo BNTS SO RAN.

Masquelier, A. (2001). *Prayer Has Spoiled Everything: Possession, Power, and Identity in an Islamic Town of Niger.* Durham: Duke University Press.

Mazin, A.I. (1984). *Traditsionnye verovaniia i obriady evenkov-orochonov* (Kon. XIX—nach. XX vv.). Novosibirsk: Nauka.

McGuire, M.B. (2002). Not all alternatives are complementary. *Medical Anthropology Quarterly* 16: 409–411.

Mcknight, D. (2002). *From Hunting to Drinking: The Devastating Effects of Alcohol on an Australian Aboriginal Community.* London: Routledge.

Metzo, K. (2003). Whither peasants in Siberia? Agricultural reform, subsistence, and the value of being rural. *Culture and Agriculture* 21(1): 1-15.

Metzo, K. (2006). Indebtedness, exchange, and morality in Buriatiia. *Ethnology*. 45(4): 287-304.

Metzo, K. (2008a). Sacred landscape, healing landscape: 'Taking the waters' in Tunka Valley, Russia. *Sibirica* 7(1): 51-72.

Metzo, K. (2008b). 'Shamanic transformations: Buriat shamans as mediators of multiple worlds,' pp. 215-246 in M. Steinberg and C. Wanner, eds., *Reclaiming the Sacred: Morality, Community, and Religion after Communism.* Washington, DC: Woodrow Wilson Foundation Press.

Mikhailov, O. (2006). Vrachi, po krupitsam sobiraiushchie chudo. *Gazeta «Inform-Polis»,* Ulan-Ude, 26 iiunia.

Mikhailov, T.M. (1987). *Buriatskii shamanizm: istoriia, struktura i sotsial'nye funktsii.* Novosibirsk: Izd-vo Nauka.

Mikhailov, T.M. (1990). 'Buriat shamanism: History, structure, and social functions,' pp. 110-120 in *Shamanism. Soviet Studies of Traditional Religion in Siberia and Central Asia.* Armonk, NY: M.E. Sharpe.

Mikhailov, T.M. (2004a). 'Obsheburiatskie, plemennie, territorial'nie, rodovie, semeinie bozhestva i dukhi,' pp. 360-366 in L.L. Abaeva and N.L. Zhukovskaia, eds., *Buriaty.* Moscow: Nauka.

Mikhailov, T.M. (2004b). 'Shamanizm—drevniaia religiia buriat,' pp. 352-390 in L.L. Abaeva and N.L. Zhukovskaia, eds., *Buriaty.* Moscow Nauka.

Mikheev, V.S. (1995). *Traditsionoe prirodopolzovanie evenkov: obosnovanie territorii v Chitinskoi oblasti.* Novosibirsk: Nauka.

Namandorj, O., Sh. Tseren, and O. Nyamdorj (1966). *Bugd Nairamdakh Mongol Ard Ulsin Rashaan.* Ulaanbaatar, Mongolia: Academy of Scientific Research.

Nemtsov, A.V. (2002). Alcohol-related human losses in Russia in the 1980s and 1990s. *Addiction* 97(11): 1413-1425.

Nemtsov, A.V. (2005). Russia: alcohol yesterday and today. *Addiction* 100(2): 146-149.

Neupokoev, V. (1926). Bol'shoi shaman—Kyndygir' (Iz predanii Severo-Baikal'skikh tungusov. *Zhizn' Buriatii* 4-5: 28-30.

Neupokoev, V. (1928). *Tungusy Buriatii.* Verkhneudinsk: Izdatelstvo zhurnala «Zhizn' Buriatii».

Nikolaev, R.V. (1985). *Fol'klor i voprosy etnicheskoi istorii ketov.* Krasnoiarsk: Krasnoiarskii gosudarstvennyii universitet.

Nikolaev, S.M., A.I. Bartanov, and D.L. Matypov (2004). *Tibetskaia meditsina (voprosy i otvety).* Ulan-Ude: Izd-vo Buriatskogo gosuniversiteta.

Ochirov, D.D., ed. (2006). *Ivolga Datsan: Fotoal'bum.* Khambyn Sume Ulan-Ude.

Okladnikov, A.P. and A.I. Mazin (1976). *Pisanitsy reki Olekmy i Verkhnego Priamur'ia.* Novosibirsk: Nauka.

Okladnikov, A.P. and A.I. Mazin (1979). *Pisanitsy basseina reki Aldan.* Novosibirsk: Nauka.

Orlov, V. (1857). Amurskie orocheny. *Vestnik Imperatskogo Russkogo Geograficheskogo Obschestva* 21(6): 193-199.

Orlov, V. (1858). Bauntovskie i angarskie brodiachie tungusy. *Vestnik Imperatskogo Russkogo Geograficheskogo Obschestva* 21(6): 180-192.

Paladimov, P. (1929). Barguzinskaia taiga. *Zhizn' Buriatii* 5: 82-89.

Parfionovich, Y.M., ed. (1994). *Atlas Tibetskoi meditsiny.* Moskva: Galart.

Petri, B.E. (1930). *Okhota i olenevodstvo u tuturskikh tungusov v sviazi s organizatsiei okhotkhoziaistva. Izvestiia Biologo-Geograficheskogo Nauchno-Issledovatel'skogo Instituta pri Gosudarstvennom Irkutskom Universitete. T. V, vypusk 2.* Irkutsk: Tipografiia izdatel'stva «Vlast' truda».

Petrov, E.V. (2004). 'O vozmozhnosti razrabotki novykh fitopreparatov na osnove printsipov tibetskoi meditsiny,' pp. 30-31 in A.I Bartanova and D.L. Martypova, eds., *Razvitie traditsionnoi meditsiny v Rossii: materialy nauchno-prakticheskoi konferentsii* (1-2 okiabriia 2004). Ulan-Ude: Izd-vo «Vita Magistra» RTSMP.

Popkov, Iu.V. and D.Dz. Anderson, eds. (2002). *Zdororov'e i zdravoohranenie.* Novosibirsk: Sibprint.

Poppe, N. (1957). An Essay in Mongolian on Medicinal Waters. *Asia Major* 6, Part 1: 99-105.

Povinelli, E. (2006). *The Empire of Love: Toward a Theory of Intimacy, Genealogy, and Carnality.* Duke University Press.

Pozdneev, A., trans. (1991). *Uchebnik Tibetskoi meditsiny.* Leningrad: Ekopolis i kul'tura.

Pozdneev, A.M. (1993 [1887]). *Ocherki byta buddiiskikh monastyrei i buddiiskogo dukhovenstva v Mongolii v sviazi s otnosheniiami sego poslednego k narodu.* Reprintnoe izdanie. Sankt-Peterburg: Elista.

Pu, Q. (1983). *The Oroqens—China's Nomadic Hunters.* Beijing: Foreign Languages Press.

Quijada, J.B. (2008). What if we don't know our clan? The city Tailgan as new ritual form in Buriatiia. *Sibirica* 7(1-Spring): 1-22.

Quijada, J.B. (2009). Opening the Roads: History and Religion in Post-Soviet Buriatiia. Ph.D. Dissertation. Department of Anthropology, University of Chicago.

Rinpoche, Ven. Rechung. (1973). *Tibetan Medicine.* Berkeley, CA: University of California Press.

Room, R. (1984). Alcohol and ethnography: A case of problem deflation? *Current Anthropology* 25(2): 169-191.

Saggers, S. and D. Gray (1998). *Dealing with Alcohol: Indigenous Usage in Australia, New Zealand and Canada.* Cambridge, UK: Cambridge University Press.

Sakharov, N. Ts-Zh. (2000 [1869]). Ob inorodtsev, obitaiuschikh v Barguzinskom okruge Zabaikal'skoi oblasti. *Ogni Kurumkana* (Jun 29): 2.

Samokhin, A.T. (1929). Tungusy Bodaibinskogo raiona. *Sibirskaia zhivaia starina* 8-9: 5-66.

Sarangerel (2000). *Riding Windhorses: A Journey into the Heart of Mongolian Shamanism.* Rochester, VT: Destiny Books.

Schultes, R.E. and A. Hoffman (1992). *Plants of the Gods: Their Sacred, Healing, and Hallucinogenic Powers.* Rochester, NY: Healing Arts Press.

Scott, J.C. (1990). *Domination and the Arts of Resistance: Hidden Transcripts*. New Haven, CT: Yale University Press.

Shirokogoroff, S.M. (1919). Opyt' issledovaniia osnov shamanstva u tungusov. Ucheniia zapiski istoriko-filologicheskogo fakul'teta v Vladivostoke. Tom 1 c. 47-108.

Shirokogoroff, S.M. (1924). *Social Organisation of the Manchus: A Study of Manchu Clan Organization. Northern China Branch of the Royal Asiatic Society*, Extended Volume 3. Shanghai: Commercial Press.

Shirokogoroff, S.M. (1929). *Social Organisation of the Northern Tungus*. Shanghai: Commercial Press.

Shirokogoroff, S.M. (1935). *Psychomental Complex of the Tungus*. London: Kegan Paul, Trench, Trubner & Co. Ltd.

Shkolnikov, V., M. Mckee, and D.A. Leon (2001). Changes in life expectancy in Russia in the mid-1990s. *The Lancet* 357(9260): 917-921.

Shrenk, L.I. (1883). *Ob inorodtsakh Amurskogo kraia*. St. Petersburg: Imp. Academy of Sciences.

Shubin, A.S. (2001). *Evenki Pribaikal'ia*. Ulan-Ude: Belig.

Shubin, A.S. (2007). *Evenki*. Ulan-Ude: Izdatel'stvo OAO 'Respublikanskaia tipografiia.'

Sirina, A.A. (2008). Chuvstvuiushchie zemliu: ecologicheskaia etika evenkov i evenov. *Etnograficheskoe obozrenie* 2: 121-138.

Sirina, A.A. and G. Fondahl (2006). Evenki Severnogo Pribaikal'ia i proekt stroitel'stva nefteprovoda «Vostochnaia Sibir»—Tikhii Okean.' *Issledovaniia po prikladnoi i neotlozhnoi etnologii*, No. 186. Moscow: Institut etnologii i antropologii.

Slezkine, Y. (1992). From savages to citizens: The cultural revolution in the Soviet Far North. *Slavic Review* 51(1): 52-76.

Slezkine, I. (1994). *Arctic Mirrors. Russia and the Small Peoples of the North*. Ithaca, London: Cornell University Press.

Smirnov, V.A. (1932 [1926]). *Arshani Mongolii: Mongol oronii arsaanuudiin tus otchet o rabotakh gidrokhimicheskovo otriada Mongol'skoi ekspeditsii*. Leningrad: Izdatel'stvo Akademii Nauk SSSR.

Smith, W.R. (1889). *Lectures on the Religion of the Semites*. Edinburgh: Black.

Solomon, S.G. (1993). The Soviet-German syphilis expedition to Buriat Mongolia, 1928: Scientific research on national minorities. *Slavic Review* 52(2): 204-232.

Souto, W.M.S., R.R.D. Barboza et al. (2009). Zootherapy in Brazil: An urgent necessity of interdisciplinary studies. *West Indian Medical Journal* 58(5): 494-495.

Sundström, O. (2007). Kampen mot 'schamanismen':sovjetisk religionspolitik gentemot inhemska religioner i Sibirien och norra Ryssland. *Studier av inter-religiösa relationer* vol. 40. Uppsalla: Uppsalla universitet.

Suslov, I.M. (1936). Shamanstvo i bor'ba s nim. *Sovetskii Sever*. No. 3–5: 89–152.

Svidorova, N.A. (1995). *Priglashaem na tuiun. Iz evenkiiskoi natsional'noi kukhni*. Krasniarsk: Fond Severynykh literature Kheglen.

Titov, E.I. (1926). *Otchet o rabote po izucheniiu olennykh tungusov*. Arkhiv Zabaikalæskgo kraevogo kravedcheskogo muzeia im. A.K. Kuznetsova. Nr. 15319.

Troshev, Zh.P. (2002). Shamany i shamanstvo. *Evenkiiskaia zhizn'*. (August 29 and September 5, 12, 26).

Tsing, A.L. (2005). *Friction an Ethnography of Global Connection*. Princeton: N.J: Princeton University Press

Tsintsius, V.I. (1975). *Sravnitel'nii slovar Tunguso-Man'chzhurskikh iazykov*. Leningrad: Nauka. T. 1-2.

Tugolukov, V.A. (1962). The Vitim-Olekma Evenki. *Sibirskii etnograficheskii sbornik* 4: 15-40.
Tugolukov, V.A. (1969). *Sledopyty verkhom na oleniakh*. Moscow: Nauka.
Tugolukov, V.A. (1977). 'Polevye issledovanie v Severnoi Priamur'e,' pp. 36-44 in M. Vainshtein, ed., *Polevye issledovanie instituta etnografii 1975*. Moscow: IE RAN
Tugutov, I.E. (1978). 'The Tailagan as the principal shamanistic ritual of the Buriats,' pp. 267-280 in V. Diószegi and M. Hoppal, eds., *Shamanism in Siberia*. Budapest: Akademi Kiadó.
Turaev, V.A. (2008). *Dal'nevostochnye Evenki: Etnokul'turnye i etnosotsianlye protsesy v XX veke*. Vladivostok: Dal'nenauka.
Turner, V.W. (1969). *The Ritual Process: Structure and Anti-Structure*. London: Routledge & K. Paul.
Turov, M.G. (1975). 'K proiskhozhdeniia i evoliutsii evenkiiskogo labaza «noku»,' pp. 193-209 in G.I. Medvedev and V.V. Sviinin, *Drevniaia istoriia narodov Iuga Vostochnoi Sibiri*. Irkutsk: Irkutsk State University.
Turtuev, Ts.D. and V.V. Boronoev (2004). 'Primenenie avtomatizirovannogo pul'sodiagnostichneskogo kompleksa tibetskoi meditsiny v poliklinike Tsentra vostochnoi meditsiny,' pp. 36-38 in A.I Bartanov and D.L. Martypov, eds. *Razvitie traditsionnoi meditsiny v Rossii: materialy nauchno-prakticheskoi konferentsii (1-2 okiabriia 2004)*. Ulan-Ude: Izd-vo «Vita Magistra» RTSMP.
Vajda, E.J. (2001). *Eniseian Peoples and Languages: A History of Eniseian Studies with an Annotated Bibliography and a Source Guide*. Surrey: Curzon Press.
Vajda, E.J. (2010a). Ket shamanism. *Shaman* 18(1)2: 131-150.
Vajda, E.J. (2010b). A Siberian link to Na-Dene languages. *Anthropological Papers of the University of Alaska* 5(1)2: 33-99.
Vajda, E.J. (2010c). 'Siberian landscapes in Ket traditional culture,' pp. 297-314 in P. Jordan, ed., *Landscape and Culture in Northern Eurasia*. Walnut Creek, CA: Left Coast Press.
Varlamova, G.I. (2002). *Epicheskie i obriadovye zhanry evenkiiskogo folklora*. Novosibirsk: Nauka.
Varlamova, G.I. (2004). *Mirovozrenie evenkov: otrazhenie v folklore*. Novosibirsk: Nauka.
Vasilevich, G.M. (1957). 'Drevnie okhotnich'i i olenevodcheskie obriady evenkov,' pp. 152-187 in S.P. Tolstov, *Sbornik Muzeia antropologii i etnografii 17*. Leningrad: Nauka.
Vasilevich, G.M. (1958). *Evenkiisko-russkii slovar'*. Moscow: Gosudarstvennoe izdatel'stvo inostrannykh i natsyonal'nykh slovarei.
Vasilevich, G.M. (1969). *Evenki: Istoriko-etnograficheskie ocherki (XVIII-nachalo XX v.)*. Leningrad: Nauka.
Vasilevich, G.M. (1971). 'O kul'te medvedia u Evenkov' pp. 150-169 in A.P. Potapov and S.V. Ivanov, eds., *Sbornik Muzeia antropologii i etnografii 27*. Leningrad: Nauka.
Vasmer, M. (1986). *Etiminologichesii slovar' russkogo iazyka*. Moskva: Progress.
Ventsel, A. (2005). *Reindeer, Rodina and Reciprocity: Kinship and Property Relations in a Siberian Village*. Berlin: Lit Verlag.
Vitebsky, P. (2005). *Reindeer People: Living with Animals and Spirits in Siberia*. London: Harper Perennial.
Voskoboinikov, M.G. (1965). Prozaicheskie zhanry evenkiiskogo fol'klora. Unpublised Doctoral thesis. St. Petersburg: Institute of A. I. Gertzen.

References

Vostokov, V. (2003). *Slaviano-Tibetskaia meditsina.* Moscow: Dilia.

Vstrecha s Khambo Etigelovym (2003). Ulan-Ude: Izd-vo OAO «Respublikanskaia tipografiia».

Waldram, J.B. (2000). The efficacy of traditional medicine: Current theoretical and methodological issues. *Medical Anthropology Quarterly* 14(4): 603-625.

Werner, H. (2006). *Die Welt der Jenissejer im Lichte des Wortschatzes: zur Rekonstruktion der jenissejischen Protokultur.* Wiesbaden: Harrassowitz.

White, S.D. (2001). 'Medicines and modernities in socialist China: medical pluralism, the state, and Naxi identities in the Lijiang basin,' pp. 171-196 in L. Connor and G. Samuel, eds., *Healing Powers and Modernity: Traditional Medicine, Shamanism, and Science in Asian Societies.* Westport, CT: Bergin and Garvey.

Willerslev, R. (2007). *Soul Hunters: Hunting, Animism, and Personhood among the Siberian Yukaghirs.* Berkeley, CA: University of Calfornia Press.

Wilson, K. (2003). Therapeutic landscapes and First Nations peoples: An exploration of culture, health and place. *Health and Place* 9(2): 83-93.

Zabianko, A.P., A.I. Mazin, and O.A. Kobyzov (2002). 'Shamanizm evenkov Priamur'ia i Iuzhnoi Iakutii (sovremenoe sostoianie),' pp. 294-304 in *Traditsionaia kul'tura Vostkoka Azii.* Blagoveschensk: Izdatel'stvo AmGU.

Zelenin, D.K. (1929). Tabu slov u narodov Vostochnoi Evropy i Severnoi Azii. In Series: *Sbornik Muzeia antropologii i etnografii* 8. Leningrad: MAE.

Zelenin, D.K. (1935). Ideologiia sibirskogo shamanstva. Izvestiia AN SSSR po otd. *Obshchestvennykh nauk* 8: 709-743

Zelenin, D.K. (1936). Kul't ongonov v Sibiri. Prezhitki totemizma v ideologii sibirskikh narodov. In Series: *Trudy institute antropologii, arkheeologii, etnografii* 14 (3). Moskva, Leningrad: AN SSSR.

Zhukovskaia, N.L. (2004). 'Neoshamanizm v Buriatii,' pp. 390-396 in L.L. Abaeva and N.L. Zhukovskaia, eds., *Buriaty.* Moscow: Nauka.

Znamenski, A.A. (2003). *Shamanism in Siberia Russian Records of Indigenous Spirituality.* Dordrecht, Boston, MA: Kluwer Academic Publishers.

Zolotarev A.M. (1938). Novye dannye o tungusakh i lamutakh XVIII veka. *Istorik Marksist* 2 (66): 63-88.

The Healing Landscapes of Central and Southeastern Siberia

Glossary

KEY: Bur. = Buriat; Ev. = Evenki Ket = Ket; Oro. = Orochen; Rus.= Russian;

A

agdyrin: (Rus.) lightning mushroom
adyl: (Rus.) lightning, thunder
ayhan tarim: (Bus.) charms and spells while wrapping a patient in the hide of newly killed animals
aiaga (Bur.) ceramic bowls for use at *arshaan*
aia-ganga: (Bur.) thyme
airag: (Bur.) fermented mare's milk
algyr: (Rus.) spirits
aloi: (Rus.) aloe
arga-bilig: (Bur.) harmony
arenkil: (Oro.) the souls of hunters or herders who did not reach the world of the dead
arkhi: (Bur.) type of alcoholic beverages
arshaan (pl. *arshanuud*): (Bur.) freshwater mineral spring/s; consecrated (or holy) water
ayurveda: medicine

B

bag emch: (Bur)
bagulnik: (Rus.) rhododendron, Labrador tea
bangoket: (Ket) earth person
bangos: (Ket) folk healers
bediaga: (Rus.) poor (man)
bit: (Ket) loon
bria zaza,: (Bur.) bone setting arts
barikha: (Bur.) to hold
baryaasha: (Bur.) bone setters
bogoroditskaya trava: (Rus.) a variety of thyme
brusnika: (Rus.) red whortleberry
bryzgat: (Rus.) 'sprinkling' - as in sprinkling vodka
buben: (Ev.) drum
buu: (Bur.) local
but: (Bur.) prayer flags

C

chabrets: (Rus.) wild thyme
cahimi: (Ev.) tea
cheremsha: (Rus.) wild leek/onion
chernota: (Rus.) black activities
chimchen: (Oro.) large animals
chiushachii bagulnik: (Rus.) Labrador tea
chumy: (Oro.) conical tents

D

dagh: (Ket) giant eagle
dangols: (Ket) spirits of dead ancestors
datsan: Buddhist monastic centers of healing
datsanud: monasteries
delaniusa: (Oro.) stone-oil
Den' Aborifena: (Rus.) Aboriginal Day (celebration)
dikii rynok: (Rus.) wild market
dogoniat: (Bur.) track (them) down
dom: (Bur.) traditional therapies
dukuvuchi : (Oro.) rock art sites ('one who drew')
durnaia bolezn': (Ev.) venereal disease
dynd: (Ket) dragonfly shaman
dzho: (Oro.) bear gall bladder

E

elaki: (Oro.) ptarmigan
emchi-lama: (Bur.) Tibetan healer, physician-monk
emtei-lama: (Bur.) a *lama* who has medicaments
ereket: (Ev.) cliff fern
esdeng: (Ket) spirits
eteng kherigde: (Rus.) heart of the thunder
eting temoeraschka: (Rus.) thunder tobacco

F

fartovaia: (Ev.) luck
fel'shery: nurse-practitionners
fel'sher-akusher: nurse-practitionner–midwife

G

ger: (Bur.) conical dwelling
grekh: (Rus.) sins
gudzhir: (Bur.) briny

H

hango: (Ket) fly agaris mushroom
has: (Ket) shaman's drum
hatbul: (Ket) shaman's beater stick
hyna sening: (Ket) minor shaman

I

ianda: (Ev.) flowering plant, bitter in taste; plant medicine
iasak: (Ket) fur tax
inorodcheskie upravy: (Ev.) indigenous administrative districts
irunda: foolishness
iurta: (Ev.) conical mobile lodge

J

K

kalendula: (Rus.) calendula
kamennoe maslo: stone-oil
kamennyi zveroboi: (Rus.) cliff fern
kamlanie: (Bur.) ceremony
kandelok: (Ket) shaman that sported bear paws instead of hands
kash: (Ket) hoop
kato: (Ev.) knife
khadag: (Bur.) white or bright blue silk scarves marking *arshaan* water sources
khaluun: (Bur.) hot
khaman: (Ev.) shaman
kha-mi: (Ev.) knowledge
khenkere: juniper
khii: (Bur.) vital functions
khorkhog: (Bur.) special soup for preventing diseases and for replenishing strength
khoziain (pl. *khoziainy*)*:* head/s of household
khubi: a *khoziin's* share of a slaughtered animal
khuiten: (Bur.) cold
kolduny: (Ev.) magicians
kolkhoz: (Ev.) nomadic reindeer farm
kolobo: (Ev.) bread
komersanty: (Rus.) traders
korenizatsiia: Soviet nationalization initiatives
kostopravstvo: broken bones
krai: (Rus.) region
krapiva: (Rus.) nettle
khurylkha: ceremony to return an absent soul
khuvaraguud: (Bur.) pupils of the *emchi-lama*
kurort:(Bur.) sanitoria
kukish: (Rus) signs (e.g., finger signals)
kuso: (Rus.) dry, rotted wood
kuznetsi: (Bur.) blacksmith shamans

L

lama: healer
lekar: (Ev.) doctor
liubopytsvo: (Rus.) curiosity
luba beriozy: (Rus.) birch buds
lung: air
lus: (Bur.) water, water spirits

M

mahabhutas: the main elements (earth, water, fire, air, and space)
malina: (Rus.) raspberry
manba-datasan: Mongolian healer
manba-datsanuud: Mongolian medical schools at monestaries
marilia: (Oro.) fence
mesta sily: (Rus.) 'places of strength'
mozhzhevelnik: (Rus.) juniper smoke

moxa: cones
mumio: (Rus.) stone-oil
m*yshlenie*: (Rus.) Asian way of thinking

N

nasheptanyi chai: (Rus.) black tea
ngelomel: (Oro.) sins
nimnanivkil: (Oro.) shamans

O

oblast': (Rus.) area
oblepikha: (Rus.) sea buckthorn
oboo: (Bur.) marker
obraz shizni: (Rus.) lifestyle
obshchina: (Ev.) p. 134
okrug: (Rus.) area

okurivanie: (Ev.) smudge
omiruk: (Oro.) doll or object in which one places his or her soul to protect well-being
ongon (pl. *ongonuud*): (Bur.) dead ancestor shaman spirit/s
onggor: holder of power; the 'soul-spoor of previous and now dead shamans
oribko: (Oro.) partridge

P

pantakrin: (Rus.) velvet antler products
panty: (Rus) velvet antler
pe-ken: phlem
plokhoe mesto: (Rus.) 'bad place'
*podorozhni*k: (Rus.) common plantain
polisy: (Ev.) insurance certificates
poniaga: (Ev.) frame backpack
porcha: (Bur.) curses; (Rus.) damage, spoil
po-solntsu: (Rus.) clockwise
potdelka: fake
pritok energii: (Rus.) 'inflow of energy'
pustyrnik: (Rus.) motherwort

Q

qa sening: (Ket) 'great shaman'
qaduks: (Ket) reindeer shaman
qossul: (Ket) storage trunk or box for family heirlooms; shaman's sled
qut: (Ket) shaman's 'gift'
qutn: (Ket) shaman's breast pendant

R

raion: (Rus.) district
rarshaan (pl. *arshanuud*): (Mong.) freshwater mineral spring/s
rodiola rozovaia: (Rus.) roseroot, golden root
rodovoe prokliatie: (Rus.) clan curses

rodovye zemli: (Rus.) clan territories
romashka: (Rus.) chamomile

S

Sagaalgan: (Bur.) white month (New Year)
sagaan dali: (Bur.) rhododendron
sakhandalia: (Bur.) wild rhododendron
savdag: (Bur.) land
semeiskie: (Bur) 'old believers'
senda boon: (Ket) shaman's gloves
senda du: (Ket) shaman's crown
senda qat: (Ket) shaman's coat
senda tesing: (Ket) shaman's boots
sening: (Ket) shaman
senkire: (Oro., Ev.): Labrador tea
shar: clay mud used for treating arthritis, heart disease, and nervous disorders
shepki: (Rus.) wood splinters
sheptunu: (Oro.) healer
sheree: (Bur.) table used for offerings (e.g., of food) to the spirits
shipovnik: (Rus.) rosehip
shiretui: (Bur.) chief *lama*
shuluun tarim: (Bus.) charms and spells using stones
slantsky: (Ev.) shale
sovkhoz: collective farm
sviniachii bagul'nik: (Rus.) Labrador tea

T

tagoks: (Ket) shaman's staff
tailgan: offering ceremony
tau: (Ket) crane
tegsh: (Bur.) balance
tarbagan: Siberian marmot
tarim: (Bur.) charms and spells
tarisun: a spirit distilled from milk
tarymte: (Rus.) psychological ailment
tengri: (Bur.) the heavens or most powerful spirits
tigh: (Ket) swan
tisiachilistnik: (Rus.) yarrow
tri-pa: bile
tselitely (Rus.): female folk healers ['one who makes whole']
tumbe: (Bur.) books of traditional remedies
tuneng: (Ket) shaman's headband

U

ugaalga: (Bur.) initiation ritual
ulus: (Rus.) kin village
ulvei: (Ket) the immortal life essence thought to animate each human being

V

valerian: (Rus.) valuerian
vrachivanie: (Rus.) doctoral practice
vragi naroda: (Ev.) 'ememies of the people'

W

X

xese: (Ket) shaman's drum

Y

yhan tarim: (Bus.) charms and spells using water

Z

zalozhit: to be built into or ' in debt to'
zalozheno: (Bur.) harnessed
zaschita: (Bur.) (first) protective initiation
zdorov'e: (Rus.) health
zglaz: (Rus.) evil eye
zelenaia apteka: plant pharmacies
shily: (Ev.) tendons
zolotoi koren': (Ev.) medicinal herb kept in bundles
zemliachestvo: homeland association
znakary (Rus.): one who knows; (Eve.) sorcerers
zveroboi: (Rus.) St. John's wort
zimov'ia: winter log houses
zoltoi us': (Rus.) golden tendril
*zverobo*i: (Ev.) p. 139

Notes on Contributors

David G. Anderson is Professor of Social Anthropology at the University of Tromsø, Norway. His interests include circumpolar ethnography, ethnoarchaeology, ethnohistory, and the history of science. He is the author of a monograph on Taimyr Evenkis and Dolgans, the editor of several collections from Berghahn Books, and Associate Editor of the journal *Sibirica*.

Donatas Brandišauskas is Lecturer and Postdoctoral Fellow at the Centre of Social Anthropology of Vytautas Magnus University and Vilnius University in Lithuania. He received his MRes and PhD in Social Anthropology from Aberdeen University, Scotland (2004, 2009). His thesis research focused on the variety of Orochen–Evenki skills and knowledge including ideas of power and luck necessary for success of hunting and reindeer herding in post-Soviet taiga in Zabaikal'e. His ongoing research focuses on the ritual practices and ecology of indigenous people of Eastern Siberia.

Janice Brummond is from Fargo, North Dakota and holds Master's and Ph.D. degrees from the University of Michigan, specializing in the freshwater ecology of the Lake Baikal region of Siberia and Mongolia. She has lived in Brazil, Indonesia, and Ukraine as well as on the Pacific Islands of Hawaii, Fiji and Tonga, working to implement freshwater protection programs that are integrated with local socioeconomic concerns and cultural heritage issues. Janice is currently serving in the Office of International Visitors at the U.S. Department of State in Washington, D.C., developing and implementing environmental and cultural exchange programs for international scholars and practitioners.

Justine Buck Quijada is a postdoctoral fellow at the Max Planck Institute for the Study of Religious and Ethnic Diversity. She received her PhD in Anthropology from the University of Chicago in 2009. Her dissertation, Opening the Roads: History and Religion in Post-Soviet Buryatia examines how Soviet anti-religious discourse shapes the current Buddhist and shamanic revival in Ulan-Ude, Russia.

Vladimir N. Davydov was an NFR Yggrasil research fellow at the Department of Archaeology and Social Anthropology, University of Tromsø at the time that this chapter was written. He is presently a senior researcher at the Peter the Great Museum of Anthropology and Ethnography, Russian Academy of Sciences. He received his graduate diploma in social anthropology from the State University, St. Petersburg, candidate of science [*kandidat nauk*] degree from the Institute of Sociology, Russian Academy of Science, Moscow, and his PhD from the Department of Anthropology, University of Aberdeen. He completed 11 months of fieldwork among Evenkis in the North Baikal area. His primary research interest is how hunters, reindeer herders and fishers move across the landscape and have changed in the context of development projects.

Vindarya Gololobova is a PhD student at the Institute of Philosophy and Law of the Siberian Division of the Russian Academy of Sciences in Novosibirsk. Her interests include the relationship between health and ethnicity, the sociology and philosophy of health, and traditional medicine. She has conducted research on the influence of ethnicity on well-being and ideas of self-preservation in the Buriat Republic.

Joseph Long is a Research Fellow in the Siberian Studies Centre at the Max Planck Institute for Social Anthropology in Halle, Germany. In 2010 he completed his PhD at the University of Aberdeen, Scotland. His thesis, which focuses on ritual, performance and cultural institutions in western Buriat communities, was based on extensive fieldwork from 2005-7, during which time he was a visiting researcher at Irkutsk State Technical University

Katherine Metzo has conducted research in Buriatiia since 1998. Her current research focuses on the transmission of traditional ecological knowledge and sacred sites in the Tunka and Oka districts. Recently, she founded Arigun Foundation, a non-profit organization that collaborates with government and non-profits in the Tunka and Oka districts, focusing on education and economic development.

Earle H. Waugh is Professor Emeritus of Religious Studies and Director of the Centre for the Cross-Cultural Study of Health and Healing in Family Medicine at the University of Alberta. In 2005, after many years in the Faculty of Arts, Professor Waugh joined the faculty at the Department of Family Medicine, where he heads up a research team on the intersection of Culture and Health. Their most recent project has been Towards Culturally-Responsive Care in the Community, a study of five ethnically-distinctive communities' views on dementia and end-of-life care. These activities have spawned a book on the interface of culture and medicine and a manual for health care professionals on cultural competence. Professor Waugh lectures and consults widely on health-care and culture and has provided seminars for hospitals, pharmacy seniors, graduate physicians and health care professionals throughout the province.

Edward Vajda is a professor at Western Washington University in Bellingham, Washington, where he directs the Center for East Asian Studies. He teaches Russian language, culture and history, as well as courses on general linguistics and Inner Asian and Siberian peoples. Dr. Vajda has conducted original fieldwork on Ket, a language spoken by fewer than 100 people in a remote area near Siberia's Yenisei River. He has recently presented evidence supporting a genetic link between Eniseian, the language family to which Ket belongs, and the Na-Dene family of North America. Vajda received his university's Excellence of Teaching Award in 1992.

Index

A

Aboriginal Day 113
acupuncture 32, 44, 57, 61, 64, 66
adaha tarim 47
adaptation 8
addiction 19
adyl 104
agdyrin 104
aiaga 70
air 33, 36, 38-39
airag 64, 69, 72
Alba 152
alcohol 72, 87-88, 92-94, 117, 143
   consumption 87, 92-94
   rituals 5
   poisoning 93
alcoholism 1, 14, 19-20, 24, 93-94, 99, 111
allergies 39, 70
aloe 41
alpine 49, 72
altered states of consciousness 65
alternative healing systems 5, 7-8, 101, 103, 108, 131
amulets 119
ancestors 17-26
ancestor spirits 13, 27, 87-91
ancient cultures 148
ancient healing practices 43
ancient narratives 78
Angara 2
angry souls 123
animal-based remedies 5, 10, 72, 102, 107
animal dung 68
animal fat 98, 107, 110
animal helpers 148, 154
animal parts, products 8, 51, 107, 108, 110, 111, 117, 120, 131, 133, 134, 144
animal tracks 120
annual blessing 65
anti-religious 62, 131
anti-shaman 157
anxiety 106
appendicitis 133
Arctic Ocean 2

arenki 123, 124, 125
arga-bilig 63
arkhi 72
arsenic 52
Arshaan Saiani 67, 73, 75, 76, 83, 84
arshan, arshaanuud 35, 36, 37, 38, 39, 42, 63, 65, 70, 72, 80, 81, 83
artesian hot sulfate spring 77
arthritis 70, 111
artifacts 149
ashes 52
asphaltum 120
asthma 70, 81
astrology 55
Atlas of Tibetan Medicine 64
autonomous healing 1, 7
ayurveda 2, 30-35, 43

B

bad dreams 111
bad energy 116-118, 127
bad luck 19-20
bad spirits 125
bag emch 64
bagulnik 41-42
Baikal–Amur Railway 140
baiunchuka 143
balance 32-33, 43, 47, 63
balneotherapy 66
bandages 104, 107
bargos 148-149, 151, 153, 157
baria 70
baptisms 157
bariashad 64
barishi 64
bark 50, 104
bar'sa 90
baryaasha 48, 62
bath 10
bear 75, 78
bear-visits 125
beater stick 153
berries 75
best practice 101
bicarbonate and carbonic gas spring 78
Big Shaman 131
Bilberry 75

bile 33, 49
biodiversity protection 82
bio-energy 34, 65
biomedical conditions, symptoms 13, 95, 101-102, 108-109
biomedical standards 101
biomedicine 2, 5-8, 10, 30, 34-37, 44
birch fungus 106, 122
birth 58, 66
black tea 118
blessing 66, 99
blood enhancer 122
bloodletting 47-48, 57, 60, 62
blood pressure 121, 133, 143
blood test 111
Bolshoi Aginskii Chzhor 52
bone-setting 47-48
Booruljuut 70
borax 52
boreal system 75
borovaia matka 143
botanists 60
brimstone 52
buben 131
Buddhism 8, 14, 25, 30, 32, 44
Buddhist monasteries, temples 19, 32
Buddhist school of Gelug-pa 45
buga 123, 126
Bugunda 119, 125
Buktokon River 125
buni 125
Buriat 45-62, 87-94, 110-118, 121
Buriat healing 8, 29, 32, 37, 40, 43-44
Buriatiia 8, 45-55, 58, 60-62, 90, 110-116, 125, 129, 144-146
Buriat offering rites 88
Buriat Scientific Centre of the Siberian Branch of the Russian Academy of Sciences 60
bustards 78
but 45, 47 49, 51, 54, 63-66, 72, 74, 78, 80-83
buu 63

C

cabin 117
calcites 52
Canadian Arctic 1
Canadian First Nations 10, 101-102, 108
candles 32
cannabis 72
capability 124
capitalist system 5-6
carbonate waters 76
cardiovascular problems 78
cauterization 47-48, 57, 62
central medical institutions 5-6
centres of learning 8
ceremonies 16, 20-25, 47, 65-66
chaga 122
Chaia River 143
chanting 65-66
charisma 34
charms 47, 118
Chernobyl 75
chilitkan 143
Chinen 124
Chinese medicine 81
Chinggis Khaan 68, 78
Chinggis Khaan spring 78
Chirinda 106
chistotel 144
Choibalsan 81
Choigan arshaan 74
Christian 45, 157
chronic illness 37
chumy 114
chzhory 48
cigarettes 121, 125
circulatory ailments 40
circumpolar North 2
cirrhosis 93, 121
clan 46, 88-91, 94, 112-116, 129
clan ancestors 20
clan curses 112
clan hearth 88, 91
clan territories 113
clay mud 78
cleansing 100, 118
climatic conditions 45, 56, 72, 80
clinical medical knowledge 101
clinics 96

coastal landscapes 2
coat and crown 153
coins 99, 109
collapse of the Soviet system 7, 113, 116, 133
collecting and using medicinal plants 36, 42
collective farm 89, 92, 126, 133
colonial structure 2
colored cloth 65
commensality rites of 87
communication with spirits 14, 19, 131
communion 88, 90, 91, 92, 151
communitas 91, 94
community health 1, 64
community health workers 95-97, 100-101
competition over resources 140
conical tents 114
coniferous 75
core elements 63
cosmology 72, 104
craftwork 120
Cree 1, 10, 95, 97-102, 109
creolisation 10
cross-cultural healing 10
crown 153
cultural context of consumption 87
cultural knowledge 17
cultural preservation 82
cultural traditions 5
culture of reciprocity 134
cultures of respect 98
cupping 32
cures 1, 47, 56, 63-66
curiosity 119, 123
curses 19, 112, 115
Customary law codices 46

D

dagh 155, 156
dairy products 36, 38
dwth ancestors,*angols* 154
dariy 152, 153
datsan 8, 48, 59
datsanuud 32
datura 72
death 21, 66

deceased's soul 127
decoctions 52
deer 51, 75, 100, 107, 117, 126
deities 25
Den'Aborigena 113
Dene 1, 10, 95- 99, 101-102, 109, 120
desiccating 103
diagnosis 18-21, 25, 27
diamond dust 105
diarrhoea 38, 121
diet and lifestyle 30
disease 47, 52, 54-58, 61, 109, 111, 115, 120, 126
disinfect 104, 107
disrespect 127, 144
divination 19, 33, 114-115
doctor 1, 32, 37-40, 46, 54, 56, 60-61, 96-97, 99, 101-102, 109, 111, 114, 118, 129, 133
Dolgan 95, 103, 108, 110
dozhdevii grib 104
dream 21-24
dream-guidance 24
drinking 64, 66, 69, 70, 72, 75, 78
drum 102, 131, 153- 154, 156-157, 181
drumming 65
dukh khoziain 112
dukuvuchi 125
dulin buga 123
Dushkachan 129, 130-131
Dzelindenski 75
Dzemchuk 77

E

earth 49
Eastern medicine 7
Eastern Siberia 2, 9
ecological knowledge 8
economic crises 11
economic potential 30
edible wild plants 47
Ekonda 100, 106
elders 104, 106-107, 109-110, 112, 116, 118, 120, 122, 124, 126
elk 75, 117, 121, 126
Elogui River 151
emchi-lamas 32, 43, 45-48, 52, 54-58, 60-62

emergency services 35
empowerment 101
emtei-lamas 58
endangered species 50
energy 63, 110, 116-118, 124-125
Enisei River 2, 10, 99, 147, 181
environmental ethics 138
ephedra 69
epilepsy 113
ermine 117
esdeng 151
Essei 106
eteng kherigde 104
ethnic groups 25
ethnologist 2
eting temperashka 104
European healing traditions 6
evacuation 7
Evenki 2, 5, 8-10, 95-110
Evenki Autonomous District 96-97
evil eye 111, 117
evil spirit 47, 57, 99, 108, 118-120, 123, 127
evil witch 150
exercise 66, 72, 79
eye ailments 77
Ezhin 64

F

fake 111
family guardian spirits 154
family recipes 35
farming 89, 91, 92
fel'dsher-akusher 96
fel'dshery 8, 95, 129, 146
female folk healers 32
fermented dairy products 36
fertility ceremony 66
fire 49
first aid 96, 133, 146
first initiation 18-19
fluorine 77
fly agaric 72
folk healers 2, 8, 32, 34, 47, 48, 62, 101, 129, 148, 182, 187
folklore 149-150
folk medicine 7, 45-49, 61, 81, 129, 132-133, 144-146
folk religion 64, 65

forest resources 29, 30, 35-36
frame backpack 136
fresh air 72, 145
fur tax 150

G

gall bladder 56, 107, 120-121
galvanometer 61
Garginski kurort 75
gastrointestinal 130
gather medicinal plants 9, 30, 38
geun 46
gems and stones 52
ger 78
ghosts 123
ginseng 75
global capitalist system 5
globalization 83
gornaia valeriana 143
Goryachinsk 75
grasses 49, 81
graveyards 126
grizzly bear 117
groza 104
guardian spirits 114
Gurvan Nuur 70, 78

H

harmony 63, 64
harvest resources 113
harvest time 52
hatbul 153
hawks 78
headband 153, 156
heal communities 99
healer 32, 34, 45-48, 51, 58, 62, 95, 97-102, 110-111, 115, 117, 127-128
healing 1, 5, 13, 47, 62, 129, 146
  knowledge 98, 102, 108
  landscapes 10, 112
  protocols 2, 5, 10
  rituals 64, 102, 111, 117-118
  rocks 10
  springs 9, 10
  strategies 6, 8, 109
  traditions 1, 2, 5-7, 9-11
  'indigenous' tradition 1
  'Western' tradition 1
  waters 65

health 47, 56, 87-88, 94--97, 99-, 101, 103, 107, 110
health and healing 1, 2, 87, 95-96, 110
health issues 14, 88, 115, 125
heart of the thunder 104
helicopter evacuation flights 7
helper spirits 152
herbal cures, medicines, treatments 7, 9, 32, 34, 39
herbalists 32, 33, 35
herbal teas 30, 32
herders 80-81
herding grounds 113, 115, 117, 120, 123
heretics 32
hergu buga 123
heritage 64, 78, 81, 83
HIV/AIDs 81
holy water 64
homeopathy 34, 61
home remedies 7, 32
horse herders 111
Hosedam 150, 151-152, 154, 156-157
hospital 5, 7, 18, 24, 35, 95, 97-104, 107, 109, 111, 118, 129, 130, 145
hot and cold 47, 63, 72
hot blood 68
hot sands 68
hot springs 58, 68, 74, 77-78, 130
household 88-89, 90
Hunnic Era 156
hunter-gatherers 5, 147, 150, 156
hunters and herders 51, 108, 113, 125, 129, 134, 138, 141, 144
hunting luck 125-126
hygienic rituals 63

I

ianda 9, 133-144
iasak 150
icons 32
idols 119, 127
Ikh Ukhgun River 77
illness 13-14, 18-19, 21, 23-27, 48, 56, 62, 87-88, 93, 97, 99, 106-109, 112-118, 120, 125-128
  spiritual cause of 27

immortal life essence 150
immune system 74
inappropriate behaviour 126
incense 32, 33
Indian *ayurveda* healing 2, 32
indigenous
  administrative districts 129
  communities 87, 96, 113
  healers 110
  kinship networks 26
  knowledge 72, 83
  peoples 9, 26, 157
  tradition 17
industrial activities 123
inebriants 72
infectious diseases 55, 96, 104, 107-108
inflow of energy 125
infusions 52, 75
inhalation 66, 72
initiation 153, 182, 186-187
injuries 112
injury 21
inner warmth 49, 56, 61
inorganic ingredients 52
institutional medical care 111
integrative medicine 61
intellectual property 82
intermarriage 25
interpretation of dreams 120
intervention 108, 151, 156, 184, 187
Irkut River 77
Irkutsk 2
iron pendants 153, 156
iurta 131
iurty 141

J

Jud-Shi 45, 49, 51
juniper 69, 99, 106, 107
juniper smoke 106

K

Kamchatka 92, 93
kamennoe maslo 10, 144
kamlanie 24
kandelok 154, 156
Karenga River 116
karmic factors 57
Kellog Village 155, 157
Kets 5
Ket shamanism 149, 150, 156, 157
Ket traditions 148
khadag 64, 66, 72
Khaju Bulag 78
Khakuses 75
khan 69
Khantaikskoe Ozero 106
Khasurtai 80
khii 63, 80
Kholodnaia 129, 131-135, 138, 140-146
khorkhog 56
Khoyto-Gol 74
khoziain 88-90, 112
khubi 89-91, 93
khurylkha 47
Khuty 88-94
khuvaraguud 54, 58
kidney 54, 81
kinship 20, 25
  networks 7, 13, 26, 29, 37
  obligation 13, 18, 23-24
  relations 87, 88
kin-village 88
kites 78
knotweed 81
knowledge traditions 7
kolduny 131
kolkhoz 133-134, 144
komersanty 121
Krasnyi Iar 125
kukish 119, 123
Kurba River 80
Kurumkan district 75
kuso 103, 104
kuznetsi 18
Kyngarga River 76

L

Laboratory for Pulse Diagnostics 60
Labrador Tea 99, 118, 142, 143
Lake Baikal 2, 5, 9, 14, 22, 130
Lake Kyren 70
lama 45-62, 111, 115, 118
landscape 55, 64, 72, 74, 107, 108-109
landscape medicine 9, 10
land spirits 5
larch 2, 75, 103, 104
lawlessness 117
legends 78
lekpom 130
libations 88, 91, 93
lichens 75
licorice 81
life-cycle rites 66
life expectancy 34, 93
lifestyle 30, 33, 94, 108
lightening 10, 104
lightening mushroom 104
livestock 81
local
  adaptation 8
  cultural traditions 5
  healers 1, 2
  healing landscape 1, 8, 10, 112
  healing protocols 2
  knowledge 61, 129, 132-133, 144
  traditions 101, 110
Local Religious Organization of Shamans, Tengeri 13
loon spirits 152
luck 99, 112, 118-120, 123, 125-126, 128, 136, 138
Lumurchen 125
lung 33, 70
lupine 81
lus 63-64, 80, 83
lynx 117

M

magic 47, 119, 123
magicians 131
mahābhūtas 49, 61
manba-datsan 45, 48, 60, 62
Manchurian Chinese Empire 2
mantras 52, 58
manual diagnostics 61
market economy 2, 96, 101, 129
marmot 78
marriage 66
Marxism 6
massage 33, 47, 57, 62, 66, 72, 74, 115, 118
master-spirits 112, 123, 125-127
matches 99
medical anthropology 5
medical
  assistant 130-133, 145
  centre 29, 118, 143, 144

colleges 101
first aid 146
insurance certificates 145
intervention 17
station 107, 129-131
traditions 1, 6
training 58, 96, 100, 109, 110
medical pluralism 5-7, 10, 95, 101, 110, 146
medical schools at monasteries 45
medication 47-49, 51-52, 54, 56-57
medicinal herbs 52, 129, 131-143
medicinal plants 9, 29, 30-44, 49, 59-60, 70, 72
medicine 45-62, 95-102, 106-110
  clinical 5
  cosmopolitan 5
  having medicine 98
medicines 1, 7, 8, 9
mental illness 13, 115, 152, 184
metabolism 121
metals 52
methane waters 77
Middle World 123
midwifery 64, 96, 130
migration 89, 90
military activities 123
mineralisation 10
mineral pitch 10, 77, 120
minerals 111, 118, 131, 133-134
mineral springs 37, 39, 47, 58
mining 123
minor shaman' 153
misdiagnosed shamanic callings 25
misdiagnosis 13
misfortune 21, 111, 113, 117, 123, 126-127
missionaries 65
mixed economy 116
mobile camps 116
mobile medical groups 129
modernity 26
modernization campaigns 17
monasteries 32, 37
Mongol 2
Mongolia 17, 18, 22, 45-46, 48, 54, 60-61

Mongolian 14, 16
Mongolian Adonis 78
Mongolian folk medicine 45, 48
Monks 66
moose 75, 116, 117, 121, 126
moral drinking 88
Morality 126
mortality rates 87
mortuary 113, 119, 120, 124-125
mortuary sites 124
mosses 65, 75
Mount Michangda 104
moxibustion 32
mozhzhevelnik 106
mud, mud pools 66, 70-71, 77-78
Muishin River 125
multivitamin 38
muneo 10, 120
munio 51
muscle pain 70
mushroom 72, 75, 104, 151, 184-185
mythology 23

N

Naadam 65
nastoika 133
National Commissariat of Public Health 129
natural foods 37
nature cults 65
neo-shamanism 17
nerve stimulant 81
nervous disorders 77, 79
new age practices 34
New Year 66
nicknames 119, 123
Nizhnaia Tunguska River 110
Nizhneangarsk 130, 131, 134, 139, 140, 144
nomadic diet 72
nomadic way of life 114, 127
nomads 63, 81, 116, 150, 156-157, 185
Nomama Lake 132, 135-137
Nomama River 133, 138
non-clinical treatments 7
non-human beings 112-113, 120, 123, 127--128
non-timber forest resources 29, 30, 35

northerly steppe zones 2
Northern Alberta 96
northern health practice 96
Northern Norway 2
Northern taiga medicine 5
Northwest Territories 96
novices 54
Novonikolaevsk 88, 89, 90, 92, 93
nurse practitioners 8, 32, 95-96, 129, 146
nursing stations 96, 98, 101, 109

O

oblast' 45, 88
oboo 66, 67, 72
obshchina 136, 138, 141
offering 21, 22-23, 87-88, 90-91, 98, 101, 109, 113, 119-120, 125
okrug 88
Olkhon Island 22, 23
omen 23
omi 119, 127
omiruk 119
ongonuud 13, 18, 20-26
open air market 36
open tundra 2
oral history 24
oral medication 48
oral tradition 32
orientalists 60
Orochen 5, 8, 111-120, 123-128
Orochen–Evenki 111, 114
ortiliia odnobokaia 143
otter 75
oxides 52

P

packaged plant medicines 9
pantakrin 120-121
panty 121-122, 144
paramedic 64
pastoralists and hunters 8
pastoralist traditions 43
'Pearl' tourist complex 77
pe-ken 33
people and land 10
perestroika 18
pharmaceuticals 5, 6, 30, 38, 39, 43
pharmacology 8, 60

pharmacopeia 9, 49
philologists 60
phlegm 33
photographs 62, 149
physical strength 124
physical symptoms of illness 13, 19, 24-26
physician 33, 64, 129, 132-133
pilgrimage 65, 78
pine 75
placings 115, 118
plant collectors 35
plant lore 150
plant medicine 9-0, 95, 102, 108
plant resins 104
plants 47-50, 52, 59-61, 101-104, 110-111, 115, 118, 120, 122
poaching 123, 126
Podkamennaia Tunguska River 149-150
poisonous 52, 72
poniaga 136-138
porcha 19, 117-119, 123
possession 13-14, 19
post-Soviet period 7-8, 14, 96, 116, 129
potdelka 111
power 98-100, 104, 108, 118, 131, 133
power of the landscape 2
prayer 32, 52, 57-58, 65, 99-100
prayer flags 66
Prebaikalsk 75
predict good fortune 151
prescription pills 1
pressure points 72
preventive medicine 33, 38, 96
prognoses 55
prohibitions 66
protect 118-120, 123, 127
protective initiation 18, 19
psychological ailment 107
psychomental complex 114
psychotherapy 47
public
  health crisis 17
  health institutions 8, 129-130, 146
  medicine 8, 10, 25, 129, 131-133

puffballs 122
pulse diagnosis 8, 32, 54, 60-61, 63, 72
punishments 127
purgative 81
purification 70
  of a dwelling 99
Putoran Mountains 104, 110

Q

qaduks 149, 154-156
qossul 153
qut 152-153, 156

R

radiography 55
radon 77
rainwater 65
raion 88, 89, 91, 94, 129, 134, 144
rashaan, rashaanuud 63, 66, 72, 74, 78
Rashanii Tsatsral 68
ratsnake 75
raw materials 48-50, 52, 54
recipes 48, 51-52, 58
reciprocity 88-94, 100, 127
  obligations of 88-91
Red Cross 129
red squirrel 117
reducing tension 72
regional center, hospital 2, 7, 35
reincarnated 151
reindeer 99-100, 104, 106-109, 111-117, 121-135, 138, 140-149, 154-156, 182, 186-189
  breath 107
  domestication 148
  farm 134, 140, 144
  herding 113-114, 125-129, 132-135, 138, 141, 143-146
  people 111
relationships between bodies of common descent 24
relaxation 72
religion 32, 45, 48, 58, 61, 131
remedy 48, 49
remote villages 111, 115
re-peasantization 29

Republic of Buriatiia 13, 14
resource redistribution 116
respiratory disorders 70
Revolution of 1917 132
rheumatism 56, 81, 130
rhododendron 143
ritual 5, 10, 17, 25, 45, 47, 52, 62, 87-88, 90-91, 99, 100-102, 106-107, 109, 111-113, 117-120, 123-125, 127
  cures 63
  events 88
  obligations 20, 25
  observances 125
  offerings 33, 65, 87
  relationship 20
  sites 64, 125
ritualized
  commensality 87-88, 92
  hospitality 88
  reciprocity 90-91
rock arches 125
rock art 125-126
rock-outcroppings 10
rodovye zemli 113
rosemary 69
Rossoshino Village 119
rue 81
rural healthcare 30
rural infrastructure 8
rural villages 6
Russian 2, 45, 46, 59-62, 88, 93, 95-98, 101, 103, 110, 112, 114-116, 118, 121
  bio-medicine 19
  colonization 2, 25
  folk healer 23, 32
  medicine 5
  state-building 2
  state-run medicine 19
  trading post 14
Russian Academy of Sciences 8
Russian America 2
Russian Federation 14, 18, 61, 62, 96
Russian Orthodox Christianity 14, 32, 77, 157

S

sable 75, 117, 122
sacred places 124

Sacred Sea 75
Sagaalgan 66
sagaan dali 40, 41, 42
sagebrush 81
Saian Mountains 37, 38, 74, 77
sakhan dalia 143
Sali River 125
salts 52
sanatoria 37, 43, 78
sap 50, 104
savdag 63
school teachers 129
scientific legitimacy 35, 43
seabuckthorn 81
séances 150, 151, 153
seasonal variations 63
second initiation 21, 23
Second Kamchatka expedition of 1740 9
secret 78
sedentarization 114
sedge 81
self-reliance 111, 113, 127
semi-nomadic reindeer herders 132
sening 148-149, 151-153, 156-157
setting of bones and muscles 48
seven layers of the sky 151
seventeen properties of food and medicinal agents 49
shale 144
shaman 7- 8, 13-27, 47, 58, 88, 97, 102, 106-107, 111, 113-115, 120, 123, 127-128, 131-133, 148-157, 179, 180, 185, 187
  ancestor shaman 20
  bear shaman 154-156
  blacksmith shamans 18
  dragonfly shaman 156
  enemy of the people 7
  great shaman 150, 153-154, 156
  initiation ritual 70
  kandelok shamans 154, 156
  qaduks shaman 154, 155
  reindeer shaman 149
  shaman's paraphernalia 149
    boots and gloves 153
    breast pendant 153
    costume 154
shamanic
  calling 13, 17-27
  gift 21, 152, 156
  healing 8, 14, 26, 151
  intervention 13, 63
  landscape traditions 5
  regalia 153
  traditions 2, 25
shamanism 13-14, 17, 20, 23, 25-26, 45, 95, 97-98, 114, 131, 149-150, 156-157, 185, 187
shamanistic
  cure 109
  practice 87, 148
  rituals 131, 148, 187
shar 63, 78
shenki 104
sheoturil 115
sheree 89
shotgun shells 99
shuluun tarim 47
Shumak 70, 78
Siberia 2, 45, 47, 88, 91, 94-95, 98, 101, 108-109, 111-112, 115, 117-118, 121, 125
Siberian Evenki 10
significant places 9
sign of the cross 32
signs 72, 119, 123, 125
sila 124, 131
siniukha golubaia 143
sins 125, 126
sinus problems 70
sites of healing 10
skin infections 107
skin irritations 81
skins of a newly slaughtered animal 47
sky people 152
sky world 154, 156
slaughter 88-91
smartweed 75
smoke 99, 100, 103, 106-107
smokes 70
smoking 99, 107
smudge 106, 141
smudging 99, 100, 102, 118, 127
smudging rituals 102
snowmelt 65
soaking 66-67, 69
social celebration 65
social institutions 5, 7
social networks 13
social tensions 88, 94
song 149-150, 152-153, 156
sopchokty 143, 144
sorcerer 131, 151, 157
soul 19, 47, 112, 119, 123, 127, 150, 181, 188
south-central Siberia 14
Soviet
  biomedicine 7
  collectivization 148
  nationalization 14
  repression 17
Soviet period 7-9, 14, 20, 24, 89, 111, 116, 120
Soviet Union 6, 43, 44
sovkhoz 89, 92
spa 10, 65, 69
space 49
specialists 7, 60, 62, 98, 111, 114-115
spells 47
spinal column 81
spirit-caused illness 19
spirit-drinking 114
spirit helpers 149, 151, 153-154, 156
spirit-masters 126
spirit possession 14
spirit possession cults 14
spirits 2, 5, 8-9, 13-14, 17-19, 22, 24-27, 47, 52, 57, 87-91, 93, 99, 101-102, 105, 107-108, 112-115, 117-121, 123, 125-127, 131, 150-155, 179, 181-184, 188-189
  benevolent 17
  malevolent 17
spiritual 17, 18, 19, 27
  cause of illness 27
  foundations of health 9
  gathering 32
  healing 148, 151, 156-157
  imbalance 17
  intervention 156
  remedies 9
  strength 124
spirit world 151-152
springs 10
staff 99, 111, 153
state farms 116
steam bath 70

steam inhalation 66
steppe 2, 5, 72, 78, 80-81
steppe nomads 156
stibium 52
stoat 117
stomach ailments 107
stone-oil 10, 51, 120, 144-145
stones 47, 51-52, 56, 58, 104-105
storage platform 117, 126
storytellers 127
street markets 9
strength of movement 124
'strong like two people' 101, 109
subsistence practices 29, 36, 112-113, 119
suffering 21, 25
sugar dust 105
sustainable harvesting 40
Suur-kharbaan 65, 84
sweetgrass 99
sweetgrass ceremony 101
system of communication 13

T

taboo 156
taiga 72, 75, 78, 98, 100, 101, 107-109, 111-113, 115-118, 120-121, 123, 126-127, 145-146
taiga medicine 5, 9, 107, 111-113, 118, 127
taiga resources 111, 116, 127
taiga-steppe borderlands 5
tailgan 22
tailgan rites 88, 89, 90
Taimyr 2, 103, 104, 106, 107, 110
talismans 151
Tantric knowledge 59
tarbagan 78
tarisun 88
tarymte 106, 107
tea 56, 90, 103, 106, 118, 122, 125, 133, 135-136, 138, 144
   commercially produced 35
tegsh 32, 63, 72
temporal and spatial rules 49
temporal and spatial rules when collecting medicinal materials 49
Tengeri 8, 13, 14-20, 22-27

tengri 64, 74
the main elements 49
therapeutic baths 77
thermal baths 69
thunder 104
thunder tobacco 104
Tibetan 2
Tibetan Book of Medicine 35
Tibetan 2
   Buddhism 14
   herbal medicine 19
   medicine 2, 5, 6, 8, 45, 56, 58, 60
   steppe healing traditions 5
   tantras 64
tincture 133, 144
Tomam 156
Tompa 129, 130, 143
Tompa Village 143
tonics 41, 43
toothaches 107
topical treatments 43
Toson Nuur 70
tourists 75, 78, 83
toxins 70
trade links 2
traders 9, 92, 121
traditional
   culture 24
   cures 8
   healing 7, 14, 32, 37
   knowledge 13, 24, 27
   medicine 48, 61-62, 100, 109-110, 120, 131
training 16, 21, 23, 129
trance 20-24, 151
trap lines 117
travel and trade 2
treatment 7, 47-48, 52, 55-58, 60-62, 66, 70, 75, 78, 81
tri-pa 33
troelistka 143
Tsarist period 129
tseliteli 101
tselitely 8, 32
tuberculosis 96, 109, 122, 130, 132-133, 143, 144, 145
tumbe 64
Tungokochen (Villlage) 111, 112, 113, 116, 117, 118, 120, 125
Tungus 108, 111, 114-117
Tunka National Park 30

Tunka Valley 2, 9
Tuva 74

U

udagan 63
ugaalga 70
ugu buga 123
Ulan-Ude 2, 8, 13-15, 17-18, 26
ulcers 81
ultrasound 55
ulus 88-90
ulvei 150-152
underworld 123, 151-152, 157
Underworld 123
UNESCO world heritage site 14
unethical interactions 126
universal health care 34
unsanitary habits 114
Upper World 123
urban-based professional elites 6
urban population 14
Ust' Avam 99, 106-107
Utaat Minj 81

V

vakhta trekhlistnaia 143
valerian 41
vapors 70
velvet antler 120, 122, 144
venereal disease 130
violence 87-88, 93-94
Vitamin C 81
vodka 5, 88-94, 98, 117-119, 121, 136, 140, 144
Volochanka 106
vrachivanie 101

W

warm and cold 49
warmed-up soil 47
wash 114, 130
wastage 126
water 47, 49, 52, 56, 58, 96, 115, 120, 123, 125, 130, 136, 142, 144-145
watershed 112
water spirits 64, 66, 80, 83
water springs 49
weasel 117
welfare state 7

well-being 62, 88, 92, 94, 112-113, 119-120, 123, 127, 150, 189
well-dressing 65
White Month 66
wild boar 117
wild market 117
wild reindeer 100, 107, 117, 121
wild thyme 70
willow 69, 104
winter log house 123, 133, 141
wolf 75
wolverine 107, 117
women 8
wood ashes 104
wood splinters 104
World Health Organization 62
world of the dead 123, 125
worldview 123
wormwood 69
wounds 104, 107
wutuoginil 115

X

Y

yadgan 63
yhan tarim 47

Z

Zabaikal Province, Region 25, 48, 50, 58, 113, 115, 116, 125
Zagulai 117
zalozheno 21, 23
zashchita 19, 21, 23
zdorov'e 101
zglaz 117-118
zimov'e 133
zimov'ia 141
znakary 8
znakhari 111, 131-133, 146
zolotoi 41
zolotoi koren' 134-135, 138-141
zolotoi us 41
zootherapy 108
  see also animal-based remedies
zveroboi 143